# Physical Therapy for Sports

Sport-Physiotherapie. English.

Edited by Werner Kuprian

With the collaboration of
Doris Eitner
Lutz Meissner
Helmut Ork

Translated by Todd Kontje

**W. B. SAUNDERS COMPANY**
PHILADELPHIA • LONDON • TORONTO • MEXICO CITY • RIO DE JANEIRO • SYDNEY • TOKYO

W. B. Saunders Company: West Washington Square
Philadelphia, PA 19105

1 St. Anne's Road
Eastbourne, East Sussex BN21 3UN, England

1 Goldthorne Avenue
Toronto, Ontario M8Z 5T9, Canada

Apartado 26370 — Cedro 512
Mexico 4, D.F., Mexico

Rua Coronel Cabrita, 8
Sao Cristovao Caixa Postal 21176
Rio de Janeiro, Brazil

9 Waltham Street
Artarmon, N.S.W. 2064, Australia

Ichibancho, Central Bldg., 22-1 Ichibancho
Chiyoda-Ku, Tokyo 102, Japan

**Library of Congress Cataloging in Publication Data**

Sport-Physiotherapie. English.

Physical therapy for sports.

Translation of: Sport-Physiotherapie.

Includes index.

1. Physical therapy.    2. Sports — Accidents and injuries.
   I. Kuprian, Werner.    II. Title.

RM701.S6613 1982        617'.1027        81–48440

ISBN 0–7216–5553–X                        AACR2

Original German Edition: Sport-Physiotherapie
© 1981 Gustav Fischer Verlag, Stuttgart

99398

Authorized English edition published 1982 by W. B. Saunders Company
Philadelphia, London, Toronto, Mexico City, Rio de Janeiro, Sydney, Tokyo

Physical Therapy for Sports                        ISBN   0-7216-5553-X

Last digit is the print number:   9   8   7   6   5   4   3   2

# Contents

## Chapter 3
**Uses of Cold** ..................................................................................... 62
*Helmut Ork*

## Chapter 4
**Hydrotherapy and Balneotherapy** ............................................... 69
*Doris Eitner*

## Chapter 14
**Foot and Leg** ....................................................................................... 224
*Lutz Meissner, Helmut Ork, and Werner Kuprian*

## Chapter 15
## Spinal Column and Torso ................................................ 262
*Werner Kuprian, Helmut Ork, and Lutz Meissner*

# INTRODUCTION

*WERNER KUPRIAN*

The constantly increasing demands of modern competitive athletics carry with them a simultaneous increase in the risk of injury and damage. The enormous stress of training and competition in today's top competitive sports results ever more frequently in serious traumatic injuries and damage to the musculoskeletal system from extreme, statically abnormal stress. Excessive straining of the spinal column, joints, ligaments, capsules, tendons, and muscles can lead to permanent damage. The danger of injury has increased not only among contenders in the top competitive sports, which are continually characterized by setting of new records but in popular sports as well. These latter, played in the schools, as a hobby, or during recreational time, show an increase in the risk and frequency of injuries. Often people who lack the slightest training are encouraged to participate in complex and physically demanding types of sports without the proper professional instruction by poorly organized fitness programs, weight control groups, jogging clubs, and the advertisements of the athletic equipment industry.

For example, consider the modern ski industry. Year after year an increasing number of out-of-condition, unprepared people who are inexperienced in mountain conditions crowd the slopes.

Riding provides another typical example. Ever since riding has become a popular sport, the number of injuries, often serious, has risen. If one examines specific incidents, it is generally found that injuries involve riders with no basic training or those who have misjudged their equestrian ability and reactions, often against the advice of experienced and qualified trainers. Experienced riders with good basic training are rarely involved in accidents entailing serious injuries.

A similar development can be observed in surfing, jogging, and other "fashionable" sports.

## A Brief Statistical Overview of Athletic Injuries

Participation in athletics causes approximately 80,000 accidents per year in the Federal Republic of Germany. Of these 75 per cent are minimal, 20 per cent moderate, and 5 per cent severe injuries. This does not include injuries caused by winter sports; in Austria, 2500 injuries are expected daily during the winter season. They generally involve broken lower leg bones and injuries to the muscles of the lower extremities and the Achilles tendon. Seventy-five per cent of all skiing injuries involve beginners.

In Europe soccer now as always is not only the most frequently played sport in the summer, but it also possesses the highest quota of injuries — about 10 per cent. Wrestling, handball, boxing, track and field, gymnastics, and other sports follow at a distance.

Among the types of injuries, the majority (78 per cent) include contusions, dislocations, sprains, bruises, and torn muscles and tendons. Fractures, torn ligaments, and meniscus injuries follow (15 per cent).

The primary cause of athletic injuries is insufficient preparation (70 per cent), followed by excessive strain, tiredness, or illness (17 per cent), and lack of discipline (13 per cent).

Sixty-one per cent of the injuries are to the legs, another 22 per cent to the arms, 11 per cent to the head, and 6 per cent to the torso.

An investigation into the extent of time lost at work conducted by Groh and Groh revealed that of 2739 injured athletes, 637 missed 1 week's work, 702 missed 2 weeks, 392 up to 3 weeks, 258 up to 4 weeks, 186 up to 6 weeks, and 110 up to 8 weeks. The time lost by the remainder ranged from 3 to 12 months. The average time lost from work through an athletic injury was 3 weeks.

Deaths are relatively rare in sports. We distinguish between deaths resulting from an external circumstance and those caused by the overextension of an athlete's personal physical limits, often connected with previously unknown organ damage.

The number of deaths resulting from organic diseases and trauma is listed at 250 per year. Incidents of deaths involving organ disease or damage, such as coronary sclerosis, are clearly in the majority. Among traumatic deaths, injuries incurred in soccer head the list.

# Injuries Caused by Athletics

Less precise statistics are available for chronic athletic injuries involving irreparable exhaustion and atrophy of tissues. Expert opinion is divided. It is often impossible to distinguish precisely between chronic, primary exhaustion of tissues and the secondary results of an accident. Groh and Groh have written in this regard: "Other than the unavoidable secondary traumatic arthritis we have hardly ever seen a primary functional osteoarthritis in top performance sports. There is essentially no primary functional osteoarthritis caused by competitive sports or long-term athletics. . . . A decisive argument against the theory that sports can cause permanent injury is the fact that osteoarthritis of the leg joints (ankle, knee, hip) has never been observed in long-distance athletes (long-distance runners, marathon runners, cross-country skiers, bicyclists).

"We may assume that there is virtually no measurable exhaustion of the musculoskeletal system for 95 to 99 per cent of the top competitive athletes, particularly in the joints. Reindall has demonstrated this for the circulatory system."

Secondary athletic injuries are generally located in the spine, the joints and the tendons. The statically abnormal stress placed on the spinal column in women's gymnastic events, for example, or in figure skating, plays an important role. Tendinitis affects the tendons and osteoarthritis the joints, but this does not result from long-term participation in sports per se but rather through injuries and trauma of the type that frequently occurs in soccer games.

# Physical Therapy and Remedial Gymnastics

Physical therapy and remedial exercises play an increasingly important role within the framework of sports medicine in the treatment of athletic injuries. These modalities are of value both in the general health care of the athlete and in the prevention of injury. The decisive renunciation of the use of drugs, particularly since the Olympic Games in Montreal in 1976, has certainly been influential, at least among official sports.

What is meant by the still imprecise term "sports physical therapy"? In modern medicine physical therapy refers to the use of natural forces in treatment. Another definition reads: "Physical therapy involves those methods of treatment that have their basis in the mechanisms of physical effects."

Examples include pressure in the form of manual, instrumental, or underwater massage, the use of heat in the form of irradiation, hydrocirculation, and whirlpool baths, the use of cold, such as cold packs, whirlpools, and the various methods of applying ice, electrotherapy in the low ranges of electromagnetic waves and currents for the stimulation of the neuromuscular structures, and others. Moreover, the various types of targeted and regulated active exercise included in both classic and modern remedial gynmastics are included among the most important forms of physical therapy.

Physical therapy is a scientifically based, medically comprehensive form of treatment, which is used in many specialized areas of medicine, but primarily in orthopedics, in pre- and postoperative treatment in modern surgery, and in internal medicine. It is not an "outsider" method, nor is it subject to speculative or abstract problems of the type encountered in the so-called paramedical methods. Physical therapy today is a firm component of scientifically oriented medicine. Sports physical therapy is a part of sports medicine. The practices and methods described earlier are applied in the case of injuries caused by sports for the purpose of healing and improvement as well as for prevention.

# The Remedial Therapist in Sports Physical Therapy

Who are the professionals who are trained, prepared, and responsible for these tasks? Persons who have completed preliminary and basic training and their clinical internship, and who have then received the necessary additional training, are termed remedial therapists; these are competent to perform the extensive physical therapy–remedial gymnastic tasks required in the area of sports medicine. The legally regulated training and recognition of remedial therapists in the Federal Republic of Germany corresponds to the training procedures for physical therapists in other countries. Remedial therapists, including members of the German Association for Physiotherapy–Central Association of Remedial Therapists, are included in and recognized by the World Confederation for Physical Therapy (WCPT).

It is obvious that remedial therapists active in sports medicine should have as much personal experience in athletics and competitive sports as possible. Only those remedial therapists with practical experience in competitive sports are in a position to understand the various problems of the athlete and the problems encountered in sports medicine and can work creatively on their solutions.

The word "therapists" in this book refers to physical therapists. The profession of "sports physical therapist" does not officially exist in the Federal Republic of Germany, although in some circles the term is used. Only the physical therapist and the masseur are legally recognized professionals in Germany.

Whereas the physical therapist has been trained in both the passive and active therapeutic treatments and practices both in the clinic and in private practice, the masseur is qualified to provide only the passive treatments. The important active methods of treatment lie beyond the capabilities of the masseur but lie within the province of the physical therapist.

It cannot be in the interests of athletes to have masseurs go through a crash course in the complex physical therapeutic methods of treatment given by an athletic organization in order to become a "sports physical therapist." Such a risky enterprise must lead to incompetence and dilettantism, because the prerequisites for the training as well as the necessary clinical time and experience are lacking. Masseurs are doubtless needed in sports, and they perform a recognized task in the care of the athlete, but in the treatment of injuries and damages caused by sports they cannot replace the physical therapist.

# Team of Attendants

It is absolutely necessary to coordinate the work of the physician, the therapist, and the trainer in the care of the athlete. Treatment with physical therapy and remedial therapy requires a doctor's diagnosis and prescription, as is the case with all other nonathletic treatment. Independently undertaken treatment by so-called "sports physical therapists," which occurs so frequently, particularly in the case of top competitive athletics, and which occasionally is even desired by the trainer and the athlete, should be condemned. The athlete, whose health and performance should always remain the primary consideration, is not served by such a practice. The rapid conditioning of an athlete, which is encouraged and striven for among certain functionaries, trainers, and attendants in top performance and professional athletics, does not benefit the athlete. Long-range freedom from injury and fitness for action cannot be expected in such circumstances. The practice is unconscionable. It is not in accordance with the ethical principles recorded in the regulations of the German Association for Physiotherapy–Central Association of Remedial Therapists.

The overall guidance of the treatment and the team of athletic attendants must lie in the hands of a professionally competent physician trained in physical medicine and rehabilitation, who is in constant contact with the therapist, whom he or she is to oversee and correct if necessary.

# Passive Treatments

This book is divided into four sections. In the first section the passive treatments of physical therapy are described. Some of these treatments go back thousands of years and were already recognized and used in ancient times both as a means of increasing performance and as therapy for athletic injuries and damage. The classic massage, which has an ancient history and still plays an important role in the care and treatment of the athlete, should be mentioned in this context first of all. Those special massages that are most important for the athlete will also be considered carefully. However, the importance of the massage is often exaggerated. All too often the "men with the golden hands" are almost viewed as magic healers, an image which should be corrected.

The other most important passive treatments, such as the uses of heat and cold, of water and baths — which also have ancient roots in traditional medicine — will also be described in accordance with their importance for athletic injuries. On the other hand, the use of electrotherapy with various currents is a more recent development, but it has doubtlessly become more important in the last two decades because of its stimulating and analgesic effect in the treatment of severe athletic damage and injury.

# Active Treatments

In the second section of the book, the active treatments of physical therapy will be discussed, which are known as "remedial therapy" in the Federal Republic of Germany. These include the various forms of classic remedial therapeutic exercises. Now as always the rebuilding of the muscular system forms one of the most important bases of all physical therapeutic procedures. The essential part of this process involves the retraining of muscles after injury and immobilization, including the development of the postural muscles, as in the case of damage to the spinal column of the athlete, and the development of balanced muscular strangth, i.e., exercises for the purpose of equalizing the one-sided developments that occur in most sports. Methods include isometric and dynamic exercises as well as eccentric and isokinetic exercises. The more recent methods are also described, including complex motions or proprioreceptive neuromuscular facilitation (PNF), based on neurophysiologic and neuromuscular functions. There are also chapters on stretching and loosening muscles, which are very important in athletics. These treatments are of greater importance in the care and prevention of athletic injuries than all of the passive treatments.

Exercises in water, manual therapy, and diagnosis each are treated in a separate chapter, as they are indispensable in today's active physical therapy.

The authors consider the active methods of treatment of physical therapy more important for prevention, therapy, and rehabilitation of athletic injuries and damage. Unfortunately, they are poorly known and frequently neglected. Many sports physicians themselves are not particularly well versed in active physical therapy methods. The antiquated standard prescription of "fango (mud applications) and massage" is still found all too often in today's practice, even in cases where such treatment is contrary to what clinical knowledge would require. Active treatment should be better known and more precisely applied by trainers, attendants, and the athletes themselves.

## Individual Descriptions

The third section of this book will include a description of the possibilities for using physical therapy and remedial exercise in the treatment of selected athletic injuries. Symptoms and their diagnoses frequently arising in practice will be briefly sketched in a series of individual descriptions. These descriptions should inform both the sports physicians and therapists, as well as the concerned athletes and trainers, about the nature and availability of treatment. They are usually presented in simple terminology. It must, of course, be understood that some treatments can only be performed by a physician or a therapist, but the interested layman may benefit from reading about them.

## Treatment for Training and Competition

Treatment for training and competition is described in the fourth and final section of the book. The primary topics for this section include the use of functional bandages and first aid, including the appropriate bandaging material, medicines, and other aids. However, a number of other fields are discussed in this section, including means to prepare for competition, such as warm-ups, stretching and special exercises, and warm-down techniques, such as jogging, relaxing baths, self-massage, sauna baths, certain exercises and sports that balance uneven muscle development, and special forms of rehabilitative training.

The book is recommended for sports physicians, therapists, trainers, physical education instructors, and especially athletes as an aid in the prevention, improvement, and cure of athletic injuries and damage, so that what has been called "the best nonessential thing in the world" does not lead to unfortunate permanent damage.

## CHAPTER 1

# Massage

*WERNER KUPRIAN*

## Introduction and Historical Development

Massage has played an important role in the treatment of sick, injured, and handicapped people for centuries. A number of experts view it as the earliest form of "treatment" altogether. People rub or stroke themselves instinctively to relieve the pain of an aching bodily part. A mother will caress her child to calm it. The massage has an instinctively relaxing effect on the psyche. Without doubt, the classic massage arose as an instinctive modality, and its popularity stretches back over a thousand years. In these days of scientifically oriented medicine, massage is offered more and more frequently as a part of medical and therapeutic treatment, and it is usually gladly accepted by the patients. Nevertheless, the knowledge of its effectiveness gained through empirical experience is only partially corroborated by science; we still lack parameters for measurements and proof of its various therapeutic values.

However, the classic massage was already in use in ancient times as one of the methods for improving the athletic performance of the athlete. This use of the massage is mentioned by Hippocrates and also Galen and Epictetus. Galen had already distinguished among 18 different variants, including hard, soft, moderate, preparatory, and warm-down massages. The trainer was to remain

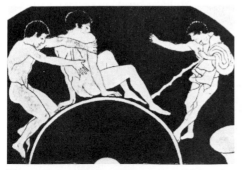

**Figure 1–1.** Back massage by athletes in ancient Greece, 480 B.C.

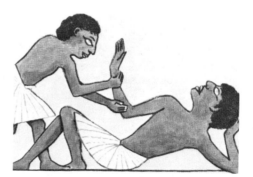

**Figure 1–2.** Arm massage in ancient Egypt.

aware of the condition of the athlete he massaged. We possess drawings from ancient Greece of backrubs and chest massages for boxers, massages of the Achilles tendon for runners, and a self-massage for the calf muscles.

Diem describes the massage as being one of the principal components of athletic care in ancient Greece, together with baths and sunbathing, in his "World History of Athletics and Physical Training." He also concludes that the athletic massages at this time, approximately 500 years before the modern era, were already extremely diverse, making use of various devices and combining massage with other treatments accompanying the training. It is notable that massage was almost always used in connection with light active and passive gymnastics and breathing exercises. In Greek antiquity, the disciplines of gymnastics and massage were still united.

The word "massage" is derived from the Greek "massein," meaning approximately "kneading," which is related to the Latin "manus," hand. The actual instrument which carries out the massage is the probing, sensitive hand of the therapist.

But the massage was well known and widely used by other ancient people besides the Greeks; the Egyptians, Persians, Romans, Japanese, and Chinese were also familiar with its use. It probably went out of common use during the Middle Ages under the influence of the contemporary religion's negative attitude toward the body. Only in modern times, for about the last 100 years, has massage been rediscovered.

The Central Institute for Gymnastics was founded in 1813 in Stockholm. The Swedish gymnastics instructor P. H. Ling taught there. He dealt with massage as his specialty. According to his interpretation, massage was a secondary branch of gymnastics. Since that time, an increasing number of doctors have devoted scientific research to the effects of massage. Metzger, Volger, Kohlrausch, Lüdge, Thomsen, Teirich-Leube, Heipertz, and others can be mentioned as making contributions in this field. Physical therapists and masseurs are also collecting and publishing the results of their experiences.

The authors mentioned wrote scientific works about the classical massage on the basis of which special methods of massage were developed; their conclusions were, incidentally, in no way unified, and some of their positions have subsequently been abandoned. The best-known special massage is the connective tissue massage, based on the segmental topography of the skin and the visceromuscular reflex. This method was developed by Kohlrausch, Dicke, and Teirich-Leube and was based on the research of the British workers Head and Mackenzie.

Vogler and Kraus developed the periosteal massage in 1953, and Vodder, a Dane, developed the controversial manual lymph-drainage technique. Further special massage techniques could be mentioned, but this would go beyond the bounds of this work, which is devoted primarily to injuries and damage caused by sports.

These special massage techniques often unjustifiably placed the classic massage into a subordinate position. Basically, however, special massages unite the most useful therapeutic elements. The classic massage, partially overvalued, but partially and unjustly undervalued too, has emerged from its earlier obscurity in the past decades as a result of efforts of scientists and practioners and today occupies a prominent position in prevention, therapy, and rehabilitation.

# Major Effects of Massage

The physiologic effects of the classic massage lie primarily in the regulatory influence of the muscle tone. Muscular hypertonia can only be lowered without danger by means of a massage. Muscular and connective tissue are only capable of withstanding loosening and stretching exercises after a massage. Research has shown that constriction of the capillaries in a muscle causes a high degree of conduction loss and cell degeneration as a result of slowing of metabolism. The massage regulates muscle tone by enhancing the circulation and local metabolism, and also by increasing the flexibility of the muscle. Heipertz has proved in his investigations that massage not only intensifies skin circulation but also leads to a true hyperemia of the muscles.

Together with the increased circulation in the muscles and the skin, an effect upon the subcutaneous fat layer and the connective tissue can also be noted. Among the incontrovertible scientific findings concerning the effects of massage include the promotion of more rapid removal of metabolic wastes, the removal of old adhesions, the effect at distant sites of reflex massage techniques, and reactive effects on the vascular system and the entire organism. Massages are also capable of quickly removing fatiguing materials from the tissues and of relieving muscular tension, soreness, and cramps. In this way they not only prevent athletic injuries such as muscle pulls and tears, but also improve the circulation and help in the transport of energy to the muscles. Massage eases the work of the heart and circulatory system. However, one of the most persistent false impressions in both professional and lay medical circles is the belief that massages are capable of increasing strength. Strengthening in the physiologic sense is solely possible by targeted active exercise and systematic training. This is true both for the muscular system and the cardiovascular system. A massage can, however, prepare the body for strengthening exercises and remove waste materials in the muscles and connective tissue that could limit performance. Moreover, the massage has a positive effect on the human psyche, if performed correctly, by promoting relaxation, calm, and a general sense of well-being.

Sperling summarizes the "certain or very probable effects of the massage" as follows:

1. General effect on the organism.
2. Local increase in capillary diameter.
3. Regulation of muscle tone.
4. Intensification of venous return and the movement of lymph, with positive effects on the muscle tone, for example.

5. Activation of neurohormones and tissue hormones (e.g., vasoactive substances).

6. Reflex effect on internal organs, but also on the surface tissues of the body.

7. A general sedative effect.

The major goal of classic massage is the support and aid of the healing process in an illness, injury, or handicap. Hamann states: "According to the state of research today, we can assume that there is no exclusively local-mechanical effect of a massage, but that the effects are always of a complex nature."

# Basic Massage Techniques

The basic techniques of the classic massage and the athletic massage are the same and have remained essentially unchanged for centuries. The use of these techniques varies according to the requirements of each individual case. We can distinguish between the following five techniques:

Stroking

Kneading and Working

Rubbing

Hacking, Thumping, and Clapping or Slapping

Vibration and Shaking

All of these techniques can be varied in a number of ways. The diverse combinations of the techniques also differ and should be used in accordance with the goals of a particular treatment.

## STROKING (EFFLEURAGE)

The primary function of stroking is to establish physical contact with the patient. The main physiologic effect occurs when stroking is begun at the peripheral areas and moves from the extremities towards the heart. The return flow of the venous and lymphatic systems is doubtlessly favorably influenced and enhanced by this process. Circulation to the skin surface is also increased by stroking. The success of cosmetic massages, which consist primarily of stroking, can be traced to the increased rate of metabolic exchange in the peripheral areas. Both one- and two-handed stroking is used. At the beginning of the massage, the pressure should be gentle, coming from the flat of the hand, with fingers slightly bent and thumbs spread. The movement should be towards the heart, and contact should be maintained with the patient as the hands are returned to the initial position. In the course of the massage, the pressure can be increased. Every massage begins and ends with stroking. Stroking should also be used between other techniques, such as kneading and working. Stroking relaxes, lessens the defensive tension against harder massage techniques, and has a mentally calming effect.

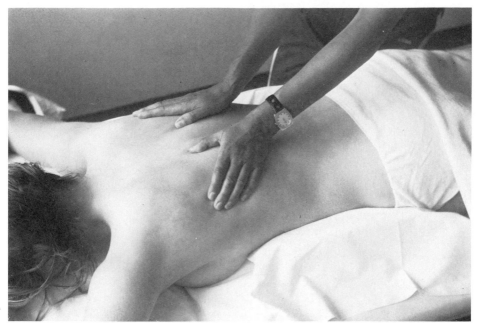

**Figure 1–3.**  Two-handed stroking of back muscles.

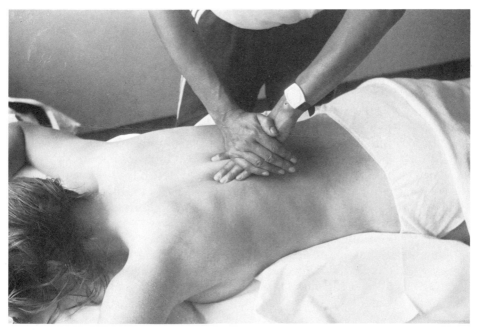

**Figure 1–4.**  Stroking of long back extensors to the left and right of the spinal column.

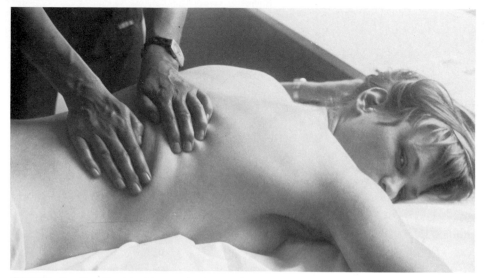

**Figure 1–5.** Traction stroking on back muscles.

## KNEADING AND WORKING (PÉTRISSAGE)

Kneading and working go more deeply than stroking and are directed primarily at the muscle system. Their goal is to press the metabolic waste products out of the affected areas through intensive, vigorous action. They have a decidedly tonicizing effect on the muscles. The most important effects include the increase in the local blood supply to the muscle and the lowering and — if the kneading becomes too vigorous — occasionally the heightening of muscle tone.

In kneading, the closed fingers and the spread thumbs work like tongs. Smaller muscles, such as the biceps, can be kneaded with one hand, whereas larger muscles, such as the quadriceps and entire muscle groups, require both hands. In kneading, the hands move from the distal to the proximal point of the muscle insertion. Varieties of kneading include: alternating kneading — for example, for the adductors and the tensor fasciae latae and iliotibial band; kneading which stretches and pulls, such as for the adductors; kneading with thumb pressure, for the gluteus maximus; and finally kneading with the fingertips, for the tibialis anterior and the erector spinae.

Like kneading, working presses more deeply into the muscle; the muscle is vigorously lifted out of position and worked across its normal course. This has a stimulating effect on the muscle receptors and the tendon fibers. Two-handed working can be used, for example, on the flexor and extensor muscles of the upper thigh. The triceps surae and the biceps muscles can be worked with one hand by pushing the muscle rapidly back and forth between sharply bent fingers and the ball of the hand.

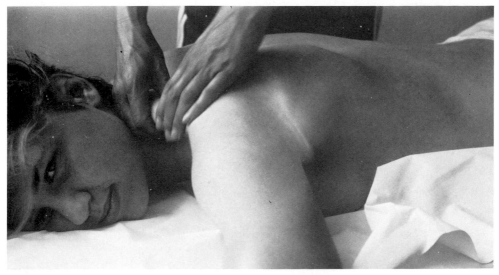

**Figure 1–6.**  Traction kneading of shoulder and neck muscles.

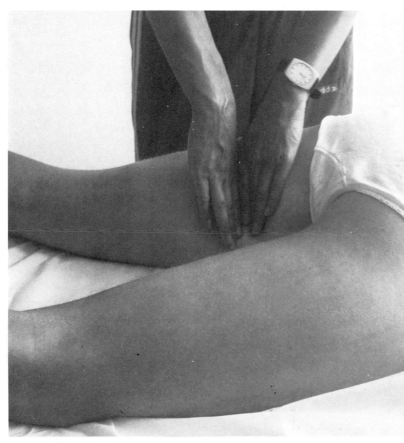

**Figure 1–7.**  Alternating kneading of knee flexors on the back of upper thigh.

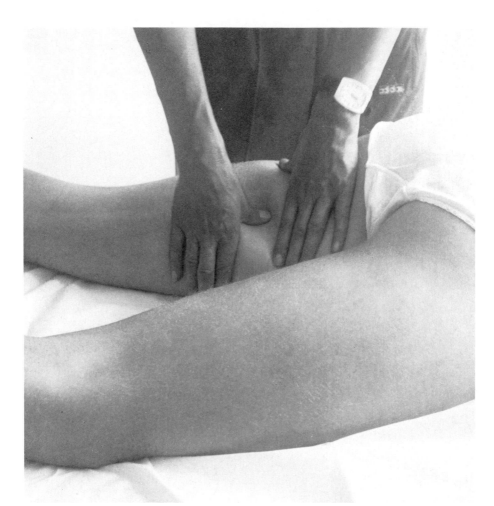

**Figure 1–8.**   Kneading with thumb pressure on the hamstrings.

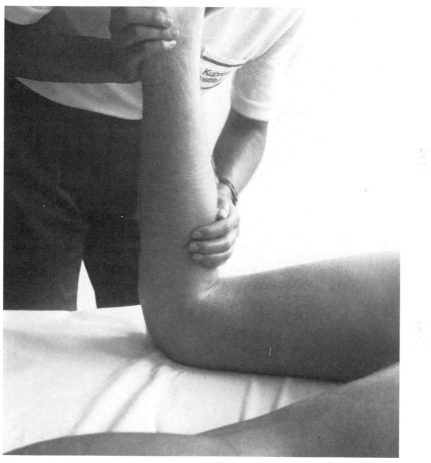

**Figure 1–9.**   Working to loosen calf muscles.

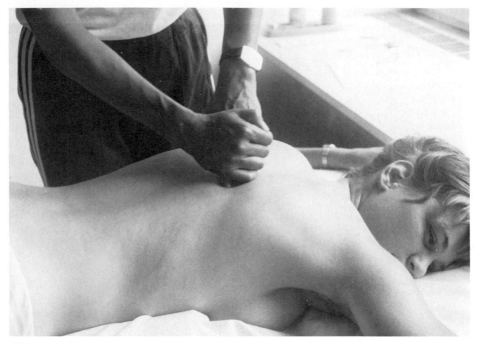

**Figure 1-10.** Fingertip rubbing of long back extensor.

## RUBBING (FRICTION)

Rubbing is used primarily in areas of local, deep-lying hardening and myogelosis. It aims to produce a strong, hyperemic effect in small surface areas of muscle. Local hardening in muscles can reduce their efficiency and flexibility. There are often adhesions as well in the hardened and tense areas of muscle. The sudden demands made on muscles that are required in many sports can easily cause damage to muscle fibers, pulls, and tears. Rubbing can therefore bring relief in tendinitis, painful muscle insertions, and adhesions. Rubbing with the fingertips around the Achilles tendon, the base of the calf, and the change from tendon to muscular tissue of the gastrocnemius may serve as an example.

Gentler rubbing over a larger area is performed with the ball and the side of the hand. More specific local rubbing is done with fingertips. The motion is circular to elliptical. The pressure varies from light circling to "Gelotripsy," the violent removal of muscle hardening, during which bleeding in the interior of the muscle can be caused by the strong local pressure. However, this procedure is somewhat controversial. An exact diagnosis of myogelosis is required for its use. When rubbing with both hands, the pressure of the one hand may be used to increase pressure on the middle finger of the other hand. The gluteus maximus, which begins at the edge of the pelvis, the long back extensors of the erector spinae, and the rhomboideus muscles are particularly well suited to rubbing treatments with the fingertips.

The Austrian therapist Strohal rejects friction entirely, however, considering it senseless and damaging, as it is unable to aid in elimination of lactic acid. On the basis of many years of experience with the use of friction massage, we cannot agree to this opinion. After all, friction is never used alone, but rather is always used in connection with other massage techniques.

## HACKING, THUMPING, AND CLAPPING OR SLAPPING

Hacking, thumping, and clapping or slapping were earlier considered typical procedures for the athletic massage. They have practically no further application for the medicinal massage. In the case of painful tissues they are in any case not recommended. Doubtlessly they can, however, create a certain preparedness for muscle tensing and contraction in relaxed muscles. Thumping the back and chest with lightly clenched fists can increase exhalation and aid in coughing up material from bronchial emphysema.

Other than increasing skin circulation, the primary effect of slapping is acoustic. A good massage can do without such theatrics. Hacking, thumping, and slapping should in all cases be used with extreme caution and restraint.

These techniques can actually adversely affect the performance of highly trained, sensitive, and tense competitive athletes, such as sprinters, hurdlers, and long and high jumpers.

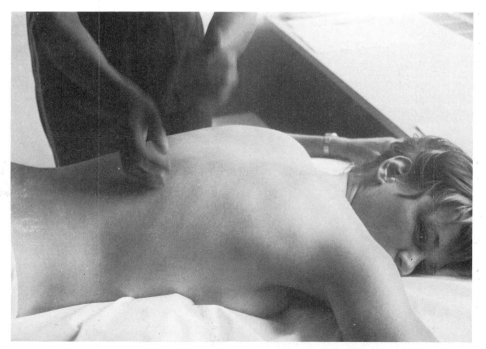

**Figure 1–11.**  Thumping of the back muscles.

## VIBRATION AND SHAKING

Manual vibration, which is particularly strenuous for the therapist, has a relaxing or occasionally stimulating effect. It can also be used on painful muscles which are as yet unable to bear kneading and working. Various manufacturers have developed an arsenal of vibration machines, as these techniques are difficult and tiring to perform manually. They are also capable of relieving certain cramped muscles. They cannot replace a good manual shaking, a technique which is difficult to learn, however. Shaking is used primarily for the extremities. It can lower the muscle tone of the arms and legs. The therapist generally stands above the patient, raising the extremity, which encourages venous and lymphatic return. Vibration and shaking are also valuable for the athletic massage as treatment for strains and the injuries caused by them.

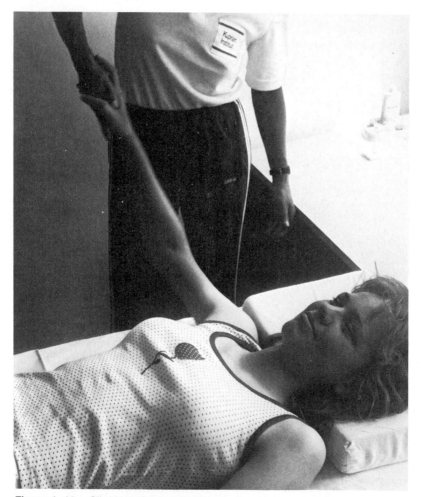

**Figure 1–12.** Shaking of arm muscles.

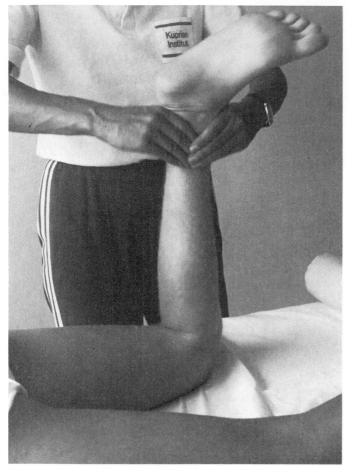

**Figure 1–13.**   Shaking of calf muscles.

# Combinations of Techniques, Variations, Treatment Programs

The techniques mentioned can be combined and varied in many ways, from calming, gentle stroking at the start of the treatment, through stimulating vibration, to the deep-working vigorous kneading, local rubbing, and shaking for the promotion of venous return and lymphatic flow. The various individual classic massage techniques alone, however, do not make for a good massage. Proper program, intensity, tempo, and rhythm, as well as the proper starting, climax, and closing of the massage, are all important too. The form of the massage depends on the individual requirements of the patient or athlete. The massage can be given daily, and should be undertaken at least two or three times per week. Partial massages last approximately 10 to 15 minutes.

*Text continued on page 29*

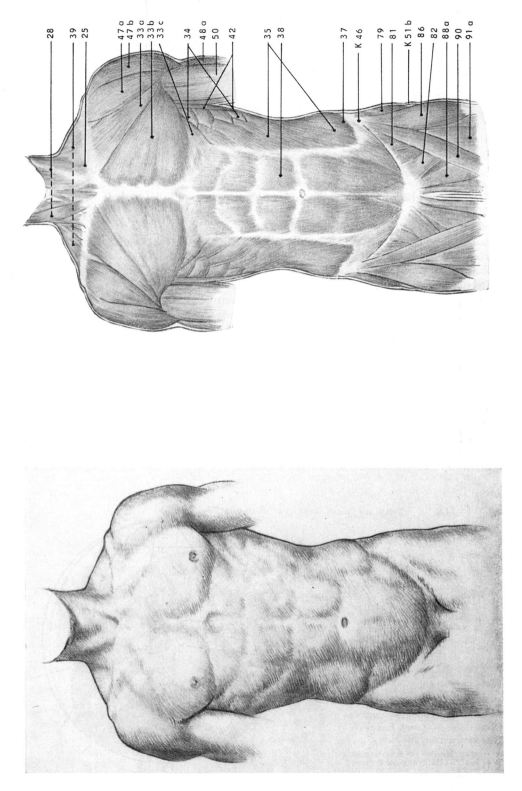

**Figure 1–14.**   Anterior aspect of torso. (Adapted from Tittel, K.: Descriptive and Functional Human Anatomy. Stuttgart, Gustav Fischer Verlag, 1976.)

*Muscles and Related Structures*

| | |
|---|---|
| K46 | Site of anterior superior iliac spine |
| K51b | Site of greater trochanter |
| 25 | Hyoid muscles |
| 28 | Sternocleidomastoid |
| 33a | Pectoralis major (clavicular portion) |
| 33b | Pectoralis major (sternal portion) |
| 33c | Pectoralis minor |
| 34 | Serratus anterior |
| 35 | External oblique muscle of abdomen |
| 37 | Lumbar triangle |
| 38 | Rectus abdominis |
| 39 | Trapezius |
| 42 | Latissimus dorsi |
| 47a | Deltoid (anterior portion) |
| 47b | Deltoid (intermediate portion) |
| 48a | Triceps |
| 50 | Biceps |
| 79 | Gluteus medius |
| 81 | Iliacus |
| 82 | Rectineus |
| 86 | Tensor fasciae latae |
| 88a | Adductor longus |
| 90 | Sartorius |
| 91a | Rectus femoris |

*Bones*

| | |
|---|---|
| 25g | 7th cervical vertebra |
| 26 | Lower thoracic vertebrae |
| 27 | Lumbar vertebrae |
| 28 | Sacrum |
| 29 | Coccyx |
| 30 | Thorax |
| 31a | Manubrium |
| 31b | Body of sternum |
| 31c | Xiphoid process |
| 32 | Clavicle |
| 33 | Scapula |
| 33b | Acromion |
| 33c | Supraspinous fossa |
| 34 | Humerus |
| 44 | Iliac fossa |
| 45 | Iliac crest |
| 46 | Anterior superior iliac spine |
| 47 | Anterior inferior iliac spine |
| 48 | Pubis |
| 49 | Ischium |
| 49a | Ischial ramus |
| 50 | Hip joint (acetabulum) |
| 51a | Neck of femur |
| 51b | Greater trochanter |

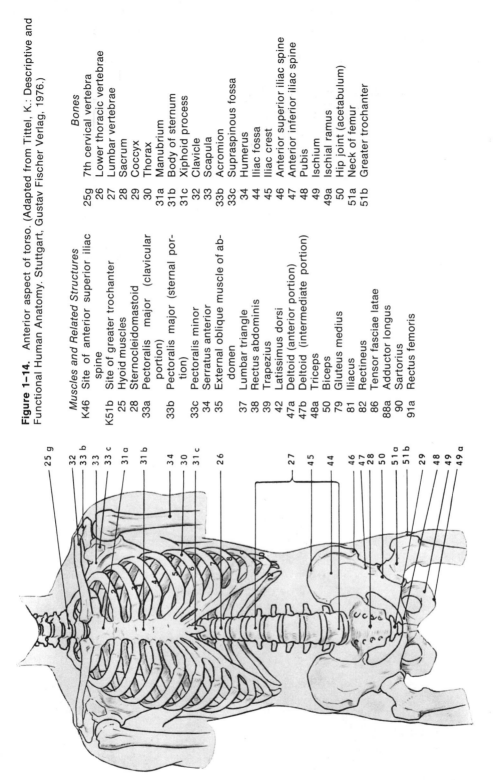

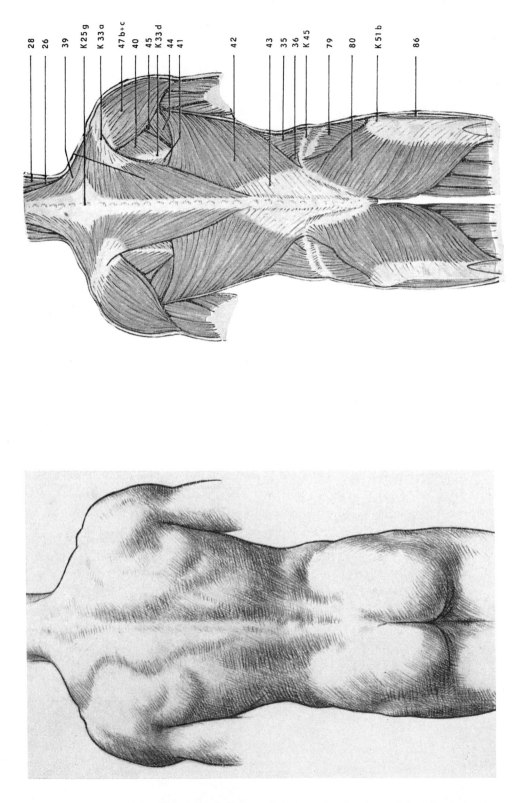

28 26 39 K25g K33a 47b+c 40 45 K33d 44 41 42 43 35 36 K45 79 80 K51b 86

**Figure 1-15.** Posterior view of torso. (Adapted from Tittel, K.: Descriptive and Functional Human Anatomy. Stuttgart, Gustav Fischer Verlag, 1976.)

*Muscles and Related Structures*

| | |
|---|---|
| K25g | 7th cervical vertebra |
| K33a | Spine of scapula |
| K33d | Medial border (scapula) |
| K45 | Iliac crest |
| K51b | Greater trochanter |
| 26 | Posterior triangle |
| 28 | Sternocleidomastoid |
| 35 | External oblique muscle of abdomen |
| 36 | Internal oblique |
| 39 | Trapezius |
| 40 | Infraspinatus |
| 41 | Rhomboideus major |
| 42 | Latissimus dorsi |
| 43 | Posterior layer of thoracolumbar fascia |
| 44 | Teres major |
| 45 | Teres minor |
| 47b | Deltoid (intermediate portion) |
| 47c | Deltoid (posterior portion) |
| 79 | Gluteus medius |
| 80 | Gluteus maximus |
| 86 | Tensor fasciae latae |

*Bones*

| | |
|---|---|
| 20 | Mandible |
| 25 | Cervical vertebrae |
| 25a | 1st cervical vertebra (atlas) |
| 25b | 2nd cervical vertebra (axis) |
| 26 | Lower thoracic vertebrae |
| 27 | Lumbar vertebrae |
| 28 | Sacrum |
| 29 | Coccyx |
| 30 | Ribs |
| 32 | Clavicle |
| 33 | Scapula |
| 33a | Spine of scapula |
| 33b | Acromion process |
| 33c | Infraglenoid tubercle |
| 34 | Humerus |
| 44 | Iliac fossa |
| 46 | Anterior superior iliac spine |
| 48 | Pubis |
| 49a | Ischiopubic ramus |
| 50 | Hip joint (acetabulum) |
| 51 | Femur |
| 51a | Neck of femur |
| 51b | Greater trochanter |

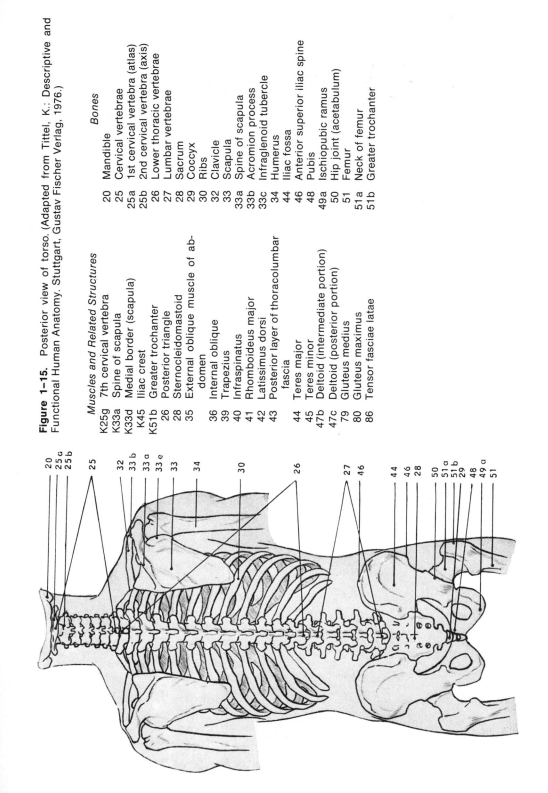

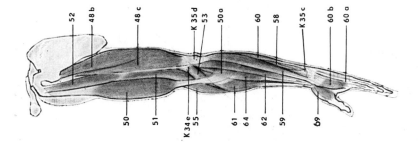

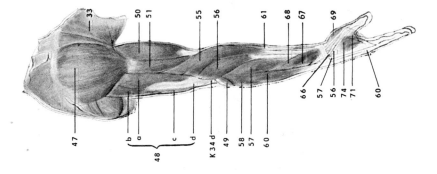

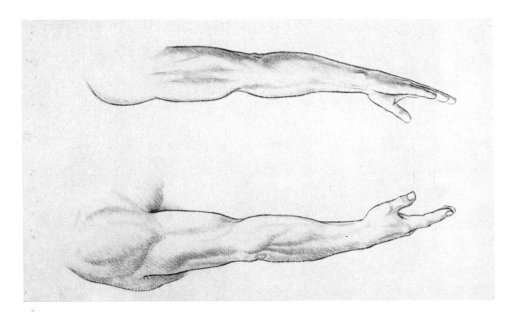

**Figure 1–16.** Upper limb, exterior and interior views. (Adapted from Tittel, K.: Descriptive and Functional Human Anatomy. Stuttgart, Gustav Fischer Verlag, 1976.)

*Muscles and Related Structures*

K34d  Lateral epicondyle
K34e  Medial epicondyle
K35c  Styloid process (ulna)
K35d  Olecranon
33    Pectoralis major
47    Deltoid
48a   Triceps — lateral head
48b   Triceps — long head
48c   Triceps — medial head
48d   Tendon of the triceps
49    Pronator teres
50    Biceps
50a   Biceps tendon
51    Brachialis
52    Coracobrachialis
53    Supinator
55    Brachioradialis
56    Extensor carpi radialis longus
57    Extensor carpi radialis brevis
58    Extensor carpi ulnaris
59    Flexor carpi ulnaris
60    Extensor digitorum superficialis
60a   Tendons of digitorum super-
      ficialis
60b   Flexor digiti minimi brevi
61    Flexor digitorum superficialis
62    Flexor digitorum superficialis
64    Palmaris longus
66    Abductor pollicis longus
67    Abductor pollicis brevis
68    Flexor pollicus longus
69    Flexor pollicus brevis
71    Adductor pollicus
74    Dorsal interosseous

*Bones*

32    Clavicle
32a   Sternal articular facet of clavicle
32b   Acromial articular facet of clavicle
33    Scapula
33a   Spine of scapula
33b   Acromion
33c   Supraspinous fossa
33e   Glenoid cavity
34    Humerus
34b   Greater tubercle of humerus
34c   Lesser tubercle of humerus
34d   Lateral epicondyle
34e   Medial epicondyle
35    Ulna
35a   Olecranon process
35b   Coronoid process
35d   Head of ulna
36    Radius
36a   Head of radius
36b   Styloid process
37    Carpus
37a   Scaphoid
37b   Lunate
37c   Triquetrum
37d   Pisiform
37e   Trapezium
37f   Trapezoid
37g   Capitate
37h   Hamate
38    Metacarpus of thumb
39    Middle phalanx of thumb
40    Proximal phalanges
41    Middle phalanges
42    Distal phalanx of thumb
43    Distal phalanges

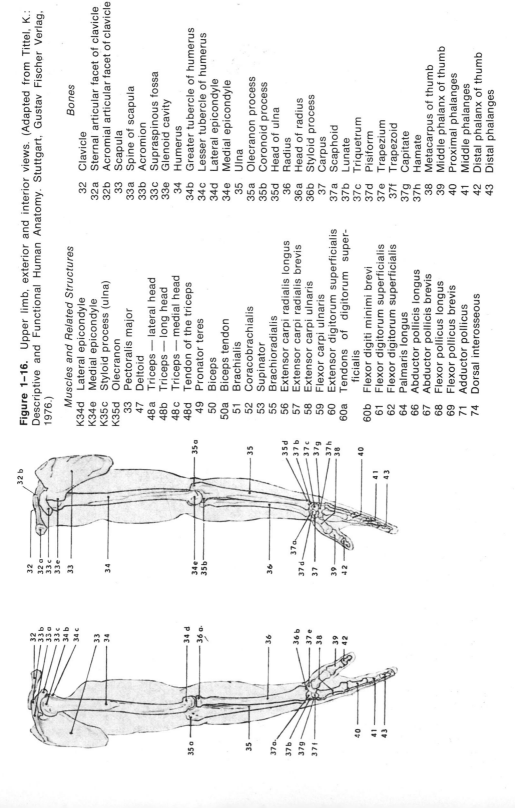

**Figure 1–17.** Lower limb, anterior and posterior views. (Adapted from Tittel, K.: Descriptive and Functional Human Anatomy. Stuttgart, Gustav Fischer Verlag, 1976.)

*Illustration continued on opposite page*

### Muscles and Related Structures

| | |
|---|---|
| K46 | Anterior superior iliac spine |
| K51b | Greater trochanter |
| K51e | Medial epicondyle |
| K53 | Patella |
| K54 | Tibia |
| K54a | Upper end of tibia |
| K56a | Head of fibula |
| K57 | Lateral malleolus |
| K59 | Calcaneus |
| 78 | Gluteus maximus |
| 79 | Gluteus medius |
| 81 | Iliacus |
| 82 | Pectineus |
| 86 | Tensor fasciae latae |
| 87 | Iliotibial tract |
| 88a | Adductor longus |
| 88b | Adductor brevis |
| 88c | Adductor magnus |
| 89 | Gracilis |
| 90 | Sartorius |
| 91a | Rectus femoris |
| 91b | Vastus lateralis |
| 91c | Biceps femoris (short head) |
| 91d | Vastus medialis |
| 92 | Ligamentum patellae |
| 93 | Infrapatellar fat pad |
| 94a | Biceps femoris (long head) |
| 95 | Semimembranosus |
| 96 | Semitendinosus |
| 97 | Insertion of sartorius |
| 98 | Popliteus |
| 99a | Medial head of gastrocnemius |
| 99b | Lateral head of gastrocnemius |
| 100 | Soleus |
| 101 | Achilles tendon |
| 102 | Tibialis anterior |
| 103 | Extensor digitorum longus |
| 104 | Extensor digitorum brevis |
| 106 | Extensor hallucis longus |
| 107 | Peroneus longus |
| 108 | Peroneus brevis |
| 109 | Origin of peroneus brevis |
| 110 | Extensor digitorum longus |
| 111a | Tendon of extensor hallucis longus |
| 112 | Tibialis posterior |
| 115 | Flexor accessorius |
| 116 | Extensor retinaculum |

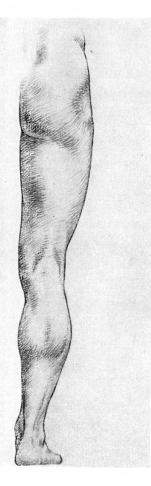

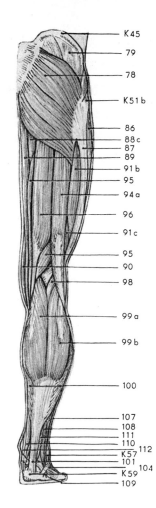

K45
79
78
K51b
86
88c
87
89
91b
95
94a
96
91c
95
90
98
99a
99b
100
107
108
111
110
K57 112
101 104
K59
109

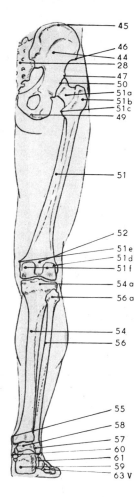

45
46
44
28
47
50
51a
51b
51c
49
51
52
51e
51d
51f
54a
56a
54
56
55
58
57
60
61
59
63 V

**Figure 1–17.** *Continued.*

*Bones*

| | | | |
|---|---|---|---|
| 28 | Sacrum | 53 | Patella |
| 44 | Iliac fossa | 54 | Tibia |
| 45 | Iliac crest | 54a | Upper end of tibia |
| 46 | Anterior superior iliac spine | 54d | Tuberosity of tibia |
| 47 | Anterior inferior iliac spine | 55 | Medial malleolus |
| 48 | Pubis | 56 | Fibula |
| 49 | Ischium | 56a | Head of fibula |
| 50 | Hip joint (acetabulum) | 57 | Lateral malleolus |
| 51 | Femur | 58 | Talus |
| 51a | Neck of femur | 59 | Calcaneus |
| 51b | Greater trochanter | 60 | Navicular |
| 51c | Lesser trochanter | 61 | Cuboid |
| 51d | Lateral epicondyle | 62l | Lateral cuneiform bone |
| 51e | Medial epicondyle | 63 | Metatarsal bones |
| 51f | Medial and lateral condyles | 63V | 5th metatarsal bone |
| 52 | Intercondylar notch | 65 | Proximal phalanges of toes |

| 9101 | Thrombophlebitis |
| 9102 | Arterial embolism |
| 9103 | Appearance of neurologic deficit |
| 9104 | Sudden cessation of pain from nerve compression |
| 9105 | Emergency situation |
| 911 | Inflammations |
| 912 | Injuries |
| 913 | Vascular disorders |
| 914 | Laminectomy of 2 to 3 vertebrae |
| 915 | Damage to corticospinal tract |
| 916 | Cerebeller damage |
| 917 | Harrington stylus massage |
| 918 | Muscles replaced with connective tissue |
| 919 | Tumors and infectious diseases |
| 921 | After operation on knee |
| 922 | After fracture of extremities |
| 9231 | After fracture of thoracic vertebra with preserved dorsal edge |
| 9232 | After fracture of cervical or lumbar vertebra |
| 9233 | After multiple fractures of spine |
| 924 | After endoprothesis of the hip |
| 924 | After endoprothesis of the hip with hepatic damage |
| 925 | After operation on lumbar intervertebral disk |
| 926 | After operation of cervical intervertebral disk (Cloward) |
| 927 | After operation for scoliosis with exception of Harrington stylus massage |
| 9281 | After metal plates or screws have been used for treating fractures |
| 9282 | After metal plates or screws have been removed |
| 931 | Confinement to bed for longer than 5 months in addition to circulatory problems in the affected area |
| 932 | Compression symptoms |
| 933 | Before puberty |

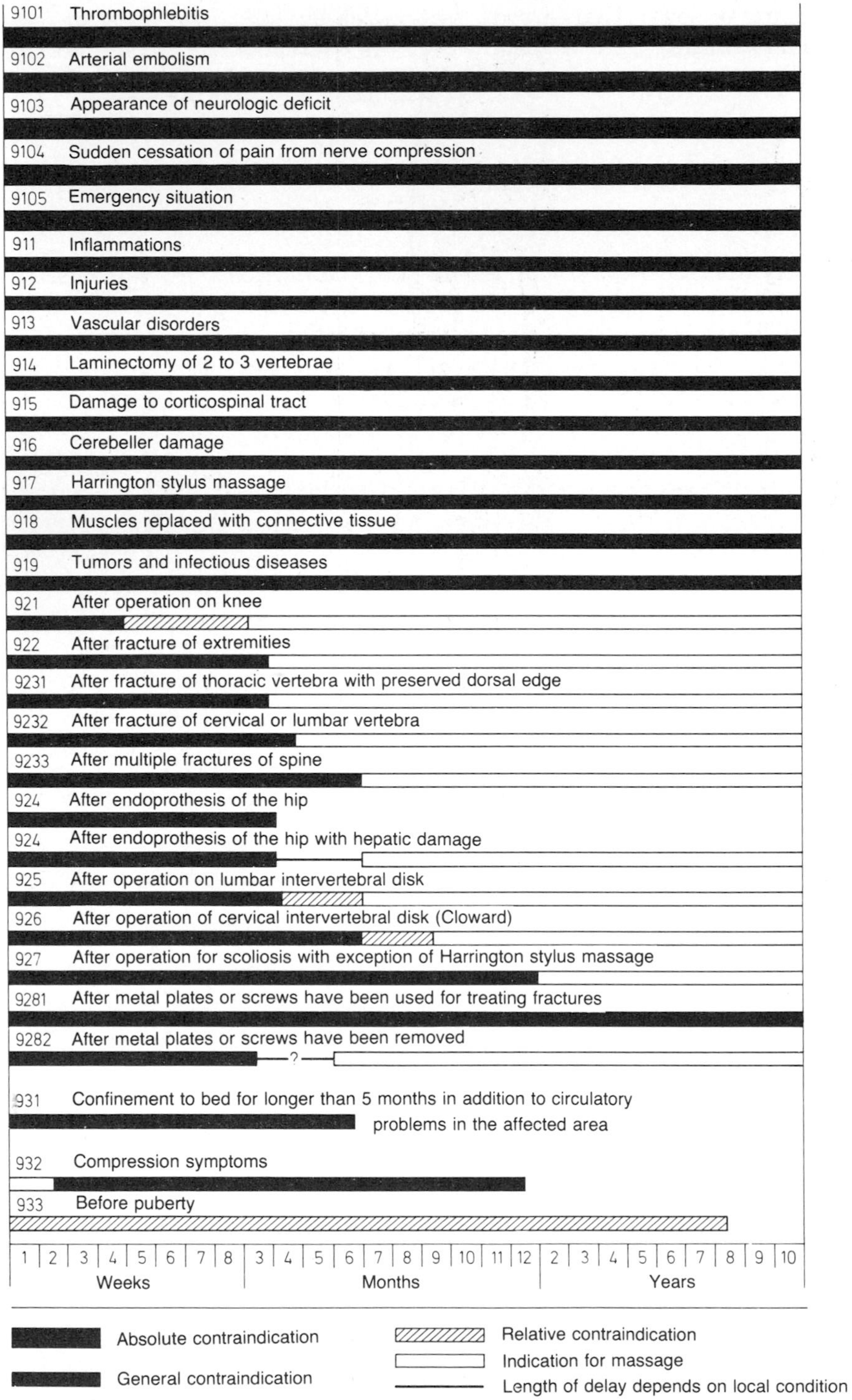

Weeks: 1 2 3 4 5 6 7 8   Months: 3 4 5 6 7 8 9 10 11 12   Years: 2 3 4 5 6 7 8 9 10

Absolute contraindication

General contraindication

Relative contraindication

Indication for massage

Length of delay depends on local condition

**Figure 1–18.** Indications and contraindications for massage. (From Hoffa, A., Gocht, H., Storck, U., and Lüdke, H. S.: *Massage Techniques.* Stuttgart, Ferdinand Enke Verlag, 1978.)

The massaging of several large body parts, such as both legs, lasts 20 to 30 minutes. The so-called "full massage," which is offered in various health spas and sauna baths, is not good policy either therapeutically or as an athletic massage.

# Lubrication

Normally the therapist's hand should not need lubricating materials. The use of talcum is out of the question, as it stops up the pores; however, in some instances, such as when a massage is necessary despite heavy perspiration, as during athletic events, its use is justified. Massage and moisturizing oils may be used for particularly dry skin, such as after plaster casts have been removed or when skin has been dried out by a combination of heavy perspiration and frequent showers. Such oils should be used sparingly, and should be placed on the hands of the therapist, not on the body of the athlete. Hyperemic lubricants are not recommended. The so-called "starting oils" (such as Ben Gay) can cause considerable skin irritation, and their effects vary according to the skin type of the athlete. They can occasionally cause allergies. They are also suspected of causing blood to drain from the muscles to the skin, which runs counter to the aim of a massage, which is to foster a good muscular blood supply. Balsam has proved to be a good material for training and preparatory massages, owing to its beneficial effect on the skin and its greaselessness. Alcoholic solutions such as rubbing alcohol or fluids used for intermediary or warm-down massages can improve their efficiency.

# Positioning

One of the most important requirements for obtaining good relaxation from a massage is the correct positioning of the body. If the patient is reclining correctly and comfortably, half of the efficiency of the massage is already provided for. In actuality, it is repeatedly made evident, on the field and during competition, that the physiologically correct body positioning is either entirely or partially neglected.

The most important aid in proper positioning of the body is the trainer's table. A soft, sagging bed is as unsuited for this purpose as a bed that is too rigid. On the field, during athletic competition, one is unfortunately often forced to work under conditions that are far from optimal for proper relaxation. One is forced to improvise with pillows, blankets, and bundled-up clothing.

Along with a proper training table, other items, such as small pillows, padding rolls, small sand and pellet bags, and pieces of foam rubber in various sizes and thicknesses, are additional necessary aids.

The training table should be equipped with an adjustable head support. The ability to make a downward adjustment of the face support, which causes a slight extension of the vertebrae in the neck and the head when the patient is

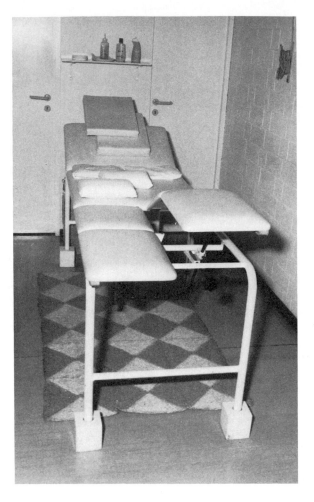

**Figure 1–19.** Training table with adjustable headrest and individually adjustable leg supports. Also used are positioning materials, foam rubber cushions, rolls, and pellet bags.

lying prone, is also a great advantage. Also strongly recommended are individual, adjustable supports for the legs, which can allow the legs to be raised with the knees slightly bent when the patient is lying on his back.

The surface of the training table should be padded and not too hard. For the purposes of cleaning and disinfection a washable plastic surface is preferred. A cotton sheet is necessary because of perspiration and because the surface of the plastic material is generally too cool.

The training table should be 200 cm long and 65 to 70 cm wide. The height should be variable, and adjusted to the height of the therapist. A moderate height of 75 cm is usually adequate, however. Sliding arm supports are also effective. Occasionally portable, folding training tables must be used. We have had consistently poor experiences with them. They are either too heavy or too flimsy.

Useful sizes for foam rubber pillows are: 30 × 40 cm, and 4, 6, and 8 cm thick. They should be covered over with white cotton or terry toweling. Support rolls should be 10 to 15 cm in diameter and 30 cm long for use with a

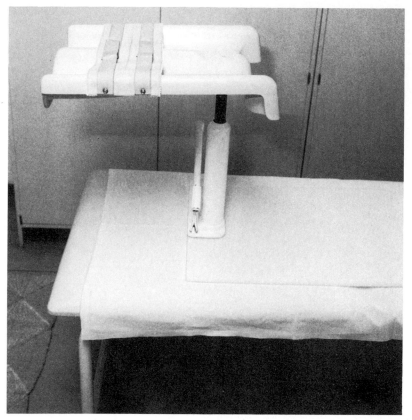

**Figure 1–20.** Positioning and extension device (after Reinhardt).

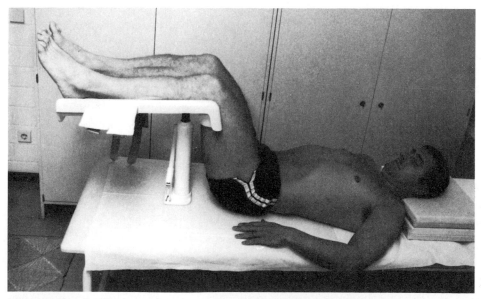

**Figure 1–21.** Positioning of legs for massage and remedial exercise.

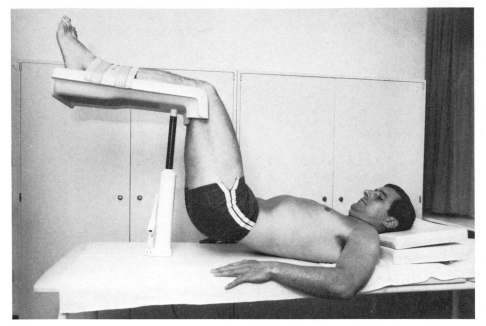

**Figure 1–22.**   Positioning for extension of lumbar vertebrae.

knee or the back of the neck, 50 cm long for use with both knees. Pillows filled with pellets are very useful for positioning knees, feet, neck, arms, and hands. The moveable yet firm stuffing permits a wide variety of individual position- ings. These pellet or sandbags should measure about 20 × 30 cm. Restraining belts with foam rubber pads in various widths should also be a part of the equipment for the training table. When a patient is being massaged in a supine position, such as during the massage of a leg, abdomen, chest, or arms, the part of the table supporting the headpiece should be raised approximately 20 degrees. A neck roll is also necessary. The knees should also be placed in the so-called resting position, at an angle of about 25 degrees with padding rolls or pellet bags.

When the patient is being treated in a prone position, as for the back of the legs, buttocks, back, shoulders, or nape of the neck, padded rolls should be placed under the ankles, so that the knees are slightly bent. The feet should hang over the end of the training table.

A 5 to 10 cm thick foam rubber cushion should be placed under the abdomen of the patient for correct positioning of the lumbar vertebrae, particularly in cases of lumbar lordosis. One should take care to place this cushion between the lower costal arches and the anterior superior iliac spine, so that the lumbar lordosis is really corrected. The arms should lie relaxed beside the torso on the training table or on the sliding arm supports, with the head either to the side or resting on the face support of the headpiece, raised to about a 25 degree angle. The muscles on the nape of the neck can be treated easily in this position, the lordosis is corrected, and the spine is slightly ex- tended.

The raising of the supine patient's legs with individually adjustable leg supports is advantageous for enhancing venous return and to ease circulation in the treatment of stases. Both massage techniques that encourage venous return and remedial exercise for the facilitation of the venous return can be carried out well in this position.

Reinhart's extension apparatus (stepstool positioning bed) is also well suited for raising the legs and for the relief and correction of the spine during a massage and remedial exercise. A light wool covering is necessary for the parts of the body not being treated to guard the patient from chills during the treatment.

# Treatment Room

The room in which the massage takes place should be clean, bright, and cheerful, and also easily ventilated. The days in which even the leading clinics relegated the physical therapy department exclusively to basement rooms should now be gone for good. The room temperature should be at least 24°C. In order to assure the confidentiality of the conversation between patient and therapist, the room should be private. Having other patients listening in is no aid to relaxation.

# Special Massage Techniques

It is beyond the scope of this book to examine all of the special techniques of massage and the various types of equipment they require. These are all treated at length in texts and professional medical journals. Moreover, they are taught and described in the training institutions for physical therapy and massage, as well as in the continuing education courses of the professional associations. We intend here only to cover in detail those special massage techniques that are particularly important for the athlete and his specific injuries and damages. These include the connective tissue massage, the stylus massage, the underwater massage, and the athletic massage.

## CONNECTIVE TISSUE MASSAGE

The connective tissue massage, developed in the 1940s jointly by Dicke, Teirich-Leube, and Kohlrausch, is a neurotherapeutic method, which is performed with a special stroking technique of the subcutaneous tissue of the torso and the extremities. This stimulates the nerve endings of the autonomic nervous system. Afferent impulses travel to the spinal cord and the brain, which causes a change in reaction susceptibility.

The connective tissue massage is the most important reflex zone massage known. It is characterized by a type of stroking that causes a sharp pain in the tissue. The limitation caused by adhesions between the hypodermis and the

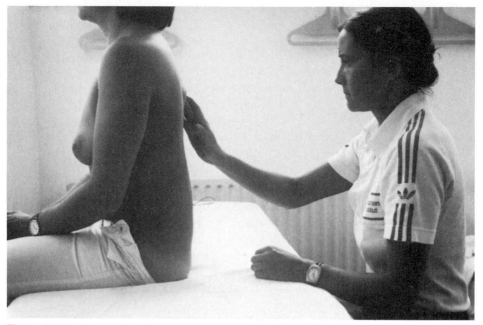

**Figure 1–23.** Connective tissue massage.

fascia is more striking than muscle tension in the case of many internal disorders. The connective tissue massage is therefore used primarily for internal disorders. Numerous disorders and ailments of this nature can be treated successfully with the techniques of the connective tissue massage.

This massage is used primarily for myocarditis, coronary insufficiency, high blood pressure, functional stomach and intestinal disorders, inflammation of the gallbladder, and hepatitis. The use of the connective tissue massage has been effective in the treatment of arterial circulatory problems, venous disorders, headaches, and particularly trauma to the head and in some gynecologic disorders.

It is usually recommended after surgery and in orthopedics in the case of persistent complaints and failure of revascularization following fractures, dislocations, and sprains.

The connective tissue massage is to be used primarily as a therapeutic or remedial massage. It cannot be considered a means of increasing athletic performance. However, in many competitive sports, athletes suffer from ailments that result from multiple trauma and can thus be treated successfully with the connective tissue massage. Experience has shown that the frequently recurring hormonal and functional disorders of the lower body which chronically affect competitive women athletes, such as amenorrhea and dysmenorrhea, can be positively influenced by the connective tissue massage.

The condition of the connective tissue should always be considered in the treatment of the athlete. Careful distinction between skin, muscle, and connective tissue is required.

In the connective tissue massage, either the surface lifting technique or the stroke technique may be used. The surface lifting technique moves the entire hypodermis against the fascia. The stroke technique creates traction with short, firm strokes on the connective tissue and the muscle insertions. By this means, a number of factors that can negatively affect athletic performance can be treated and relieved. The combination of connective tissue massage with classic massage has proved particularly effective for athletes.

A connective tissue massage generally is carried out in a sitting position, or occasionally in a lying position, and lasts between 15 and 25 minutes. After 12 to a maximum of 15 treatments, which are carried out two to three times per week, there should be a rest period of at least 4 weeks.

The athlete should rest for half an hour after each connective tissue massage to recover from the generally severe stress placed on the autonomic nervous system.

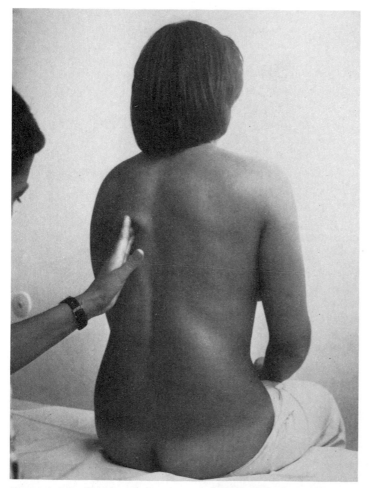

**Figure 1–24.**  Stroke technique for connective tissue massage.

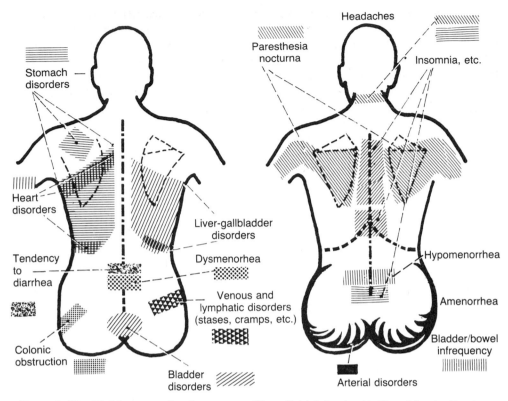

**Figure 1–25.** Visible connective tissue areas. (From Teirich-Leube, H.: Grundriss der Bendege-websmassage. Stuttgart, Gustav Fischer Verlag, 1968.)

## STYLUS MASSAGE

The stylus massage has been the subject of considerable discussion in professional circles recently. Astounding results have been reported, particularly by masseurs active in treating athletes. Deuser, who was the masseur for many years for the German National Soccer team, first made it known through his publications. He himself adopted the method from Schult, a masseur who was active in the 1936 Olympic Games in Berlin. Schult, for his part, learned the method from the Japanese. Schoberth had qualified physical therapists and masseurs test the method on a large number of patients in the Orthopedic University Clinic in Frankfurt am Main in 1970–1971 and came to the conclusion that the treatment could be beneficial if correctly prescribed and properly executed.

There are, however, strong opponents of the method in the profession, who maintain that they have observed serious damage caused by the stylus massage, including inflammatory irritations, myositis ossificans, and Sudeck's disease (reflex sympathetic dsytrophy). Many doctors doubtlessly continue to reject the stylus massage.

The stylus massage utilizes a 12 cm long smooth-surfaced hardwood stick to intensify the local mechanical effects of the therapist's fingers. In form it is similar to a miniature Indian club. On its narrow end it has a spherical bulge that supports the tip of the therapist's middle finger during the massage. This crown permits the effects of treatment to reach into deeper muscle layers and tissues and enables the pressure to remain constant over an extended period of time. The discovery of the precise extent and size of even the smallest hardenings, myogeloses, and tissue disorders is possible because of the close proximity of the crown to the fingertip. A further advantage is the ability to reach areas that would otherwise remain inaccessible to the fingers, such as under the shoulder blades.

The relative lack of sensation transmitted to the therapist during a massage carried out with such an instrument, as opposed to when the fingers are used, is the major argument against its usage. Indeed, nothing can replace the perceptions of the sensitive hand of the therapist. However, the stylus massage is not meant to replace the hand massage; it reinforces and supplements it when the hand becomes tired.

The thicker end of the stick can also be used for gentler treatments. When

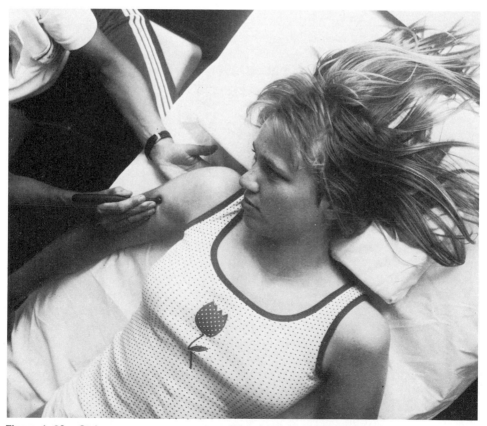

**Figure 1–26.** Stylus massage at the edge of the deltoid for a tennis player.

treating larger muscle groups, longitudinal, diagonal, and transverse strokes should be used. Circular friction is also useful. The stylus massage is usually only a part of a manual massage and is only used on particularly hardened areas.

The stylus massage is recommended primarily for adhesions in single deep tissue layers, especially between muscles and fascia. Hematomas arise frequently after contusions, sprains, and so forth, which often lead to adhesions in the course of their resorption. These can be removed well with a stylus massage. The stylus massage is also indicated for adhesions between the joint capsules and subcutaneous tissues, and also for connective tissue and the tendon sheaths. Schoberth and Treumann particularly recommend the stylus massage as a possible means of treating inflammations of the sheath of the Achilles tendon (peritendinitis achillea) conservatively, before an operation must be considered.

This method is, of course, contraindicated for all recent injuries and acutely inflamed areas. The stylus massage is absolutely forbidden for bone spurs, the spinous processes, lymph nodes, veins, and breasts. The stylus massage should be performed with extreme care. It demands even more sensitivity in the fingertips than the manual massage and is capable of producing beneficial therapeutic effects in certain cases, but it can also aggravate the injury. It is a special massage and should only be administered by therapists with many years of experience in manual massage. The stylus massage should by no means be undertaken by inexperienced laymen.

In remedial treatment after athletic injuries and in the normal treatment of athletes, during which large muscle groups and muscular hypertonia are generally being treated, the properly indicated and correctly performed stylus massage can be a good supplement in cases in which the strength of the therapist's hand alone is not sufficient.

## UNDERWATER MASSAGE

Besides the manual massage techniques, the underwater massage, or, more precisely, the "underwater pressure massage," is the most widely used massage that is performed with an implement.

It is a standard piece of equipment in clinics and institutions. Deuser reports its use and positive results in the treatment of the athletes at the world soccer championships. In the physical therapy section of the Olympic Village in Munich in 1972 it was also used successfully. It is very popular with injured and spent athletes of all disciplines.

The therapeutic effect of the underwater massage on the patient comes from the relaxing effect of the warm water and the ability to direct a high-pressure stream of water of greater or lesser force on the muscles, particularly on deep-lying muscle layers, subcutaneous tissues, the skin, and, if need be, the abdominal organs (intestines).

In the underwater massage the patient lies relaxed in a large tub with a capacity of 400 to 600 liters, which is filled with warm water. A stream of

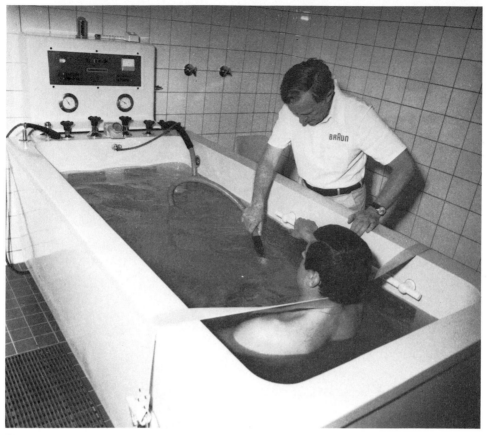

**Figure 1–27.** Underwater massage.

water under a pressure ranging from 0.5 to maximum 7.0 bar (absolute pressure units) (kg/cm²) is brought to bear on the part of the body being treated by means of a movable hose, which has a changeable nozzle.

The high-pressure stream of water is created by a pump. Most of today's units use a recirculating process, in which the water needed for the massage is drawn out of the tub and then returned under pressure through the massage hose.

The temperature of the water in the tub should be 36 to 38°C. The temperature of the pressurized stream can be regulated; it can also be at a higher temperature than the water in the tub. In the same way, cold or warm water can be added to the circulating water as needed. The water temperature should be precisely controlled by means of a thermometer built into the apparatus, as the underwater massage puts a large strain on the circulatory system.

Various extracts, which either stimulate the metabolism or relax the body, can be added to the water such as hayseed, pine needles, spruce needles, rosemary, bromine, valerian, sulfur, and so forth.

Pressure is regulated by a manometer. It should be noted, however, that

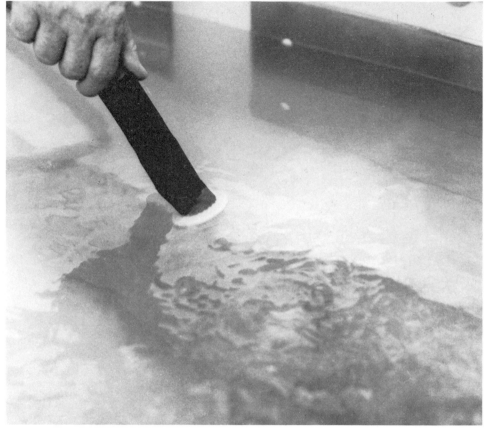

**Figure 1–28.**   Stream of water at 3 bars pressure.

the pressure of the water stream is reduced and slowed by the water in the tub, and therefore it is not the same as the pressure registered by the manometer. Within the 10 to 15 cm separating the nozzle from the body surface there is a breaking action on the water pressure. The diameter of the nozzle is between 80 and 140 mm.[2] Narrower nozzles increase the pressure of the water stream and make it more forceful and smaller. They are used for local myogeloses. However, if the water pressure causes a stabbing pain, the muscles react with an increased defensive tightening, the opposite of the effect intended. Nozzles with medium and larger diameters are generally preferred. They have a gentler, broader effect at an equal force and are usually more comfortable for the patient. There are also nozzles that can mix air in with the water, which also helps decrease the water pressure. For those patients who have very painful tissues highly sensitive to pressure, such as slender runners and track and field athletes, one must begin with low water pressure (0.5–1.5 bar), and raise the pressure slowly.

Athletes with large masses of muscle, such as heavyweight wrestlers and boxers, can usually withstand higher water pressure (2.0–4.0 bar). The prescribed treatment is always individualized, however. It must take into consideration the subjective feelings of the patient and should never be painful.

The massaging stream can be directed along or across the muscle, or it can be moved in a circular rotation. The angle of the water stream to the muscles, whether perpendicular or acute, is also important.

The front of the legs, the chest, and the arms are treated with the patient in a supine position. The head rests on a neck support. A support for the feet is necessary for short patients.

A massage of the upper thighs begins with a centripetally directed stream. The massage of the calves and the feet follows. In this way better venous and lymphatic drainage is encouraged. The same is true for the arms. Here one begins on the upper arm and only then moves to the forearm and hand.

The massage of the back of the legs and of the back is always carried out with the patient lying on his side. In this position, the hips and knees are slightly bent. The neck and the head rest on a belt which is stretched over the surface of the water. A massage with the patient in a prone position is not recommended because it places the patient in a hyperlordotic position. The back should be treated from the pelvis, gluteus maximus, and sacrum upwards along the spinal column. The muscles of the back — the erector spinae, latissimus dorsi, and trapezius — should be massaged with either a diagonal or a circular motion. The intercostal areas should be stroked out from the spinal column to the sternum. Rotating and diagonal motion is suitable for the neck and shoulder muscles, the trapezius, rhomboideus, and the scapulae.

The thorax and abdomen are treated with the patient in a supine position. The large thoracic muscle, the pectoralis major, should be treated with a gentle, circulating stream, except for the armpits. The female breasts should also be avoided. The abdominal region should be massaged with a gentle, circular stream along the course of the large intestine.

The length of a general treatment is 20 to 30 minutes; a partial treatment lasts 10 to 15 minutes. Three minutes are necessary for the patient to get used to the water before commencing treatment, and half an hour should be allowed afterwards for rest. A cool or cold affusion stimulates the circulation favorably at the conclusion of an underwater massage.

Particularly sensitive body areas, such as the spinous processes of the spinal column, bone spurs, genitalia, anus, backs of the knees, and the female breasts should be omitted during the underwater massage. Similarly, the method is not recommended for all recent athletic injuries, open wounds, hematomas in an acute state, effusions in the knee joints, acute muscle, ligament, and tendon pulls, and recent fractures.

The underwater massage is contraindicated for cardiovascular insufficiencies, venous disorders, thromboses, and varices.

The underwater massage is indicated for fractures, osteosyntheses, dislocations, sprains, and contusions in the subacute stages after the patient has been released. Also, it is used in sciatica, lumbalgia, brachialgia, joint and scar contractures, myogeloses, degenerative spinal disorders, chronic joint and muscular rheumatism, Bechterev's disease (ankylosing spondylitis), scoliosis, and flaccid and spastic paralyses.

The underwater massage can be put to good use in the case of muscular hypertonia and for uninjured athletes as a warm-down massage after hard training and competition; in these situations it is helpful in the removal and breakdown of waste materials and also as a treatment for improving muscular performance. The underwater massage should never be used before competition, however, because of the strain it puts on the circulatory system. In addition, there should be at least 2 days between a treatment and scheduled competition.

## ATHLETIC MASSAGE

There are few publications about the athletic massage at the present time. Equally noteworthy is the fact that there is no school or curriculum specifically devoted to the athletic massage, which could provide a scientific basis for empirical knowledge and experience. One repeatedly finds conflicting statements by practicing athletic masseurs. A prominent heavyweight boxer reports that eight different athletic masseurs have treated him and that each gave him different advice and suggested differing methods of treatment, some of which were completely contradictory.

However, on comparing the statements of various professionals in the field of athletic massage some areas of consensus are found along with the opposing and contradictory opinions.

### Increase of Performance Produced by the Athletic Massage

Whereas therapeutic or remedial massages are primarily concerned with aiding the healing process after an injury or in a functional disorder, the athletic massage has other aims. In this case we are dealing with a healthy, usually young person whose physical and athletic abilities generally are far above average. The athlete expects that the trainer's massages will help him or her to run faster, jump higher or farther, throw or put farther, kick more accurately, or be a better gymnast, rider, swimmer, or skier. An objective, measurable increase in performance is expected.

That the athletic massage is only one of many means to increase performance is clear to anyone who has ever participated in competitive athletics. Furthermore, the fact that the massage as a passive treatment is only an adjunct in the much more important active training methods is the unanimous opinion of all professionals.

Only a few years ago the players on a prominent professional soccer team received an extensive full massage and a heat-lamp treatment before the game, on the advice of the trainer and the team doctor. This is different today. An extensive massage before a game or competition has been replaced universally by an active, loosening warm-up program, which increases circulation about five times more than can be achieved by a massage. But, in spite of the emphasis on active methods, the massage has retained its place among the treatments of the athlete. To do without it completely would be akin to throwing out the baby with the bathwater.

## Psychologic Aspects of the Athletic Massage

A further important aspect of the athletic massage should be mentioned here. It not only improves the way the athlete feels and his reaction time, but also affects his general sense of well-being. Of two athletes whose physical, technical, and tactical preparation is equal, the one who is in the optimal psychic condition at the time of the competition will always win. The athletic massage can be an important part of the psychologic preparation for competition. The psychologic condition of the athlete should be such that his performance is as good as his physical conditioning will permit. In this way, a tense athlete can be calmed down before the start of his event with the proper treatment, just as a sluggish one can be stimulated.

The athletic massage has an energizing influence on the psyche, which can, however, produce the opposite effect if falsely applied. The athletic massage can therefore have positive effects not only on the body, but also on the psychological state of the athlete. The therapist's familiarity with the principles of psychological preparation for competition is required.

## Types of Athletic Massage

Types of athletic massage include the following:
1. Training massage.
2. Preparatory massage.
3. Intermediary massage.
4. Warm-down massage.

The *training massage* is a massage which is used before a training period to support and prepare the body for the considerable conditioning it must undergo in order to reach top form. This task should be undertaken at the resumption or start of a training program. After initial gentle treatment, one can soon begin rubbing more powerfully and deeply, to accustom the body to deep-reaching kneading and working and thereby to prepare it for a vigorous massage. Treatment soreness can be expected. After all, when this form of massage is given, the athlete is not going to compete the next day.

The *preparatory massage* before competition is different. It should be light, relaxing, and warming. It must be pleasant, should not be painful, and should stimulate; therefore, it has an important psychological function. Active warm-ups, however, such as jogging, calisthenics, and active stretching, are more important.

The *intermediary massage* is used during intermissions of a game, between events for an athletic discipline involving several separate competi-
*Text continued on page 50*

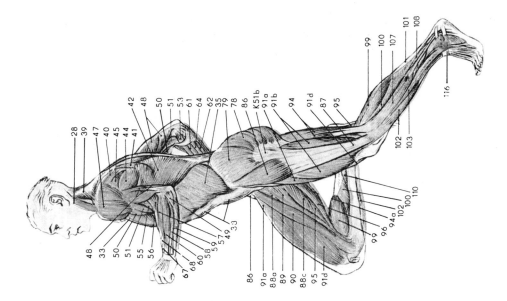

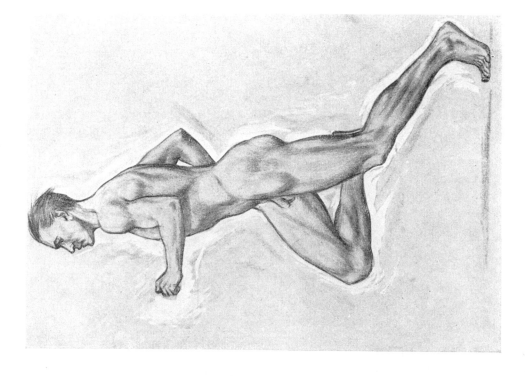

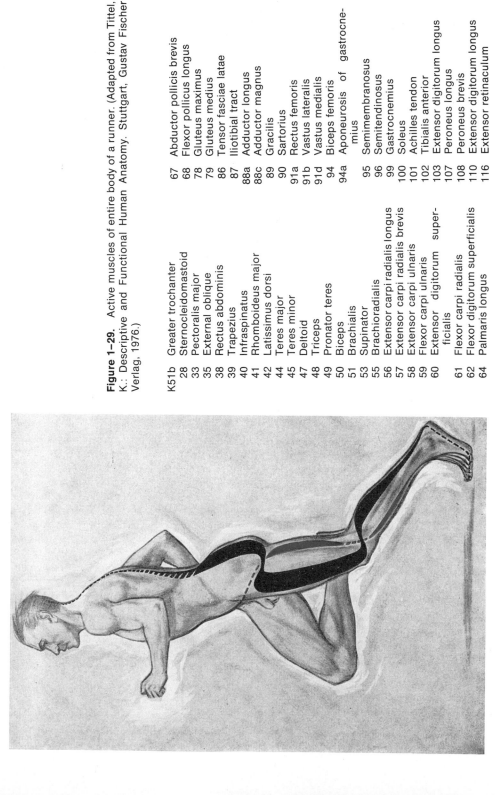

**Figure 1-29.** Active muscles of entire body of a runner. (Adapted from Tittel, K.: Descriptive and Functional Human Anatomy. Stuttgart, Gustav Fischer Verlag, 1976.)

| | | | |
|---|---|---|---|
| K51b | Greater trochanter | 67 | Abductor pollicis brevis |
| 28 | Sternocleidomastoid | 68 | Flexor pollicus longus |
| 33 | Pectoralis major | 78 | Gluteus maximus |
| 35 | External oblique | 79 | Gluteus medius |
| 38 | Rectus abdominis | 86 | Tensor fasciae latae |
| 39 | Trapezius | 87 | Iliotibial tract |
| 40 | Infraspinatus | 88a | Adductor longus |
| 41 | Rhomboideus major | 88c | Adductor magnus |
| 42 | Latissimus dorsi | 89 | Gracilis |
| 44 | Teres major | 90 | Sartorius |
| 45 | Teres minor | 91a | Rectus femoris |
| 47 | Deltoid | 91b | Vastus lateralis |
| 48 | Triceps | 91d | Vastus medialis |
| 49 | Pronator teres | 94 | Biceps femoris |
| 50 | Biceps | 94a | Aponeurosis of gastrocnemius |
| 51 | Brachialis | | |
| 53 | Supinator | 95 | Semimembranosus |
| 55 | Brachioradialis | 96 | Semitendinosus |
| 56 | Extensor carpi radialis longus | 99 | Gastrocnemius |
| 57 | Extensor carpi radialis brevis | 100 | Soleus |
| 58 | Extensor carpi ulnaris | 101 | Achilles tendon |
| 59 | Flexor carpi ulnaris | 102 | Tibialis anterior |
| 60 | Extensor digitorum superficialis | 103 | Extensor digitorum longus |
| | | 107 | Peroneus longus |
| 61 | Flexor carpi radialis | 108 | Peroneus brevis |
| 62 | Flexor digitorum superficialis | 110 | Extensor digitorum longus |
| 64 | Palmaris longus | 116 | Extensor retinaculum |

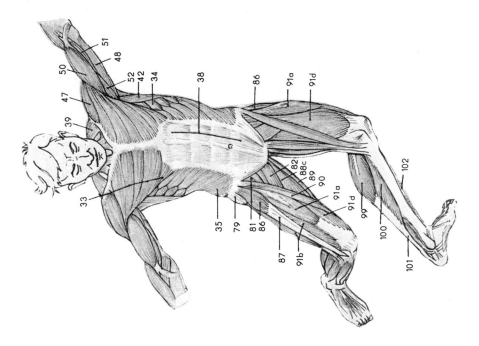

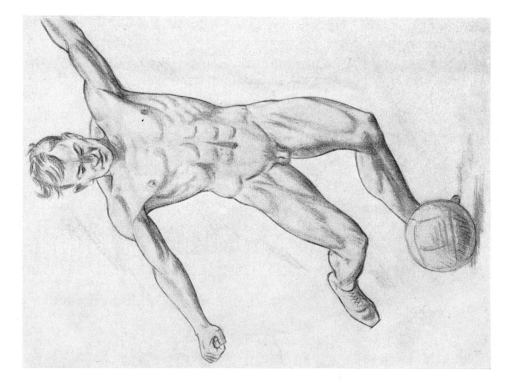

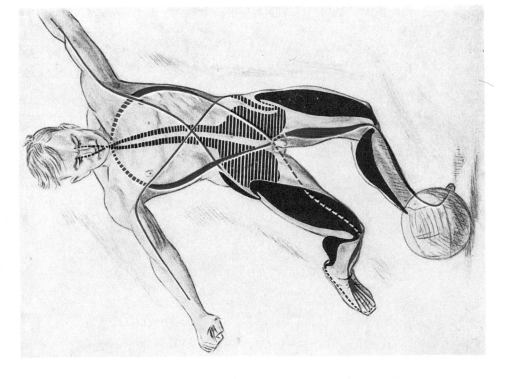

**Figure 1-30.** Active muscles of soccer player while leaning to the side and twisting. (Adapted from Tittel, K.: Descriptive and Functional Human Anatomy. Stuttgart, Gustav Fischer Verlag, 1976.)

| | | | |
|---|---|---|---|
| 33 | Pectoralis major | 82 | Pectineus |
| 34 | Serratus anterior | 86 | Tensor fasciae latae |
| 35 | External oblique | 87 | Iliotibial tract |
| 38 | Rectus abdominis | 88c | Adductor magnus |
| 39 | Trapezius | 89 | Gracilis |
| 42 | Latissimus dorsi | 90 | Sartorius |
| 47 | Deltoid | 91a | Rectus femoris |
| 48 | Triceps | 91b | Vastus lateralis |
| 50 | Biceps | 91d | Vastus medialis |
| 51 | Brachialis | 99 | Gastrocnemius |
| 52 | Coracobrachialis | 100 | Soleus |
| 79 | Gluteus medius | 101 | Achilles tendon |
| 81 | Iliacus | 102 | Tibialis anterior |

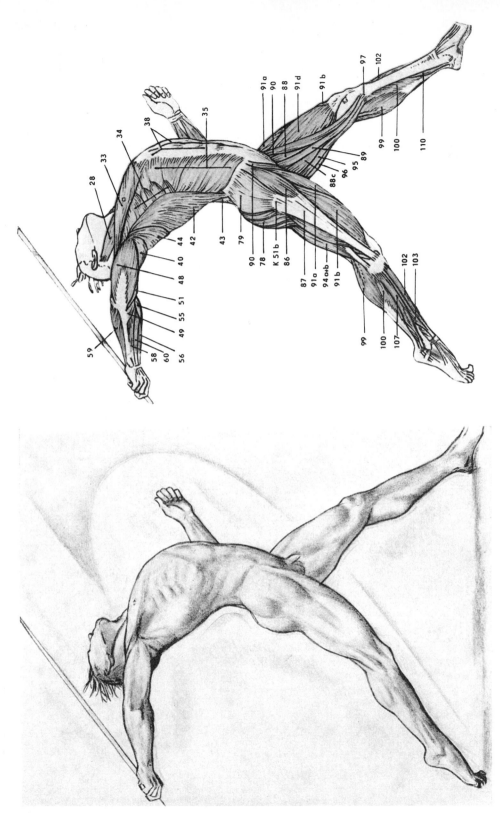

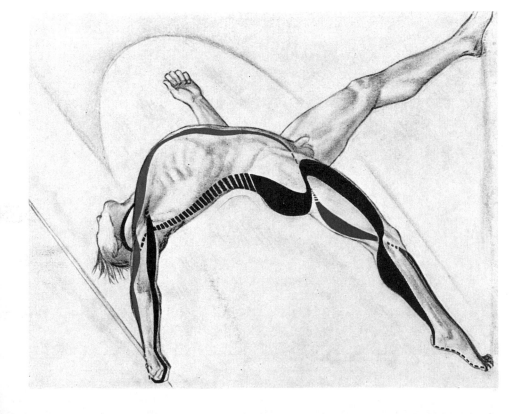

**Figure 1–31.** Active muscles in entire body of javelin thrower. (Adapted from Tittel, K.: Descriptive and Functional Human Anatomy. Stuttgart, Gustav Fischer Verlag, 1976.)

| | | | |
|---|---|---|---|
| K51b | Greater trochanter | 78 | Gluteus maximus |
| 28 | Sternocleidomastoid | 79 | Gluteus medius |
| 33 | Pectoralis major | 86 | Tensor fasciae latae |
| 34 | Serratus anterior | 87 | Iliotibial tract |
| 35 | External oblique | 88 | Adductor longus |
| 38 | Rectus abdominis | 88c | Adductor magnus |
| 40 | Infraspinatus | 89 | Gracilis |
| 42 | Latissimus dorsi | 90 | Sartorius |
| 43 | Posterior layer of thoraco-lumbar fascia | 91a | Rectus femoris |
| | | 91b | Vastus lateralis |
| 44 | Teres major | 91d | Vastus medialis |
| 48 | Triceps | 94a + b | Biceps femoris |
| 49 | Pronator teres | 95 | Semimembranosus |
| 51 | Brachialis | 96 | Semitendinosus |
| 55 | Brachioradialis | 97 | Insertion of sartorius |
| 56 | Extensor carpi radialis longus | 99 | Gastrocnemius |
| | | 100 | Soleus |
| 58 | Extensor carpi ulnaris | 102 | Tibialis anterior |
| 59 | Flexor carpi ulnaris | 103 | Extensor digitorum longus |
| 60 | Extensor digitorum super-ficialis | 107 | Peroneus longus |
| | | 110 | Extensor digitorum longus |

tions, and between the rounds in boxing. It, too, should be short, light, and loosening. It must not be painful and should only treat those muscles that either are in use or are going to be used. It also has a relaxing psychologic effect.

The *warm-down massage* is used after hard training or a tough game or competition. The hypothesis is that the residue of metabolic wastes is not yet fixed in the tissues directly after the physical exertion. The idea is to cause them to be excreted as soon as possible. Deep penetrating techniques that encourage venous and lymphatic return are recommended. Hard, painful massage techniques are contraindicated, as there is still a lack of oxygen in the muscles. The use of heat is necessary before the warm-down massage. The heat aids in dissolving and flushing out waste materials and increases the effect of the penetrating massage techniques. A hot, long shower, a hot bath, or a sauna is the best means of accelerating their elimination. The length of the recuperation time after a strenuous competition can be reduced with a good warm-down massage.

The whirlpool baths popular today, with water temperatures of 28 to 30°C, combined with an active warm-down with light jogging and rhythmic stretching calisthenics, are at least as good as the massage.

### Variations in the Athletic Massage for Particular Sports

The massage of the healthy athlete is less than a remedial or therapeutic massage; instead it is a massage of individual muscles. It focuses on functional units of connective and muscular tissue, muscle groups, and entire segments of the body as required by the specific demands of each sport. Thus, the athletic massage of a runner is quite different from that of a shot-putter or javelin thrower. The massage of the tennis player is different from that given to the rider. Further distinctions are often made within a particular athletic discipline. There is a difference in the type of massage for a dressage rider and a jumping rider. Joch, an expert in track and field disciplines, makes the assertion that "there is only a relatively slight connection between the various track and field disciplines." There is likewise little connection between types of massage of track and field athletes. Whereas the muscles of runners and long and high jumpers should be massaged from the foot to the thigh, the muscles of the hand, arm, and shoulder, as well as the upper and lower back, should be the primary sites of treatment for shot-putters, javelin throwers, and hammer and discus throwers. This does not mean, however, that the legs should be completely ignored among the latter athletes — Joch, for example, suggests that between javelin throwers of the same strength, the faster runner will throw further. For soccer players and skiers, the legs are to receive the primary attention, of course. Again, muscles of the arms and shoulders should be treated symmetrically for rowers, whereas the strain is only on one side for tennis players or fencers. These examples should suffice to give an indication of the principal differences in the use of massage for various sports.

# Summary

1. The athletic massage has been used since ancient time as a means of increasing athletic performance.

2. In the past the effects of the athletic massage have been exaggerated, and this still occurs frequently today.

3. In addition to the athletic massage, active methods of increasing performance have become prominent, which often fulfill the functions of preparation, warm-up, loosening, and warm-down better than the athletic massage; examples are the whirlpool bath, warm-up exercises, and active stretching.

4. Nevertheless, the athletic massage cannot be completely rejected as a means of increasing performance. In addition to a number of objective, positive physiologic effects, it can also have a strong psychologic, motivating, generally relaxing function, which is urgently needed by many athletes under the stress of top competitive sports.

5. As all manipulation with medications in top competitive sports should be condemned, the athletic massage, together with other physical therapeutic treatments, is a means of increasing the athlete's performance without risking his health.

## CHAPTER 2

# Uses of Heat

*DORIS EITNER*

## Introduction

Heat treatment, also called thermotherapy, involves simply the use of heat in various forms for therapeutic purposes.

The transfer of heat to the skin can occur by either conduction or radiation. Heat transfer by conduction, such as with mud baths and fango, requires direct skin contact with the heat source. The heat of the poultice works on the treated part of the body until the temperature difference is evened out. This process depends on the conductibility, capacity, and the rate of exchange of the heat.

During heat treatments with radiation, such as with infrared and ultraviolet light, the part of the body being treated is not in direct contact with the heat source. The rays merely penetrate the air, without heating it; only the body that absorbs the rays is heated.

## Physiologic Effects

Heat dilates blood vessels, causing the "resting" capillaries to open up and increasing the circulation. Beside the local vascular expansion, there is also a dilatation of the blood vessels on the surface of the skin triggered by the autonomic nervous system.

The hyperemia created by heat has a beneficial effect on many chronic irritations. This is based on increases of antibodies and on the improvement of the metabolic processes. However, recent hematomas must never be treated with heat, as the flush of blood and the subsequent expansion of the blood and lymph vessels occurring with this treatment can easily cause a resumption of bleeding.

These characteristics and the great variety of possible applications make heat therapy a valuable tool in physical therapy. The various heat applications are particularly indispensable as a preparation before massage and active remedial exercise for athletic injuries and damage.

Heat applications will be considered under two subheadings: dry heat and moist heat.

# Dry Heat

Dry heat includes the following methods:
1. Infrared/red light.
2. Incandescent light/hot air.
3. Ultraviolet irradiation.
These are the most common heat sources used for therapy.

## INFRARED IRRADIATION

There is no direct contact between the source of heat and the body in this modality. The infrared rays penetrate the air without heating it. After their absorption into the skin, they are converted back into heat.

The infrared rays do not penetrate deeply, only about 3 cm. The irradiation is effective only if it is carried out long enough and at a high enough intensity. The treatment lasts 20 minutes. It can be followed by a massage or remedial exercise.

## RED LIGHT IRRADIATION

Red light works more deeply with less heat than white light, which stimulates the heat sensors of the skin more intensely. Red light has a soothing effect on inflamed areas.

## INCANDESCENT IRRADIATION

Although incandescent heat does not cause chemical changes as short wavelength radiation can, it still has considerable therapeutic importance. This is because it penetrates deeper into the tissue than ultraviolet or infrared rays. Incandescent heat increases the blood supply to the deeper regions of the skin and tissue without irritating the skin surface.

The incandescent bulb consists of an apparatus in the shape of an arch with rows of carbon filament lamps on the inner side. There are incandescent bulbs that can treat the entire body and others for local areas, such as the extremities, the back, and the head. Because it is easy to employ, incandescent heat is in widespread use.

Treatments of the entire body last about 15 to 20 minutes. Perspiration begins after approximately 5 to 10 minutes. The treatment is followed by a lukewarm bath ending with a final cold burst of water. This complete treatment is recommended in cases in which a full body sweat is desired in the gentlest and most comfortable way — for example, in the case of colds, rheumatic disorders, circulatory problems, and skin diseases.

Partial treatments of 15 to 20 minutes are used after athletic injuries, such as fractures, sprains, and contusions in the later phases, and as a preparation for active remedial exercises.

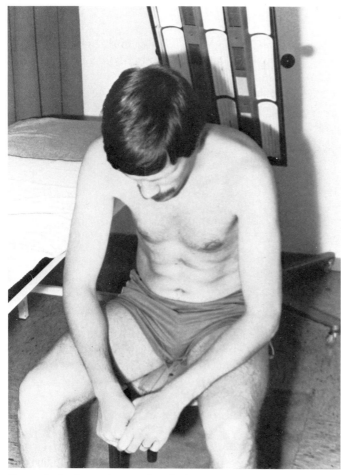

**Figure 2–1.** Incandescent irradiation.

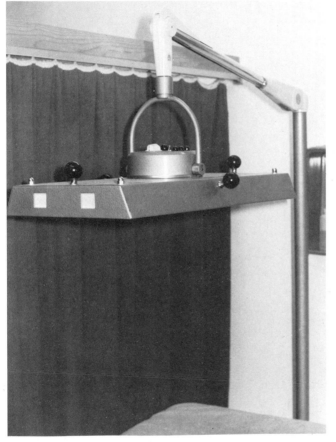

**Figure 2–2.**  Incandescent lamp.

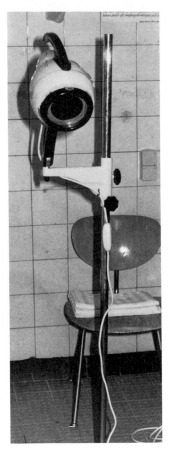

**Figure 2–3.** Sollux lamp.

## SOLLUX LAMP

Local radiotherapy, which causes a deep local hyperemia, can be administered with the aid of a Sollux lamp. These lamps are equipped with red and blue filters. Sollux lamp irradiation is used for rheumatic disorders, neuralgias, bronchitis, the after-treatment of contusions and sprains in connection with massages, and remedial exercise.

The Aquasol lamp is a Sollux lamp which has a water filter in front of it. The long-wave infrared rays are absorbed and the thermal tolerance level is thereby decreased.

## ULTRAVIOLET IRRADIATION

The ultraviolet rays are the part of the electromagnetic spectrum most important for life. They have a variety of advantageous general features. They convert ergosterol into vitamin $D_3$. The defense mechanisms of the body are strengthened and they increase the regeneration of the blood. They also kill bacteria. Ultraviolet (UV) radiotherapy has proved valuable in the treatment of athletes' skin, bones, joints, and abdomen. During the winter months or between competitions complete body UV radiotherapy treatments strengthen the defense mechanisms.

On the average, these treatments are administered every other day, and not more than 20 times. The second series should begin only after a rest period. The room should be well ventilated during the treatment, as UV rays create poisonous gases in the air, which can cause headaches and nausea. The eyes must be protected from the UV rays with opaque glasses. The distance from the skin to the apparatus must be at least 1 meter. An overdose given to an exhausted athlete evokes complaints of heart palpitations, insomnia, and irritated skin. There is also a danger of burning of the skin.

# Moist Heat

Moist heat includes the following treatments:
1. Peloids, mudpacks, bog soil
2. Hot rolled towels

## PELOIDS

Broadly speaking, these are inorganic and organic fine-grained materials, which have been created through geologic processes. These materials occur naturally both in a dry state and mixed with water. In therapeutic practice they are known as mud, ooze, and fango. A further division of the peloids includes the therapeutic sediments, which are underwater deposits and medicinal soils created by the decomposition of minerals.

Peat and bog soils have primarily organic origins. They are created in the course of time from plant material submerged in water.

On the other hand, the muds from hot springs, such as fango, and the silt that gathers in rivers and river mouths are largely inorganic. The important thing about peloid poultices is that they utilize high temperatures. The heat capacity of the materials they contain is very high — that is, the heat is expended slowly and therefore lasts for a long period of time. Mudpacks are recommended for many rheumatic illnesses, as long as they are not in the acute stages. All chronic gynecologic inflammations can also be treated with heat. It has been shown that bog soils contain hormone-like substances that are absorbed by the body.

These poultices are also excellent treatments for the later stages of athletic injuries and chronic ailments, such as after fractures, sprains, contusions, and contractures. All back disorders, such as kyphosis of adolescence, hunchback, lordosis, osteochondrosis, spondylosis, and spondylolisthesis, can be prepared for active remedial exercises with fango poultices.

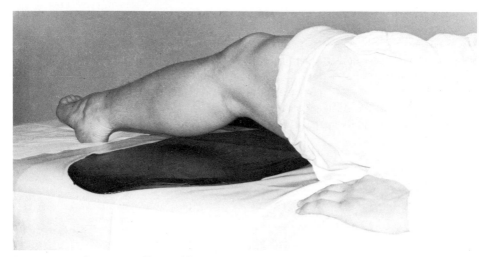

**Figure 2–4.** Fango-paraffin poultice.

## PARAFFIN

Paraffin is used as a method of heat treatment similar to that with peloids. However, paraffin poultices are, strictly speaking, not a therapeutic treatment; their effect is solely thermal. Paraffin also is a poor heat conductor, and it conducts its heat only very slowly to the body. It therefore can be used at higher temperatures than water. There is no water in paraffin. Dampness in connection with the paraffin can cause serious burns. Skin moist with perspiration must therefore be dried in advance of treatment. Paraffin is frequently mixed with fango, in a combination termed "parafango."

Fango-paraffin poultices have the great advantages of not being messy and of being easy to apply. In combination with a massage or directed remedial exercise they can have a positive influence on residual damages from an injury, often completely removing them.

## MUD BATHS AND POULTICES

Volcanic mud has been brought to the surface by thermal springs and is therefore very hot. River, lake, and ocean mud deposited at river mouths must be heated.

Mud is used for baths and poultices. Baths are given only at the sites where the therapeutic mud originates. Poultices are applied locally or over the entire body. The mud is placed directly on the body. The poultices last about 20 to 30 minutes. Afterwards the body is cleansed with warm water.

For athletic injuries and especially in the case of old, chronic residual damage, local application of hot mud poultices is recommended. The use of hot mud is also recommended as a preparation for and in addition to other physical therapy treatments.

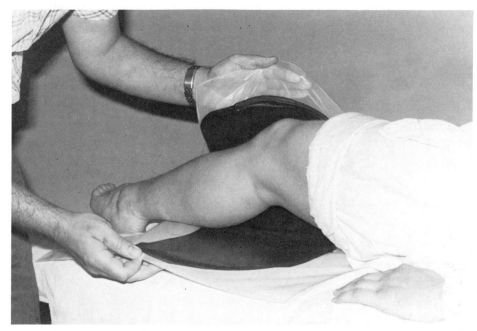

**Figure 2–5.**   Fango-paraffin poultice applied to knee.

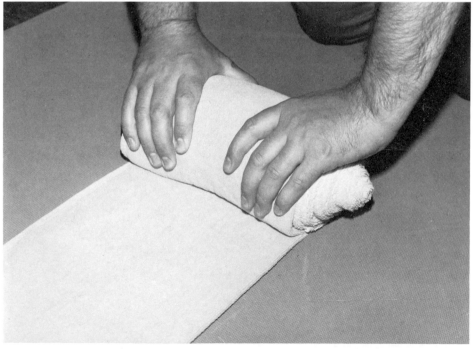

**Figure 2–6.**   Method of rolling the towels.

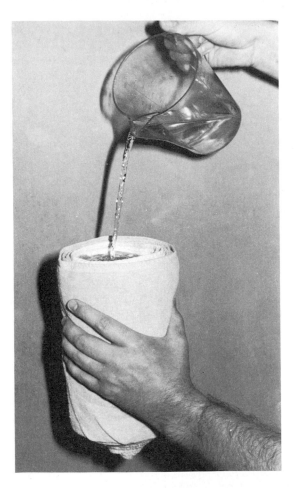

**Figure 2–7.** The boiling water is poured into the funnel-shaped depression.

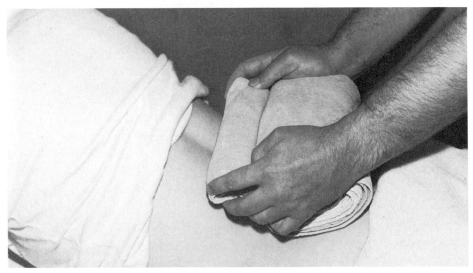

**Figure 2–8.**    Treatment of muscles along the lumbar vertebrae with hot rolled towels.

## HOT ROLLED TOWELS

A hot rolled towel is a very practical means of applying heat to a small area of the body. This is a popular treatment for athletic injuries because the necessary materials are always at hand.

Five medium-sized towels are necessary. First, four of them are folded lengthwise. Then the first towel is rolled up like an elastic bandage, in such a manner that a spiral-shaped point protrudes along at one edge and a funnel-shaped hollow is formed on the other side. Then the second towel is wrapped cylindrically around the first, but with edges even with the final turns of the first towel, so that the point and the funnel are not enlarged. The third and fourth towels are then wrapped around these first two. The fifth towel is not yet used. It is important that the towels be rolled up as tightly as possible, so that later no water drips out. When this has been prepared, a liter of boiling water is poured into the funnel-shaped depression.

The four towels completely absorb the water. Now the fifth towel is wrapped around the roll, so that a bit of the towel extends on all sides. This is important, so that the therapist can get a good grasp on the towels. Their use is then relatively simple. The pack is placed against the area to be treated using a gentle pressure. After a brief period of contact, it is removed for a moment and then replaced. The process continues in this rhythmic form until the body has become accustomed to the heat. After this point has been reached, the towel roll is left on the body for longer periods of time and finally no longer is removed. Gentle massaging movements are included in the treatment. There is no chance of cooling, first because the skin maintains a high temperature and, second, because the towel roll is repeatedly run over the entire surface even though smaller areas are treated at short intervals throughout the treatment. After even a short time, the skin becomes deeply flushed, and remains so for quite some time. When the outer towel is no longer hot enough, it is slowly unwrapped.

The hot rolled towel maintains its temperature practically unchanged in the interior throughout. Gradually the towels are unrolled. The rate at which the towels are unwrapped depends on how fast the outer layer cools and on the sensitivity of the individual patient. The last towel is not rolled up completely; rather, the therapist spreads it over the treated area and leaves it there until the patient no longer feels its warmth. A treatment with hot rolled towels lasts about 15 minutes. Among the advantages of this form of treatment is that it permits individual variations. It also permits treatment in a wide range of temperatures.

The hot rolled towel is an excellent treatment for athletes with over-strained spinal columns.

Treatment with incandescent irradiation and hot, moist towels is similar to the treatment of hot rolled towels. Athletes prefer this treatment, because it is simple to administer. The warm, moist towel is laid on the treated body part. Then the incandescent lamp is placed over it. The length of application is 15 to 20 minutes.

## CHAPTER 3

# Uses of Cold

*HELMUT ORK*

## Introduction

Cold is used in various forms such as cold towels, poultices, rub-downs, and dabbing with ice, snow, and cold water. Along with these natural cooling materials chemical cooling sprays and manufactured cold poultices are available. Various athletic injuries can be treated successfully with the use of cold. The type and the form of the application of cold depend on the location and extent of the injury. Historically, cold has been used for treating athletic injuries for a long time. Ice and snow have been used since antiquity for stopping blood flow. Around the turn of the century ice was used primarily as an anesthetic. In recent times cold has been used more and more frequently after trauma and for athletic injuries as chemical means of cooling have become readily available. Cold applications supplement active remedial exercises. They have proved themselves valuable in the prevention and the treatment of athletic injuries both alone and in connection with other physical therapy treatments.

## Physiologic Effects

In the effort to maintain a constant temperature, the human body has developed a regulating mechanism that balances temperature loss and gains. According to Aschoff, the body is divided into central and peripheral areas. The central areas include the chest and abdominal organs, as well as the head, and the surface of the body, including the skin and muscles.

The following reactions result from cold treatments:

The first reaction is a constriction of the vascular system. An expansion of the vessels, or vasodilatation, follows this reflexly. This is known as reactive hyperemia. Sensitivity to pain is also decreased. An immediate application in the acute phase of an athletic injury quickly reduces the pain. This is caused by the effect on the heat-sensitive receptors, which lie close to those for pain sensitivity. If the surface of the skin is lowered to 12 to 13° C or below, there is an analgesic effect during this coldest part of the treatment.

The neurophysiologic effect of cold treatments on the muscle and tendon fibers varies according to the length of application and is of particular importance. Cold has a general effect on the autonomic nervous system, which is related to a lowering of the muscle tone. The decisive factors in determining the effects of cold treatments include the length of application and the constancy of particular temperatures.

# Acute Phase

The application of ice in the acute stage of an injury lessens or prevents changes in the tissues, such as edema and hematoma. This effect is produced by vascular constriction. A stoppage of the blood flow is achieved, which limits or prevents the development of hematomas.

The vascular constriction lasts only about 15 minutes, however. Twelve minutes has proved to be a good application time for ice in treating recent athletic injuries. Then the cooling is interrupted for 10 minutes. During this time, the strain on the injured area should be eased as much as possible; the area should be elevated, and have a compression bandage applied. Then this process should be repeated in intervals. The entire length of time for treatment with cold depends on the extent of the damage in an acute injury. Two to 4 hours are necessary to cause local stoppage of blood.

The length of the cold treatment is primarily limited by the pain from the cold. The pain threshold should by no means be crossed, since a vascular spasm can result. This danger is particularly great with submersion in ice baths.

For the relief of pain, resolution of hematomas, and increasing mobility, the cold treatment should be repeated as frequently as possible in the two days following the acute phase. After the second day, the ice treatment is a preparatory and supplementary treatment along with active remedial exercise.

# Rehabilitative Phase

The rehabilitative phase follows the acute phase. Preeminent in this area is the combination of cold treatment with active remedial exercises. In this way the pain is relieved, so that normal stresses and later the full special stresses of the athlete's particular sport can be sustained. Passive exercises are not recommended, as they can cause microtrauma.

In contradistinction to the acute phase, a strong reactive hyperemia is caused during the rehabilitative phase by the vascular dilatation. The increased rate of absorption accelerates the healing, and adhesions in the soft parts of the body are also reduced.

The treatment consists primarily of repeated applications of cold for short periods of time, which are combined with remedial exercises.

After a long period of rest, applications of ice are a good preparation for remedial exercises. The affected areas are completely wrapped up in ice packs or cold towels for this treatment as well.

# Preventive Use of Cold

An ice massage is recommended for the elbow of javelin throwers and tennis players; cold treatments in the region of the Achilles tendon and the hamstrings are also helpful for sprinters, middle and long distance runners, and gymnasts. Ice rubs are recommended for the prevention and treatment of muscle cramps and to limit tiring and tension.

# Methods of Application

*Ice Cubes.*   This form of cold application is suited for injuries to the hand, fingers, elbow, and feet. The treated area is massaged in a circular motion.

*Ice Sticks.*   These are made by pouring water into a plastic tube about 10 cm long and 1 cm wide. The ends are then sealed and the sticks are frozen. Ice

## TABLE 3–1.  APPLICATIONS OF COLD

| Form of Application | Area of Application | Type of Injury | Method of Use |
|---|---|---|---|
| Ice cube | Small joints and small surfaces | Bruises, sprains, and closed injuries to soft parts | Circular motion on and around the injury |
| Ice stick | Medium-sized surfaces | Bruises, sprains, and closed injuries to soft parts | Local application on hard-to-reach body parts |
| Ice block | Large joints and large areas | Bruises, sprains, and closed injuries to soft parts | Circular motion on and around the injury |
| Ice bag | Large joints and large areas | Bruises, sprains, and closed injuries to soft parts | Lay on large surface areas; can be used as compress |
| Cold towel | Joints, extremities | Bruises, sprains, and closed injuries to soft parts | Lay on large surfaces and wrap around injured area as a compress |
| Ice bath | Body parts, entire body | Bruises, sprains, and closed injuries to soft parts | Large surfaces; submersion of body parts or entire body |
| Cooling spray | All areas besides face and open wounds | Bruises, sprains, and closed injuries to soft parts | Spray onto skin |
| Chlorethyl | All areas except face and open wounds | Bruises, sprains, and closed injuries to soft parts | Spray onto skin |
| Chemical Cool Pac | Joints and surfaces | Bruises, sprains, and closed injuries to soft parts | Lay on affected areas |

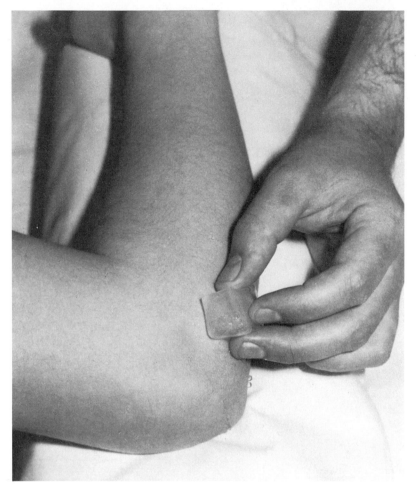

**Figure 3-1.** Ice massage with ice cube on the elbow, such as for epicondylitis humeri.

sticks are used for hard-to-reach parts of the body, such as between the fingers and toes.

**Ice Blocks.** The ice block is used for medium and large hematomas, which require cold application over a large surface. Large bruises, of the type that occur in soccer games, can be treated with ice blocks. Blocks can be made by freezing water in plastic or cardboard containers with a stick in the middle.

**Ice Bags.** Ice cubes are put in a plastic bag. The bag can be laid across a large surface area of the body or used together with an elastic bandage.

**Cold Towels.** To make a cold towel you will need to dissolve about a pound of table salt into about 5 liters of water and then soak the towels in this

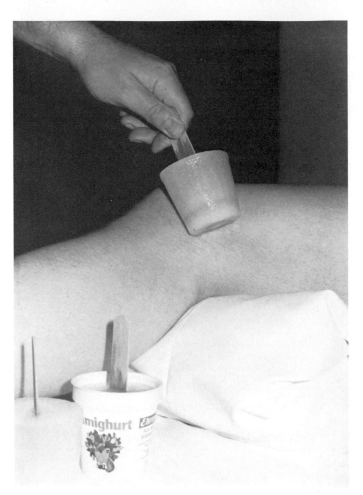

**Figure 3–2.** Ice massage with ice block on outer knee ligament. The ice block is made in a paper cup and has a wooden holder.

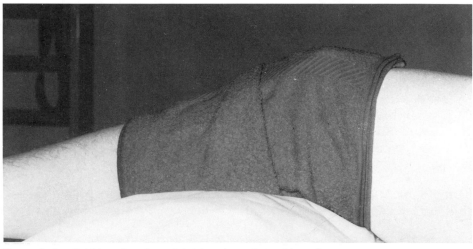

**Figure 3–3.** Cold towel on knee joint for circumferential cooling.

solution. The salt prevents towels from becoming rigid. The cold towel is particularly suited for joints, because it conforms perfectly to the shape of the body and thus has the advantage of circumferential cooling. Towels chilled in a pail full of ice cubes can also be used.

**Ice Bath.**    Dipping the surface of the extremities into a container filled with ice and water is known as a partial ice bath. A full ice bath is possible in a tub; this requires a large quantity of ice.

**Chemical Means of Cooling.**    Cooling sprays can be used on large surface areas of the body and ethyl chloride is good for local cooling. These two means of cooling are used for blunt traumatic injuries, such as to the feet, legs, arms, and shoulders. A rapid cooling can be achieved by this means, particularly for injuries that occur in games like soccer, handball, basketball, and hockey. The application of ethyl chloride in spray form through a protective material, such as a soccer knee sock, lessens the danger of a possible skin burn.

The thermal effect of the cooling spray is similar to that of ethyl chloride, but the danger of skin irritation is less with the aerosol spray.

**Cool Pac.**    This is a chemical cold pack. Cooling results from crushing the various compartments in which the chemical agent is stored. The bag is laid on the injured area or held in place by an elastic bandage.

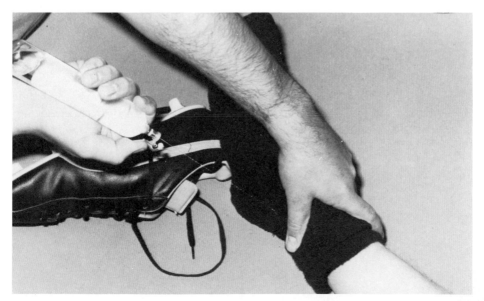

**Figure 3–4.**    First aid treatment: local cooling of sprained ankle with chlorethyl through soccer sock.

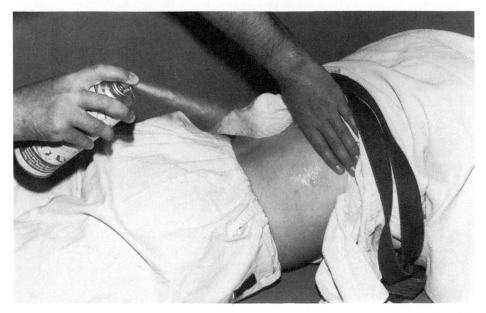

**Figure 3–5.**    Large area sprayed with cooling spray for a large bruise on the back of a judoka.

# Indications/Contraindications

The described applications are indicated for soft tissues and bone injuries, for contractures, and for postoperative treatment. They are contraindicated for people with sensitivity to cold, inflamed kidneys, blisters, and open wounds.

# Summary

The use of cold has proved its effectiveness in the treatment of athletic injuries. It can be successfully combined with active remedial exercise and other physical treatments. This depends on use of the proper types of cold application.

## CHAPTER 4

# Hydrotherapy and Balneotherapy

## DORIS EITNER

## History

The early Romans were already familiar with both hot and cold baths. The young Romans were in the habit of refreshing themselves with a swim in the Tiber after their gymnastic exercises on the field of Mars. In the years A.D. 129 to 201. Galen, a doctor at the gladiator school in his native city Pergamon and later in Rome, enriched the development of medical science with his comprehensive pathologic teachings. He frequently mentions baths, already distinguishes between full baths and partial baths, is familiar with cold affusions, and provides explicit instructions for their use.

In modern times physicians have recognized cold water as an important method of treatment. Hydrotherapy received a new impetus from the English doctor John Floyer (1649–1714). Floyer maintained that bathing in any cold water, not just in holy springs, promised salutary results.

In Germany it was Johann Gottfried de Berger who in 1694 first called attention to the baths that had been introduced by Floyer. Around 1700 Siegmund Hahn and his son Lorenz, both physicians, began to use hydrotherapy in Germany. Hahn wrote extensive instructions and described the various baths and their use for specific illnesses. In 1845, during his time at school, the minister Sebastian Kneipp discovered a booklet about hydrotherapy. As he himself was sick, he tested the described applications on himself. In 1880 he became a minister in Wörishofen. In that city, in 1889, the first public baths were established. Kneipp became one of the major figures in the development of hydrotherapy.

## Introduction

By hydrotherapy is meant all external applications of water for therapeutic purposes. Water functions essentially as a conductor of heat and cold in this process. Along with these thermal stimuli, various mechanical and chemical stimuli also play a role. Hydrotherapeutic measures are in many instances a good preparation, supplement, or accompaniment to active remedial exercise. They act on both the body surface and the entire organism. Not only are blood flow and heat balance affected, but metabolism, the nervous system, the composition of the blood, the secretion of various glands, and the psyche are influenced as well.

As we understand it today, heat represents kinetic energy — that is, it is due to the motion of the smallest particles, molecules and atoms.

Coldness cannot be defined physically, for any temperature above absolute zero, $-273°C$, is a measure of warmth, which fluctuates only in the degree to which the temperature is higher or lower. Coldness is instead a physiologic concept, the expression of a certain (usually unpleasant) sensation, which occurs due to the effects of low temperatures.

What, then, does one experience as warm or cold? Everything that is colder than the skin is considered cold, and everything warmer than the skin is considered warm. However, this is only partially accurate. If one undresses in a room heated to $22°C$, this temperature is experienced as neither warm nor cold. But it is different if one steps into a bath of $22°C$. It seems noticeably colder, although it is the same temperature. Water is a better heat conductor than air. Thus, more heat is drawn away from the body in a given time. Therefore, it is not merely the absolute temperature of the surrounding medium that is decisive, but its heat conductivity as well. The better the heat conductivity of a body one touches, the colder it will seem, should its temperature fall below the neutral point. Water seems colder to people than air at the same temperature. On the other hand, such a body will seem warmer if its temperature is above the neutral point. A bath at $40°C$ will thus seem warmer to a person than the air at the same temperature. The neutral point is therefore that temperature which seems neither warm nor cold. This point is not fixed; it depends on the following factors: skin temperature, constitution, and chemical and mechanical factors. For these reasons the neutral point is subject to considerable fluctuation. It would, therefore, be better to speak of a neutral range, rather than a neutral point.

### Guidelines for Water Temperatures

| | |
|---|---|
| Very cold | 10–12°C |
| Cold | 12–30°C |
| Mild or cool | 30–33 C |
| Neutral | 34–36°C |
| Warm | 36–38°C |
| Very warm | 38–40°C |
| Hot | 40–45°C |

The tolerance point is the highest temperature that can be withstood without suffering injury. Under normal conditions it is 45 to 46°C.

## Thermal Effects

Hot and cold stimuli primarily affect the heat and cold receptors in the skin and lead to a stimulus response of the body, whose intensity depends on the extent of the initial stimulus. The human body strives to maintain an optimal temperature for the completion of all processes important to life by means of a stable heat balance in the organism.

Physiologically, we can explain the effects of hot and cold stimuli on the body in the following manner: metabolic processes create heat in the body. Should the body be threatened with overheating from within, it begins to perspire. Sweat evaporates on the skin and thus accomplishes the cooling. But if the natural regulatory mechanisms are impeded in such a way that, for example, both the heat radiation and the evaporation of perspiration are prevented, the body temperature rises immediately. The same would occur if one were to subject the body to external heat, as is the case with heated baths.

The body reacts differently to a loss of temperature. In this case the production of heat is increased by an increase in the metabolic processes and by muscular movements in the form of shivering. In this manner the body seeks to regulate the heat balance. To return to the formation of perspiration once again, it not only is important as a factor in the regulation of temperature but also plays an important excretory role. The major portion of the excreted material in perspiration is, of course, sodium chloride; furthermore, it contains urea, uric acid, lactic acid, fatty acid, and other constituents. One liter of perspiration would contain approximately 5 gm of sodium chloride and the same amount of other excreted materials. Should the loss of minerals be too great, however, as occurs in high performance sports, the body reacts with muscle cramps.

A healthy vascular system responds to heat and cold with a vascular reaction. Heat dilates the blood vessels; cold, on the other hand, constricts them. However, a prolonged application of cold also dilates the blood vessels, increasing circulation, which is known as reactive hyperemia. The dilatation of the blood vessels extends to the capillaries, arteries, and veins. It results further in the reopening of closed capillary beds and causes reddening of the skin, during which time the blood vessel tone remains constant, despite the expansion.

# Mechanical Effects

## HYDROSTATIC PRESSURE

Hydrostatic pressure is the water pressure upon a particular surface. In a column of water, the hydrostatic pressure depends on the height of the column, the density of the medium, and the acceleration due to gravity. Hydrostatic pressure increases linearly with the height of the water column, and reaches the pressure of 1 atmosphere, 760 mm Hg, at a depth of 10 m.

In relation to the human body, this means that the pressure on the surface of the body increases steadily as one descends into water. If a person stands approximately half-submerged in water, the hydrostatic pressure aids venous return in the blood vessels in his legs. Full submersion causes pressure to affect the heart and the blood vessels. For the swimmer, the water pressure not only facilitates exhalation but also affects inhalation by creating resistance. This promotes the development of the muscles of the swimmer's chest. It should be mentioned in this context that hydrostatic pressure and water temperature can work against one another. That is, the pressure produces a slight constriction, whereas warm water temperatures cause a dilatation of the blood vessels. Should the pressure decrease, the temperature will exert its effects without hindrance. This results in a dilatation of the blood vessels and a "sinking" of the blood into the peripheral zones, leading to circulatory collapse. This often occurs when getting out of a full bath. People subject to circulatory problems should therefore remain seated in the tub until the water has run out.

## BUOYANT FORCES

From a physical perspective, the buoyancy of a solid body submerged in liquid is equal to the weight of the liquid volume displaced — Archimedes' principle.

In a simple full bath, the actual weight of a person weighing approximately 70 kg is only about 7 kg if his head remains out of water.

Because of the apparent reduction of bodily weight in water, buoyancy is a particularly important factor, especially for exercise in water.

## FRICTIONAL RESISTANCE

Along with buoyancy, the frictional resistance of water represents a considerable therapeutic aid. It depends on the working surface — the size of the body and the speed of motion carried out in the water.

The larger the working surface and the faster the movement, the larger the frictional resistance, and contrariwise.

Frictional resistance is utilized therapeutically for the strengthening of weakened muscles. Furthermore, its effects can be coordinated with those encountered during movements carried out in water.

# Baths

Baths are divided into full, three-quarter, and half-baths. Partial baths represent a further group. Here one distinguishes between sitz-, arm-, leg-, and footbaths. The water temperatures for the baths vary as follows:

| | |
|---|---|
| Cold baths | Below 30°C, usually used together with hot air or steam treatment |
| Cool baths | 30° to 33°C, such as brushbath, effervescent bath, carbon dioxide bath |
| Neutral baths | For underwater massage |
| Warm baths | Almost always used with supplements |
| Hot baths | Above 40°C, usually of short duration |
| Contrast baths | Partial baths with alternating hot/cold water |
| Rising temperature baths | Beginning at the neutral zone |

Simple baths, contrast baths, and rising temperature baths are the ones primarily used in therapeutic practice.

## SIMPLE BATHS

Simple baths involve virtually no change in water temperature — that is, the initial temperature hardly differs from the final temperature. All commonly used temperature ranges are possible (from cold baths to hot baths on the range listed previously).

## CONTRAST BATHS

Contrast baths involve the effects of repeated fluctuations between hot and cold water. They are used primarily with partial baths. In this form of

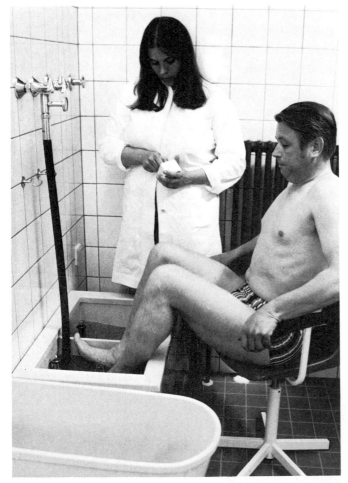

**Figure 4–1.** Contrast foot bath.

treatment increased stimulation is achieved. The degree of change can be controlled extremely precisely. It depends on the duration of the bath, the temperatures of the hot and cold waters, and the frequency of the changes of immersions. The general rule is: begin with warm, end with cold.

### Example: Contrast Foot-bath

| | | |
|---|---|---|
| *Temperature:* | Hot | 38–42°C |
| | Cold | to 20°C |
| *Duration:* | Hot | about 3 minutes |
| | Cold | about 30 seconds |

This bath is indicated for cases of chronic peripheral circulatory disturbance, as a strong reactive hyperemia is achieved, without the lowering of vascular and muscle tone. It is contraindicated for paradoxical vascular reactions.

## RISING TEMPERATURE BATHS

Rising temperature baths involve a gradual increase in the water temperature, starting in the neutral range. The slower the temperature increase, the gentler the treatment. The final temperature should be reached in about 15 to 30 minutes. The therapeutic goal of a rising temperature bath is generally the inducement of changes in the autonomic nervous system. Partial rising temperature baths are beneficial for peripheral circulatory problems, as narrowing of the primary blood vessels does not occur.

The overheating bath may be seen as a particular form of the rising temperature full bath. The goal of this bath is the generation of a body temperature in the fever range. This condition can be reached because the body, aside from the head, is submerged in water, which occasions an immediate rise in temperature.

The overheating bath causes maximal vascular dilatation. The increase in blood supply which this creates in particular organ systems stimulates the metabolism. The initial temperature is neutral, approximately 36°C. An elevation in temperature, at the rate of 1 to 2°C, occurs approximately every 5 minutes. The final temperature is about 42°C, which, however, is in accordance with the clinical picture.

This bath is indicated for chronic rheumatic joint/muscle disorders and spinal defects; it is contraindicated for heart and circulatory disorders, coronary circulation problems, when there is risk of infarction, and in arteriosclerosis.

## BATHS WITH ADDITIVES

The full baths with additives can be classified according to the materials added to the water. There are three large groups: aromatic baths; mineral baths; and physical baths.

## AROMATIC BATHS

These are baths with extracts from aromatic herbs and various types of woods, which stimulate the skin. The effect depends on the presence of essential oils. The best-known aromatic bath is the spruce-needle bath. This bath treats insomnia, nervous disorders, rheumatic complaints, and decreased skin circulation.

The camomile bath is used along with the spruce-needle bath for its relaxing influence, and for the acceleration of the healing process in poorly healing injuries. Camomile steam may also be inhaled at the onset of a cold.

## MINERAL BATHS

Mineral baths include those baths that contain primarily sodium, potassium, and magnesium as cations, and chlorine, sulfur oxide, and carbonic acid as anions. The chemical materials dissolved in the water are deposited on the skin surface, and some even penetrate. These materials are reabsorbed by the bloodstream. On the other hand, materials are lost in perspiration. This process of exchange gives rise to a change in the balance of mineral constituents in the skin, known as transmineralization.

The best-known medicinal bath is the sodium chloride or brine bath. Brine baths contain primarily chloride or sodium ions. Sodium chloride springs contain at least 1 gm of sodium chloride per liter of water; brine baths have more than 15 gm per liter. Moreover, most sodium chloride springs contain a large number of other mineral salts, particularly calcium magnesium chloride. Sodium chloride and brine baths encourage better circulation in the skin as well as a lowering of the susceptibility to colds. The autonomic nervous system is affected as well. In this context it should be mentioned that brine baths are taxing. It is advisable to rest for an hour afterwards.

For athletes, such a bath in the warm temperature range is an ideal warm-down after training or competition. Sulfur baths have likewise proved to be excellent for this purpose. Such baths contain a combination of sulfur and potassium carbonate. A full bath can be expected to contain approximately 125 gm of these minerals. Sulfur has numerous effects. It is excreted in increased amounts in the urine in cases of chronic joint disorders. The rebuilding of articular cartilage can be influenced by a substantial influx of sulfur. In general, sulfur baths cause an improvement in skin circulation, an increase in the metabolism, and finally a mobilization of the defenses against disease. Baths can be recommended, for example, during the regenerative period following a competitive season.

## PHYSICAL BATHS

For this type of bath, only temperature and water pressure are important. The chemical constitution of the water is irrelevant. Full cold baths are not common in the treatment of athletes. Full hot baths as well as overheating baths are likewise not advisable for healthy athletes, as this results in an increase in body heat. There is no objection to a brief hot shower for the purpose of loosening up the muscles before competition, if it is concluded with a short burst of cold water. Brief, strong hot and cold stimuli are both invigorating and refreshing. These short stimuli increase the tone of skeletal muscle, stimulate the motor nerves, and improve the performance of the muscles.

## HYDROELECTRIC BATHS

Hydroelectric baths utilize the ability of water to conduct an electric current. Through the connection of the cathode and the anode, the water surrounding the body becomes equal in electrical conductivity to the electrodes. In this way there is no danger of cauterization.

Hydroelectric baths conduct a galvanic current to the body. Certain medications can be diffused into the body through the skin with the aid of the galvanic current. This is called iontophoresis. At the same time, the thermal effects of a full or partial bath are exploited. Hydroelectric baths are indicated for circulatory problems of various kinds, rheumatic illnesses, and ailments of the central and peripheral nervous systems.

The most common hydroelectric baths are the four-celled bath and the Stanger bath.

## FOUR-CELLED BATH

During the four-celled bath both arms of the athlete are submerged separately in water, as are both lower legs. Then the electric current is run through the extremities, using several possible variations. The four-celled bath is well suited for iontophoresis with histamine. This histamine iontophoresis dilates the blood vessels in the skin and increases the permeability of the skin, the capillary wall, and the cell membrane. Iodine iontophoresis is used along with the histamine iontophoresis, particularly for scarred adhesions. The most important of the iontophoresis treatments is the choice of the correct terminal in each individual case. Medicines which contain primarily positive ions will drift toward the cathode, and therefore are placed on the anode. Medicines with primarily negative ions drift towards the anode and are put on the cathode. Histamine is placed under the positive pole, and potassium iodide below the negative pole.

## STANGER BATH

Stanger baths are administered in tubs constructed specially for this purpose, which have built-in electrodes both along the edge of the tub and on the swivel arms. The current can be selectively directed through the individual electrodes. In this bath the body can assume a wide variety of positions.

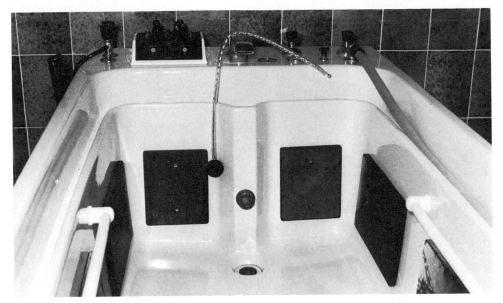

**Figure 4–2.**  Tub for Stanger bath.

The Stanger bath is used primarily for persons with paralysis, circulatory problems, rheumatic disorders, and athletic injuries.

## WHIRLPOOL BATHS

The whirlpool bath has become an increasingly valuable means of athletic treatment. It has become extremely popular in the United States. The principle is to combine the thermal stimulus of the water with further mechanical stimuli. One way in which this occurs is with the aid of a rotating propeller, which moves the water. In addition, a jet of warm air is injected into the water through a small nozzle. Depending on the size, the whirlpool bath can be used either as a partial bath for the lower legs or the arms or as a full bath for the entire body. The whirlpool bath should not be compared to the underwater massage, as the mechanical component is weaker. Furthermore, it cannot be applied to specific areas. Whirlpool baths are used primarily after injuries and for patients with circulatory problems and rheumatic disabilities, including rheumatic muscle and joint disorders, as well as for relaxing after practice and competition.

# Other Uses of Water

In addition to the wide range of baths included in hydrotherapy there are further treatments available such as affusions, showers, brushings, slap-downs, and rub-downs.

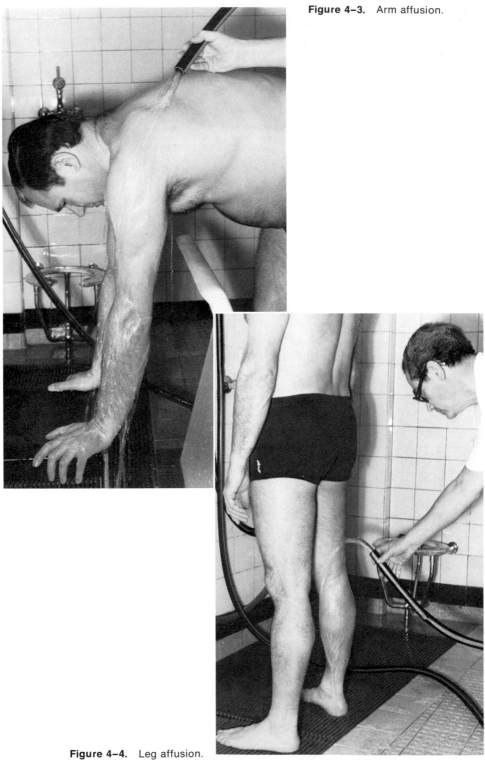

**Figure 4–3.** Arm affusion.

**Figure 4–4.** Leg affusion.

## AFFUSIONS

Kneipp considers affusions a characteristic hydrotherapeutic treatment. One typical feature of affusions is the precise regulation of the direction of the water stream on the body. Affusions have a tonic effect. There are both simple affusions, making use of a stream of water without pressure, and affusions under a pressure of 1 to 3 bars. Thus, there are two factors to consider in calculating the amount of the stimulus, thermal and mechanical. Kneipp claims that the water should surround the body like a coat. The primary effect of an affusion under pressure is mechanical. In simple affusions the temperatures used are extremely cold. In certain circumstances there can be an alternation of lukewarm and hot affusions. As is the case for all hydrotherapeutic uses of water, the patient's body and especially the feet should be warmed before and after cold affusions. The length of the affusion depends on the individual reaction of each part of the body. A uniform reddening of the skin should take place.

## AFFUSIONS UNDER PRESSURE

Affusions under pressure have a strong mechanical effect along with the thermal effect. They are administered from a hose with a nozzle, which narrows the stream of water to about 5 mm. The affusion under pressure is administered from a distance of 3 m. The temperature is usually cold, as for simple affusions, but it can also be hot or alternating cold and hot.

Not only are these "Kneipp affusions" an excellent vascular exercise for the athlete, but they also help produce a general toughening and reviving effect on the entire body. The influence of the cold water — 10 to 15°C — creates a hyperemia. Cold affusions are particularly effective following extreme exertions, especially in warm weather with accompanying heat buildup, both in the breaks between individual events in sports involving several separate competitions and during endurance events.

## RUB-DOWNS

The stimulus that the thermal affect produces is supplemented by the mechanical effect of a vigorous rubbing. A cold, wet towel is rubbed with the palm of the hands against the particular part of the body until it is warm.

## BRUSHING

Both dry and damp brushes are used. For dry brushing two brushes are used in even, rhythmic strokes. The pressure is divided evenly over the individual parts of the body until there is clear reddening of the skin. Damp brushings involve either brushes dipped in hot water or brushing carried out in connection with a shower. Begin the brushing farthest away from the heart on the extremities. Then move to the upper extremities, the chest, and the back. The treatment always moves towards the heart.

This treatment is indicated for the improvement of circulation and for general tonicizing. Other hydrotherapeutic treatments are often combined with the brushings, such as a brushbath.

## SLAP-DOWNS

Slap-downs provide a cold stimulus to the body and have a strong mechanical effect. The most common form is the slap-down of the back. A towel is folded, dipped into cold water, and wrung out to the desired degree. Then the section of the body is lightly slapped with circular motions coming from the wrist.

## SHOWERS AND STEAM SHOWERS

Showers include all applications of water or steam that are administered under pressure.

Showers are divided into cold, neutral, warm, and hot. Hot showers and extended showers are preferred for rheumatic disorders.

For the athlete, warm showers after training or competition have a

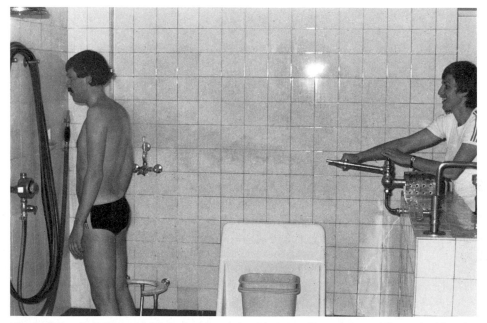

**Figure 4–5.**  A distance of 1.5 to 2 meters is kept between the nozzle and the patient for steam shower.

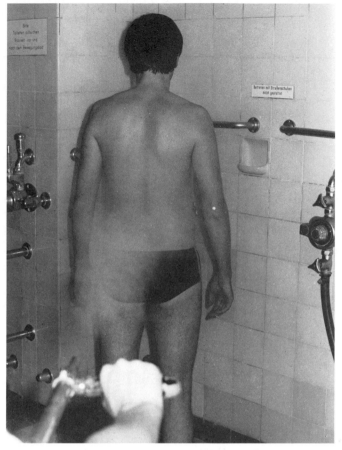

**Figure 4-6.** Treatment of the back with steam shower.

generally loosening and relaxing effect, in addition to being cleansing. Cold showers have a tonic effect on the blood vessels and are a good way to conclude a warm shower. Steam showers can be used to improve muscular recovery after competition.

In this case, the steam is sprayed onto the skin at a pressure of 1 to 2 bars and a temperature of about 48°C. The therapist should take care to keep a distance of 1.5 to 2 m between himself and the athlete, as the steam can otherwise scald the athlete.

The steam shower is also suited for the treatment of residual damage, such as occurs in contractures, scars, and rheumatic disorders.

## CHAPTER 5

# Electrotherapy

*HELMUT ORK*

## Introduction

Electrotherapy involves all those methods of treatment in which electricity itself is used directly. The subdivision of electromedicine uses electrical energy for the treatment of disorders and injuries.

Electrotherapy is divided into three main groups, on the basis of technical and physiologic considerations: low frequency, 0 to 1 kHz; middle frequency, 1 to 300 kHz; and high frequency, about 300 kHz.

## Low Frequency Therapy

This is divided into galvanization and stimulus or impulse current therapy, according to Bernart and Träbert.

### GALVANIZATION

Galvanization is a treatment using constant, direct current that continues in the same direction and at the same strength.

The electrical conductivity of the human body depends on the watery solutions of salts, bases, and acids, which are found in all vascular fluids. When the electromotive force, as in this case the galvanic current, affects such solutions, positively charged sodium ions are driven from the positive pole and pulled towards the negative pole. The organism experiences the change in ion concentration caused by the galvanic current as an external stimulus. When the direct galvanic current is used within the therapeutic dosage range it does not cause muscular contraction. The resulting decrease in pain is due to the raised pain threshold of the sensitive nerve fibers, which are assumed to register pain.

An intensive increase in circulation arises in the form of a long-lasting, reactive hyperemia on the surface and deep in the soft tissues.

Treatment is possible in a Stanger bath and in the four-celled bath (see Chapter 4) and with iontophoresis. When placed on the proper pole, medications pass through the skin in ionized form, driven by the electromotive force.

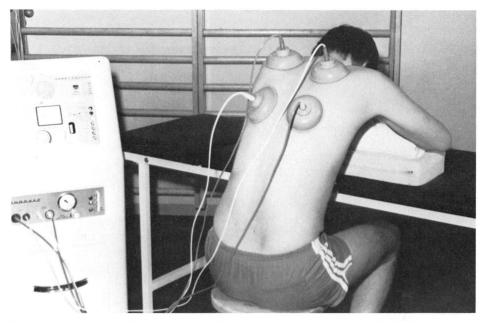

**Figure 5-1.** Galvanization. Constantly flowing direct current treatment with four paravertebrally placed suction electrodes.

Such medications are capable of having a local and deep effect without damaging the skin.

The deep-reaching effects influence the subcutaneous tissues, tendons lying near the body surface, ligaments, muscles, and the periosteum.

The treatment lasts between 5 and 30 minutes and can be administered daily for sports injuries.

The unpleasant, often painful muscle contraction caused by the turning on and off of the apparatus should be avoided by increasing and decreasing the intensity of the current gradually.

*Indications.* Galvanic currents are used for degenerative and inflammatory disorders, for peripheral circulatory problems, and particularly for postoperative and posttraumatic states following athletic injuries and damage. Sprains, contusions, dislocations, and hematomas can be treated in this way, as can inflammations and joint disorders.

*Contraindications.* Treatment with galvanic current is ruled out for acute inflammations, various dermatologic ailments, malignant tumors, and metal implantations. One should also bear in mind that there are individuals who cannot tolerate this treatment.

## STIMULUS AND IMPULSE CURRENTS

Faraday and exponential impulse currents are among the low frequency currents; also included are diadynamic and ultrastimulus currents (Träbert).

## Faraday Currents

The "classic" Faraday current was originally obtained with the help of a coil system and a circuit breaker (Wagner's hammer) during faradization. The optimal stimulus on healthy muscles was a frequency of 50 Hz (50 interruptions per second). The stimulus varied at higher or lower frequencies. At a stimulus of about 5 to 10 Hz the muscles vibrated (vibration current). At higher frequencies the patient often experienced a "rippling" sensation (rippling current).

This original form revealed certain problems, however, and was further developed in the course of time. At the present time there are devices by which the forms of impulse and the series can be regulated at will. This method is termed neofaradization and uses (see later) "triangular" impulses with an impulse length of 1 millisecond (ms) and an interruption of 20 ms. This extremely short effective period of the individual impulse and its brief interruption is only suited for the stimulus treatment of healthy or only slightly damaged muscles, however, as only these are capable of reacting to such a brief impulse and interruption time with a tetanic contraction. A further insufficiency of this type of current lies in the reaction time of the healthy muscle to the impulse. Healthy muscle reacts quickly and strongly to the stimulus treatment, whereas degenerated muscle reacts slowly, which can be recognized as a strong reaction of the antagonist muscle.

Modern electrotherapy has meanwhile allowed for the adaptation to physiologic and pathologic states, with the use of a gradual increase in the current, which permits extensive variation of the length of both the impulse and the interruption, along with the ability to reproduce them exactly.

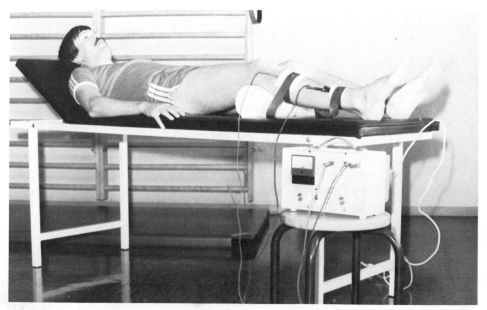

**Figure 5–2.** Stimulus and impulse current treatment for a perineal lesion.

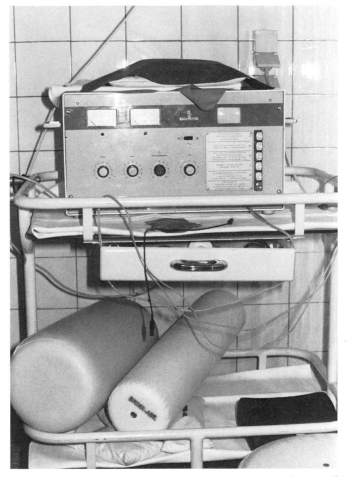

**Figure 5–3.** Stimulus current apparatus with modulation possible to DF (diphase), CP (short period), and LP (long period).

## Exponential Currents

The basic improvement lies in the ability to increase the current impulses gradually. When represented graphically, these impulses display a similarity to a triangle, which is why this form of current is referred to as triangular current. As the current does not increase in a straight line, but rather in a flat curve, which is in accordance with a mathematical exponential equation, the current is also called exponential current.

This stimulation of a nerve or a muscle with the help of an electric current occurs whenever the electric stimuli are given for a sufficient length of time and at a strength sufficient to reach a certain threshold value. The height of this threshold depends essentially on the electrophysiologic characteristic of the muscle or nerve; it is not constant, and can be displaced by the electric current.

A sufficient stimulus lowers the rest potential. When the threshold value is reached, the action potential comes into play, which, however, displays no change after the threshold value is surpassed (all-or-nothing law), but which rather responds with a heightening of the repetition frequency of the action potential, that is, the stimulus frequency. A coding of the stimulus effects is thus the result. Four factors are essentially responsible for the electric stimulus of a nerve or a muscle:

1. Density of current, that is, the strength of the current per electrode surface area.
2. Direction of current.
3. Rate of current increase.
4. Extent of time (usage time).

## Diadynamic Currents

Diadynamic currents, also named Bernard currents after their discoverer, are sinusoidal, direct current impulses with a frequency of 50 to 100 Hz. There are six different types of currents, which are each used for different purposes.

The MF (monophase) is a half-sinusoidal alternating current, which is created by a one-way DC converter of 50 Hz, with an impulse length and interruption of 10 ms each. The primary effect of this type of current is a motor stimulus; it can be termed a muscle stimulator.

The DF (diphase) type of current is created by an alternating current of 50 Hz by means of a two-way DC converter, so that a current of 100 Hz is achieved. The patient feels a stabbing oscillation in the treated area. The stimulus is less than that of the MF and primarily affects the autonomic nervous system in the sense of lowering the increased sympathetic tone.

The short-period current (CP) involves a sudden alternation between MF and DF currents. The patient senses the abrupt change between the tensing MF current and the relaxing DF current.

In the long-period (LP) current, the MF current is mixed with a second modulated MF. The gradual raising and lowering of the amplitude is experienced by the patient as a more pleasant sensation than that produced by CP.

In the syncopated rhythm (RS) the current is interrupted by a pause of 0.9 second after a current flow of 1.1 second. This type of current is used for the electrical stimulus of the muscles.

The modulated monophase (MM) current is not listed by Bernard, but it is a logical extension of his series of currents. In the MM the RS is gradually reduced in stepwise fashion. Like the RS, the MM is suited for the treatment of muscular atrophies, but the faradic excitability of the particular muscles must be maintained.

The therapeutic effects of the diadynamic currents have been researched and established in numerous studies (Bernard). The results obtained, particularly in their application in sports medicine, differ slightly. However, two

## DIADYNAMIC CURRENTS (AFTER BERNARD)

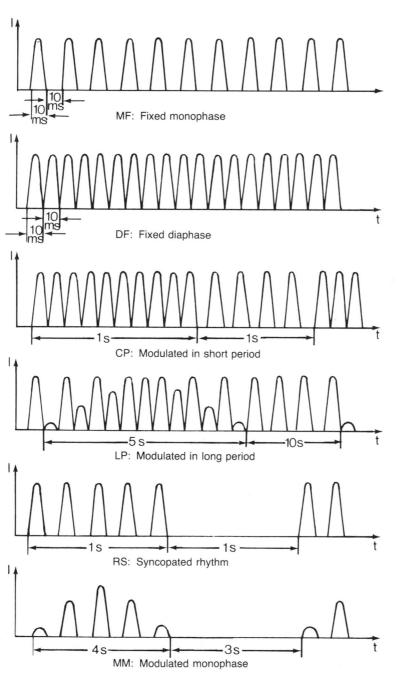

**Figure 5–4.**  Modulation for various phases of diadynamic currents.

types of effects can be distinguished — the analgesic and the hyperemic. It is not exactly clear, however, how the analgesic effect arises. Some authors explain the analgesic effect as a blocking of a particular area of the reflex arch, similar to that caused by Novocain.

DF is used for a brief analgesic effect, CP for a lasting one. Furthermore, CP is the type of current best suited for trophic disorders. The LP also reduces pain.

In the areas affected by the current, blood vessels are dilated, and the blood supply and metabolic rate in the tissues increases. Thus, favorable conditions for the rapid reabsorption of edemas and swellings are created and the process of recovery is hastened.

The hyperemic effect of the diadynamic currents is nevertheless restricted primarily to the tissues lying directly below the surface of the skin. Until this time, it remains uncertain to what degree the diadynamic currents cause a reflex increase in circulation in the deeper lying tissue layers as well. The same is true for its possible effects on inner organs.

The method and technique of treatment with the diadynamic currents are the same as those for the galvanic current. Indications vary, however, owing to the differing way in which they work. The strength of the current is gradually raised to the tolerance level in the course of the treatment. The patient must remain comfortable. The length of the treatment ranges from 2 to 15 minutes according to the type of current, and therapy is generally given in a series of six applications. Serious cases may be treated up to three times daily.

Some authors claim that the pain is already diminished after three treatments. Treatment with diadynamic currents can occur both alone and in connection with microwaves, ultrasound, or medications. Soviet doctors have ascertained that the diadynamic currents can also be used for iontophoresis with both anesthetics and other medicines. It is the relatively short length of the treatment and its rapid effects that have made the use of diadynamic currents prominent, particularly in the treatment of sports injuries. Muscle and joint pains, contusions, sprains, and dislocations, which occur frequently in athletics, are beneficially affected by this treatment. When treating acute, blunt trauma, such as injuries of the type that occur in soccer and ice hockey, a CP treatment is recommended after beginning for 1 minute with DF. A later transition to LP, with its long-lasting analgesic effect, is recommended.

The treatment with diadynamic currents is contraindicated in the same disorders as for the galvanic current.


## Träbert's Stimulus Current

This current involves a stepped series of impulses with a frequency of 140 Hz, with an impulse length of 2 ms and an interruption of 5 ms.

Tense muscles and strains in athletes participating in strenuous sports and gymnasts are benefitted.

Indications for use of this modality are similar to those for diadynamic currents, that is, for analgesic and hyperemic effects and as a muscle relaxer.

# Middle Frequency Therapy

Middle frequency therapy involves the use of alternating current up to 100 kHz. The best-known treatment is Nemec's interference current therapy. Two electric currents of moderate frequency are used — for example, 3900 and 4000 Hz or 4000 and 4100 Hz. The currents are supplied separated and each is led into the part of the body to be treated individually in a crossed direction. It has been noted that the crossing of the two individual currents in the stimulated tissues causes an interference effect. This produces a new biologically effective low frequency current in these tissues and organs, with a frequency corresponding to the difference between the two crossing currents. That is, the actively effective current is not led in from outside the body, but rather is developed endogenously within the tissues and organs of the human body. The deep-penetrating effect created by this method is a substantial advantage from the therapeutic standpoint. As the frequency increases, the stimulation of the sensitive nerves of the skin lessens, and a painless application is possible. In this way, higher intensities can be tolerated and thus deeper lying bodily tissue reached. Skin irritations, cauterizations, or possible burns are prevented by the constant rapid changes in the direction of the current. It has a hyperemic, reabsorbing, and muscle-relaxing effect similar to that of the lower frequency currents. It is contraindicated for the same disorders as low frequency electrotherapy.

# High Frequency Therapy

High frequency therapy can be divided into short waves of 27.12 mHz, decimeter waves of 433.92 mHz, and microwaves of 2450.00 mHz.

The high frequency current creates deep heat, which has an analgesic effect. It aids circulation and metabolism and causes relaxation of the muscular system.

Short waves can be classified into capacitor, coil, and radiation fields.

*Capacitor Field.*    The part of the body to be treated is placed between two capacitor electrodes. Those tissues with high electrical resistance, such as fat and bone marrow, are greatly warmed, whereas those tissues with low electrical resistance, such as muscles and organs, are only slightly warmed (ratio, 9:1). This depends on the distance from the electrode to the skin. A distance of 1 to 2 cm warms the surface more, and a distance of 2 to 6 cm causes a relatively deeper warming.

*Coil Field.*    The treatment in the coil field is carried out with an induction electrode. The exchange of energy occurs best in muscles that have a good blood supply. The fatty tissues are not warmed, in contradistinction to the treatment in the capacitor field.

*Radiation Field.*    The tissues lying in the radiation field are warmed with a dipole. In this case, fatty tissues are warmed less than the muscular system.

| Distance of electrode from skin | Warming of the knees | Inducted current |
|---|---|---|
| 0,2 cm | 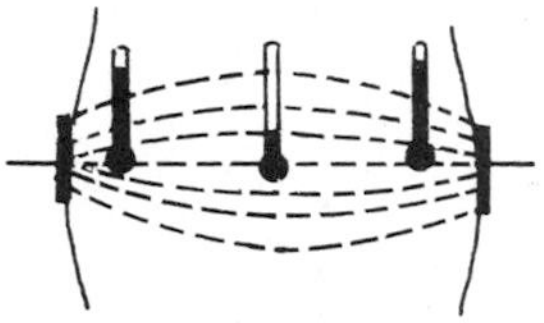 | 70 Watt |
| 2 cm | 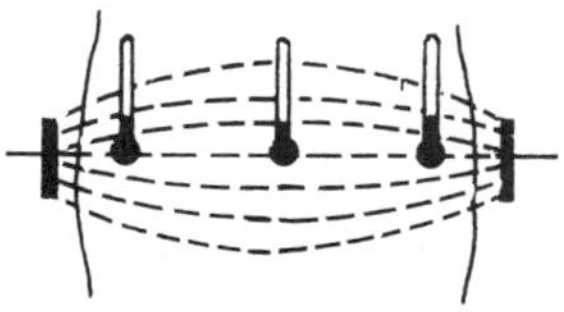 | 70 Watt |
| 2 cm | 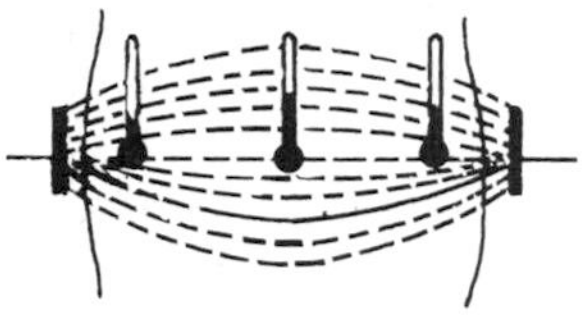 | 200 Watt |

**Figure 5–5.** Warming of the skin surface and below with electrodes at various distances from the skin.

The depth of penetration is determined by the degree of absorption, reflection, and refraction. The closer these levels are to the border zones, the lower the depth of the penetration, and the opposite. Circular and long-field electrodes warm superficially, with the exception of fatty tissues; Mulden radiation warms deeper layers, also with the exception of fatty tissues.

Various emitters are used, depending on the size of the body part to be treated. Minode, monode, and diplode can be used for short wave treatments; circular and long-field emitters for decimeter and microwave treatments. The Mulden emitters are well suited for large areas with good depth penetration.

Active conditions are treated carefully, briefly, and frequently, whereas chronic disorders are treated intensively, extensively, and at longer intervals.

The following dosage levels should be heeded:
Level I     unnoticeable heat.
Level II    slightly noticeable heat.
Level III   more noticeable heat.
Level IV    very noticeable heat.

High frequency therapy is indicated for disorders of the musculoskeletal and motor systems and in postoperative and postinjury treatment.

The possibility of creating both surface and internal warmth with high frequency current therapy has made its use prominent in the treatment of athletic injuries and damages.

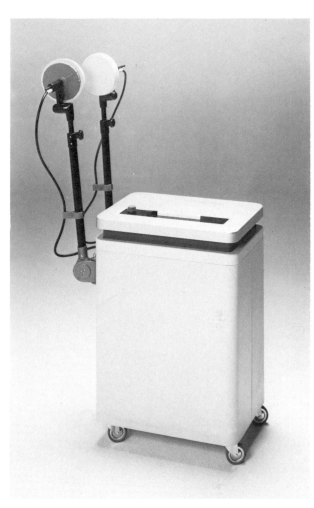

**Figure 5–6.** Shortwave apparatus with diplode.

The treatment is absolutely contraindicated when there are metal objects in use such as rings, watches, and metal implants, as irreversible tissue damage can result. Care should be exercised when treating arterial circulatory problems and acute inflammations, particularly of the inner organs, as well as when treating pregnant women and patients with tumors.

## Ultrasonic Therapy

Ultrasonic therapy is included in the high frequency range of electrotherapy, although electrical energy is no longer used directly. The effect is varied, both general and local, and can occur both immediately and after a delay. A combination of ultrasound with stimulating currents is possible. Statistics show that ultrasound is among the most frequently used electrotherapeutic treatments for athletic injuries. This is especially true of the

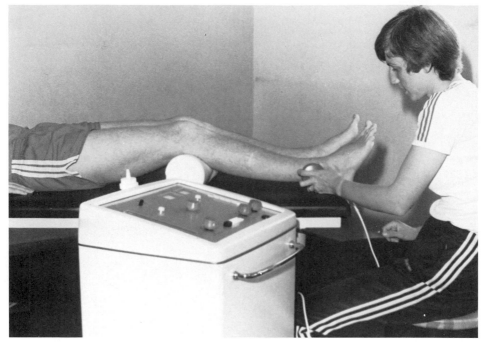

**Figure 5–7.** Ultrasound treatment after sprained ankle.

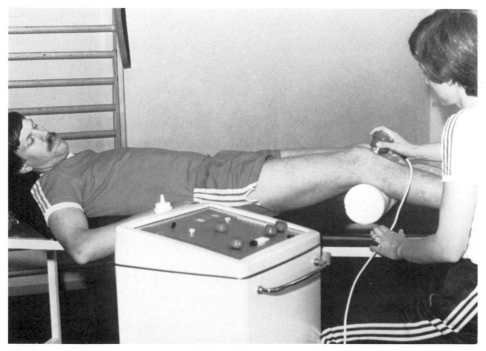

**Figure 5–8.** Ultrasound treatment of irritated knee.

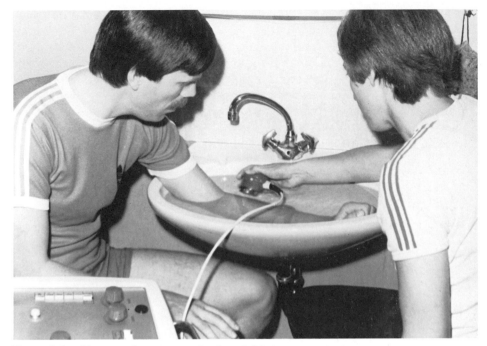

**Figure 5–9.** Ultrasound treatment of epicondylitis in a water bath.

combined use of ultrasound and diadynamic currents. This combination permits the rapid alleviation of pain, as it treats the causes of the pain. A distinct reddening of the skin appears at the triggerpoint of pain. Treatment in water has proved excellent for acute or chronic athletic injuries and damage. Various possibilities exist for the use of this treatment for epicondylitis in tennis players and javelin throwers and for insertion tendinitis, which occurs in soccer players and track and field athletes. The pain is relieved and the muscles are detonicized. Ultrasound is a better treatment than most of the other electrotherapeutic treatments because of its penetrating effects, particularly in the case of the periosteum. A variety of sizes in apparatus permit localized treatment.

Ultrasound is indicated for the treatment of traumatic injuries, such as tears, bruises, sprains, dislocations, hematomas, contractures, and scars. Peripheral circulatory problems, tendinitis, myogelosis, and joint disorders of the spinal column and the extremities are other areas of possible usage.

Excessive dosages and static sonic treatments are to be avoided.

## Summary

The increasing use of electrotherapy in the remedial treatment of athletic injuries and damage is linked to the short length of the treatment, the rapidity of analgesic, hyperemic, and stimulating effects, and the fact that the treatments are generally easily tolerated.

The success of the treatment depends not only on proper administration, but also on the subtle adjustment of the type of electrical stimulus to the type of injury, its stage of healing, and the individual reaction of the patient.

The compactness of many available electrotherapy devices makes it possible to bring them along on trips to the site of competition, so that they can be used with no loss of time for injured athletes. Their direct use is beneficial to the healing process for most athletic injuries.

# PART II Active Treatments

## CHAPTER 6
# Strengthening Exercises

### *WERNER KUPRIAN*

Strengthening exercises for the muscular system play an essential role in physical therapy and in retraining after all types of athletic injuries. Knowledge of the various training methods is thus among the most important requirements for effective treatment.

The strength of a muscle depends largely on its diameter. Systematic exercise results in the adjustment of the muscle to the training stimuli. The muscle hypertrophies — that is, it grows in thickness and increases in diameter. In this process, the number of muscle fibers does not increase; rather, each individual fiber increases in mass. The stimulus for increase in muscle diameter is thought to be the tension during contraction.

Lehmann, Hettinger, Müller, and others have divided strengthening exercises into two fundamental groups of muscular work, static and dynamic. Usually the two are mixed, and in this case they usually have a focal point.

Two other types — eccentric and isokinetic strengthening exercises — can be distinguished. The maximal strength of a muscle can be achieved by the use of all types of exercise. The degree, intensity, length, and frequency of the muscular tension produced are decisive for the growth of strength.

All types of exercise must be used in the correct proportion in athletics. The focal points should vary according to the athlete's individual constitution, condition, and type of sport. Equalizing and compensatory factors should also be considered in establishing a balanced training program. This is particularly true for athletic disciplines that require the unilateral patterns of motion or stopping which are repeated thousands of times, such as in gymnastics, shotputting, javelin throwing, and tennis.

Isometric exercises form the first part of active physical therapeutic treatment after athletic injuries, as after sprains, contusions, dislocations, torn tendons, osteosyntheses, or fractures that were conservatively treated.

## Isometric Exercise — Static Muscular Work

Exercises that cause contraction of individual muscles or muscle groups but no motion in the joints adjacent to them are called isometric exercises. No work is done in the physical sense in this type of muscular work. In the

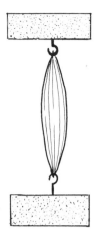
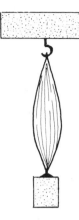
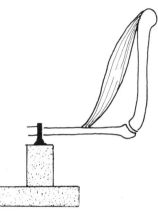

| ISOMETRIC | ISOTONIC | MIXED |
|---|---|---|
| Only development of strength (no work done in physical sense—"static work") | Work = Force × Distance (physical definition of work) | Isometric: Up to the point at which the force exerted by the muscles exceeds that of the weight<br>Isotonic: Lifting of weight |

**Figure 6–1.**   Forms of muscular work.

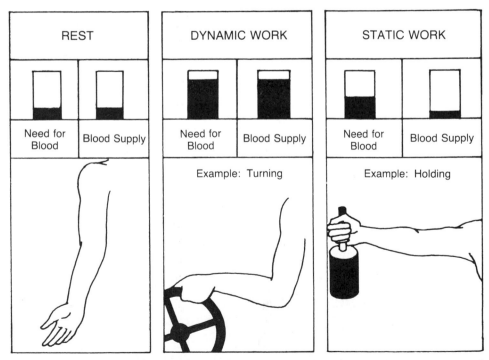

**Figure 6–2.**   Blood supply of muscle during dynamic and static work. (From Lehmann, G.: Praktische Arbeitsphysiologie. Stuttgart, Georg Thieme Verlag, 1953.)

physical formula, work = force × distance, and the isometric exercise lacks the component of distance. However, a high degree of tension is achieved. This is termed static muscular or holding work, which can be very strenuous and tiring for the person performing it. The relatively rapid tiring from static holding work is caused by the compression of the capillaries during the contraction of the muscle, which prevents the sufficient supply of oxygen and the removal of metabolic wastes. The work must be accomplished anaerobically.

Sitting upright without support and maintaining good posture in general are examples of typical static holding exercise for the long back extensor muscles, the erector spinae.

Hettinger recommends a muscular contraction with about 40 per cent of maximal strength as a favorable training stimulus for the muscle. If one contracts a muscle even for a few seconds daily the muscle will hypertrophy, that is, there will be a measurable increase in the muscle mass. The length of tension should be between 6 and 10 seconds. The training should be repeated 3 to 5 times daily for optimal results. Isometric training is thus capable of increasing muscular strength without joint movement and therefore without dynamic muscular work. This fact is of great importance for remedial therapy after athletic injuries, and also for the maintenance of muscular strength during a period of immobilization.

It is generally known that when a muscle is immobilized in a cast after a fracture, or even during partial immobilization in an elastic bandage after a muscle pull, a greater or lesser degree of muscular atrophy occurs even after only a few days. The lack of exercise caused by the immobilization results in the loss of muscle tone; it becomes thinner and can no longer fulfill its normal function.

The interruption of training leads to a loss of strength not only in the muscles of the damaged extremity but also in those of the noninjured extremities. This loss, however, can be largely avoided with the proper use of isometric muscular exercises. In most cases, the noninjured extremities can be exercised even on the first day of the immobilization of the injured part. This helps to improve the blood supply in the injured extremity by achieving a consensual hyperemia. The injured and immobilized extremity can also be isometrically tensed and thus exercised while still in a cast or in a splint after the immediate pain has subsided, 3 to 4 days later, such as after a meniscus operation. In this way the loss of muscular strength can be avoided. The muscular atrophy already setting in can thus be countered and training can be resumed. This must, of course, be done under the proper supervision of a therapist.

It has been our experience that it is also difficult for patients to move individual muscles separately. Particularly after long periods of immobilization, even athletes with well-developed coordination and motor skills have difficulty in tensing and relaxing specific muscle groups. This weakness in responding to stimulation must be overcome early and reconditioning undertaken.

Isometric training is easiest for the lower extremities, such as the

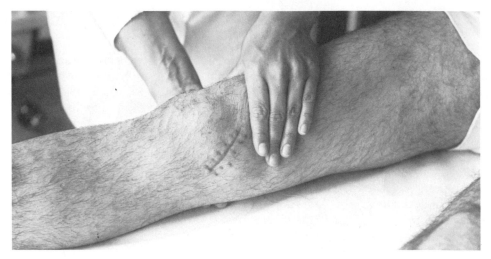

**Figure 6–3.**   Isometric strengthening exercise of quadriceps after meniscus operation.

quadriceps, gluteus maximus, and the gastrocnemius, and all static leg muscles. The muscles of the upper arm, biceps and triceps, are also relatively easy to stimulate and exercise isometrically. Bending and stretching the upper arm are motions familiar to everyone. For this reason, isometric contraction is learned more easily and quickly for these muscle groups.

The situation is different for muscle groups whose contractions are usually performed unconsciously — for example, the muscles supporting the shoulders and the upper body, the rhomboideus and trapezius. In these cases it is more difficult to learn the isometric exercises. Greater patience, more precise directions, and, if necessary, the application of other methods, such as

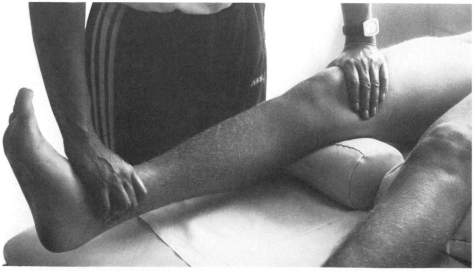

**Figure 6–4.**   Isometric strengthening exercise of entire leg.

facilitation techniques and a longer period of therapy, are required. Protective mechanisms, such as the pain of an injury to a joint or to soft parts, can have a hindering and blocking effect on the nerves of innervation.

The primary advantage of isometric training in remedial therapy after athletic injuries lies in the opportunity for localized muscle exercise without moving the joints. Strength increases more rapidly in isometric exercises than in dynamic exercises. On the other hand, strength is also lost more rapidly after cessation of exercise. Further disadvantages include: the muscular coordination necessary for many types of sports is not integrated in this treatment, which is why isometric exercises must in time be combined with dynamic exercises in the treatment of athletic injuries. Isometric exercise places great strain on the cardiovascular system; people in danger of heart attacks should not engage in isometric training because of the danger of compression, which narrows the blood vessels.

## Isotonic Exercise — Dynamic Muscular Work

In contradistinction to isometric exercise, isotonic exercise does involve work in a physical sense. This work is also called dynamic muscular work.

When, for example, the biceps contracts and shortens under stimulus and the lower arm is bent or a weight is lifted, movement is accomplished. The physical formula, work = force × distance, is fulfilled.

Dynamic muscular work does not involve lengthy contractions but instead is distinguished by the rhythmic alternation between contraction and relaxation. In the contraction phase, the muscle is pulled together, its origin and insertion approaching one another. In the relaxing phase, the tension is relaxed, the origin and insertion moving apart. In each motion, the agonistic and antagonistic muscle groups are involved together. By this means, each motion is precisely regulated and guided. At the moment of contraction, the intramuscular pressure increases. Even one fifth of the maximal contraction ability forces blood into the veins. During relaxation, the increase in the capillary bed is then so extensive that the circulation is 15 to 20 times stronger than when the muscle is at rest. The number of opened capillaries increases during muscular work. This involves about 15 per cent of the muscle volume under maximal stress. In this way, the circulation can both supply the tissues with oxygen and remove metabolic wastes. Dynamic muscular work thus promotes circulation and metabolism and eases the pumping work of the heart. The dynamically working muscle system itself does not tire as rapidly.

Isotonic exercise results in maximal gains in strength, in the same way as does static holding work. In addition, however, muscle coordination and speed are improved. The amount of force depends on the amount of resistance. The motion of the legs during bicycling is a typical example of dynamic muscular work.

The rhythmic alternation between tensing and relaxing the muscle aids the cardiovascular system at the same time. Oxygen is supplied better to the

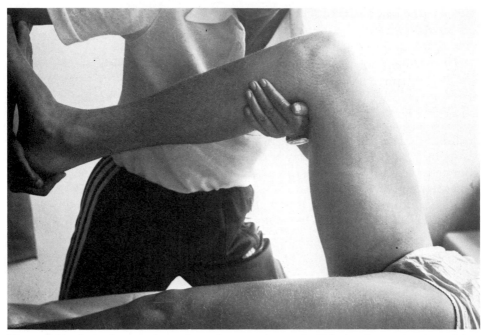

**Figure 6–5.** Isotonic exercise — dynamic muscular work. This involves extension of knee against manual resistance.

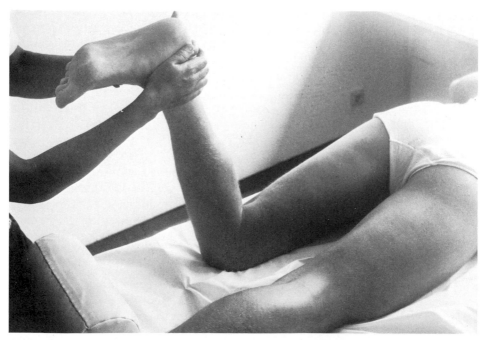

**Figure 6–6.** Eccentric exercise — dynamic negative work. The patient holds the flexion while the therapist tries to extend the knee.

muscle tissue owing to the flexion and extension. The muscle tires less rapidly than during static holding work. Dynamic muscular work is accomplished aerobically.

Isotonic exercise involves work against resistance. In the realm of athletics there are various ways of creating resistance, such as weights, dumbbells, leg-weights, running in soft sand, or swimming against rubber restraining bands or against an artificially created current. The Universal Gym should also be mentioned as an apparatus that makes possible a large variety of muscular resistance workouts.

In physical therapy the primary "tools" are the patient's own body weight and the manual pressure of the therapist against the patient. Other devices can be employed as well, however, such as sandbags, weights, chest expanders, and the "Bali-device."

Dynamic exercise begins in the second phase of physical therapy, after the immobilization of the injured part is no longer necessary and after nerves innervating the local muscle have been prepared in advance with isometric exercises. As soon as motion is allowed after a period of immobilization, dynamic exercises should begin to supplement isometrics. Static muscular work alone can be supported by the skeletal muscles only for a short time. The dynamic forms of training offer great advantages for the blood supply to the muscles, metabolic processes, and the cardiovascular system and heart.

At first one- and two-dimensional exercises should be used. Later three-dimensional exercises can be used, the so-called neurophysiologic methods (see Chapter 7). When retraining to full athletic ability, intensive work on elasticity and motor skills should be included along with the three-dimensional exercises.

It should, however, be repeated that strengthening exercises doubtlessly increase muscular performance. Without them, an improvement in performance in any sport is impossible. A properly carried out system of exercise is necessary for the preservation and restoration of muscles after athletic injuries. This must be operational from the period of immobilization through the early resumption of motion up to full recovery and resumption of competitive activity. In no phase of the physical therapy of the athlete can the proper use of strengthening exercises be neglected. However, the efficiency of the heart and circulatory system cannot be improved by strength exercises. Strength exercise alone does not benefit the cardiovascular system. An athlete trained solely for strength would leave much to be desired in the way of endurance.

## Eccentric Exercise

Eccentric exercise involves the repeated stressing of a muscle against maximal resistance. It can be termed dynamically negative work; however, during it muscular tension two to three times greater than normal can be created. Strength and muscular endurance can be increased in this way, as the patient has a partner against whom resistance exercises are performed. In the physical therapy the therapist takes the role of the partner.

## TABLE 6-1. THREE PHASES OF MUSCLE STRENGTHENING IN PHYSICAL THERAPEUTIC TREATMENT AFTER ATHLETIC INJURIES

*1st Phase: During Immobilization of the Injured Extremity*

1. Isometric and isotonic exercise of the noninjured, heathy extremity
2. Careful isometric exercise of the injured extremity. Isotonic exercise on the neighboring joints of the injured extremity. Begin after cessation of pain.
3. Circulation–respiration–metabolic training to maintain these functions during immobilization.

*2nd Phase: After Movement Is Permitted; Partial Stress*

1. Isometric exercise of the injured and the healthy extremities.
2. Isotonic exercise against strong resistance for the healthy extremities.
3. Isotonic training of the injured extremity, first with no weight, then against its own weight, then against manual resistance.
4. Mixed isometric and isotonic muscle exercises, such as exercises in water, remedial walking in water.
5. Vigorous circulation, breathing, and metabolic training.

*3rd Phase: After Full Stress Is Permitted*

1. Maximal stress with isometric and isotonic exercise of both extremities, concentrating on the injured extremity.
2. Mixed isometric and isotonic exercises for both extremities with concentration on the injured extremity. Also as exercise in water with resistance against buoyant devices.
3. Three-dimensional complex motions.
4. Remedial walking, running, and jumping for injuries to the lower extremities. Remedial exercise with devices for injuries to upper extremities (balls of various sizes and weights, bars, dumbbells, etc.), Universal Gym, training to increase elasticity, and coarse and fine motor skills.
5. Exercises for particular sports—first partial stress, then maximal stress—and resumption of conditioning training, merging with normal training in time, within limitations imposed by the advice of trainer.

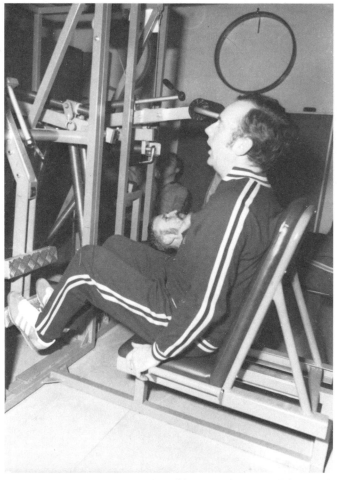

**Figure 6–7.**   Isokinetic exercise of knee extensor on Universal Gym.

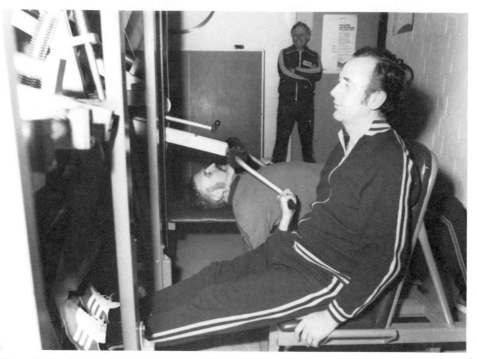

**Figure 6–8.** Knee extension on Universal Gym. This exercise is useful in training of quadriceps.

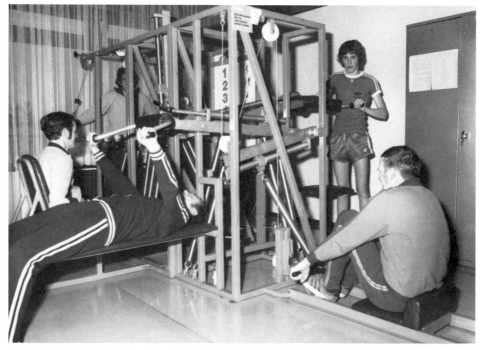

**Figure 6–9.** Group may work on the Universal Gym at the same time. Various muscles are being exercised.

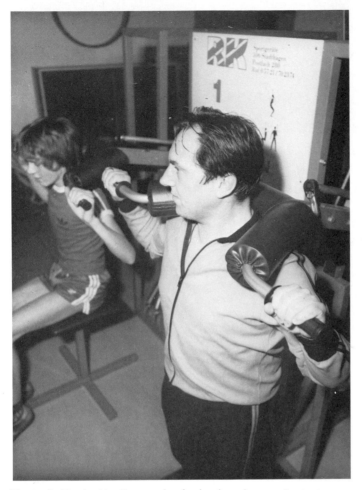

**Figure 6-10.**  Isokinetic exercise for back and arm extensors.

# Isokinetic Exercise

During isokinetic exercise, the pressure remains constant throughout the movement. A machine (Universal Gym) regulates the amount of resistance and also its rapidity. It quickly and thoroughly improves muscular strength and is a good supplement to other forms of exercise. It has become indispensable in today's top competitive sports.

For physical therapy after athletic injuries, isokinetic exercise is well suited for the transitional phase from the reattainment of normal strength to the reaching of full strength by the athlete.

## CHAPTER 7

# Proprioceptive Neuromuscular Facilitation — PNF Complex Motions

## LUTZ MEISSNER

## History

The concept of complex motions was developed by Dr. Hermann Kabat in America in the years 1946 to 1951. The work of the American therapist Sherrington and others provided the basis for this method. In subsequent years the method was improved and its area of application expanded. In this process two American physical therapists, Margaret Knott and Dorothy Voss, made outstanding contributions. In modern physical therapy treatment, use of complex motions has become an indispensable component of the treatment, particularly for disorders of the musculoskeletal and nervous systems, improper development, and trauma.

## Introduction

The method of complex motions is also termed the PNF Technique, "proprioceptive neuromuscular facilitation." This means roughly self-induced neuromuscular promotion and facilitation, thus entailing the opposite of blocking. In this process, the reactions of the neuromuscular mechanism are improved, smoothed, and accelerated through the stimulation of the proprioceptors. The use of complex motions is based on the principles of maximal stimulation of the neuromuscular apparatus with the additional help of an entire movement. The receptors in the muscles and joints are important elements in the stimulation of the motor system.

## Basic Principles of the Technique

The following basic principles enhance the desired reaction and are employed to achieve optimal functioning.

## GRASPING TECHNIQUE

The proper and precisely employed grasping technique of the therapist determines the strength of the complex motion produced.

## VERBAL AND VISUAL STIMULATION

Simple, clear instructions ease the work of the therapist. The patient should see and participate in what the therapist is doing.

## PRESSURE AND TRACTION

Pressure brings the joint surfaces closer together; traction moves them apart. The receptors are stimulated. Traction on the muscle system facilitates movement; pressure increases stability.

## MAXIMAL RESISTANCE

The all or nothing law of muscular contraction obtains. Isometric or isotonic resistance, or both, are employed. The maximal resistance is determined by the muscular strength of the individual patient.

## PROPER SEQUENCE OF MUSCULAR ACTION

When muscles contract in proper sequence, the stressed muscle group overcomes the demand made on it with optimal effectiveness. The correct timing plays an important role both in the complex motions and in sports.

Three components of motion, relating to all joints and focal points, take part in each spiral and diagonal pattern of motion: flexion, adduction or abduction, and outward or inward rotation. Outward rotation takes place with supination, inward rotation with pronation. Variations of the complex motion technique improve the implementation and effectiveness of the musculoskeletal system.

## DIRECT RESISTANCE

In direct resistance, maximal resistance occurs over the entire course of motion; this is geared to the various segments of the motions.

## REPEATED CONTRACTIONS

Static and dynamic contractions are involved alternately. Muscle strength is improved, particularly in the areas of holding strength, range of motion, and endurance.

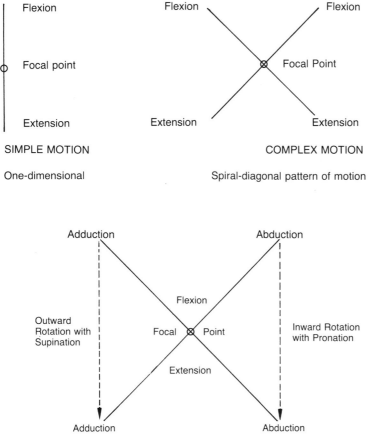

SIMPLE MOTION

One-dimensional

COMPLEX MOTION

Spiral-diagonal pattern of motion

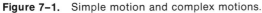

**Figure 7–1.**   Simple motion and complex motions.

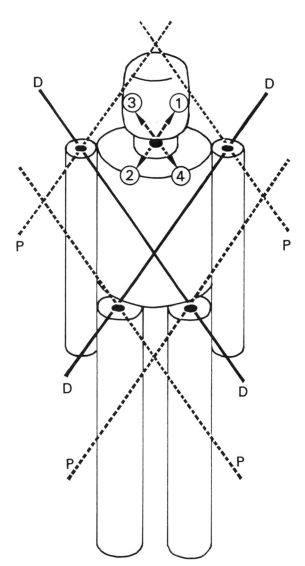

**Figure 7–2.** Direct body diagonals (*D*) and their variations, including parallels (*P*) as orientation for direction of motion.

## SLOW TURNING

In slow turning, an isometric, static contraction of the antagonist is followed by an isotonic dynamic contraction of the agonist muscle.

## SLOW TURNING — HOLDING

In this exercise, an isotonic, dynamic contraction of both the antagonist and the agonist is followed in each case by an isometric, static contraction of both muscles.

## RHYTHMIC STABILIZATION

Rhythmic stabilization is an isometric, static contraction of the antagonist followed by an isometric, static contraction of the agonist, which can be increased to a co-contraction, that is, multiple contraction of the antagonist.

# Complex Motions as Prevention and Rehabilitation for Athletes

In the second revised edition of the book *Complex Motions — Motion Facilitation after Dr. Kabat,* Margaret Knott and Dorothy Voss write in the preface: "Somewhere and sometime we hope that these still imperfect methods for the facilitation of motor skills and the prevention of injuries will also be used in athletic training programs."

In 1973 the author spent several months in California at the Kabat-Kaiser institute in Vallejo under the direction of Margaret Knott to learn the method of complex motions. In the succeeding years, he has trained many injured and healthy athletes with this method. He attempts to sketch here the difference between this technique and the "pure technique with complex motions." The use of complex motions in the physical therapy of athletes is certainly not yet sufficiently researched. There is no uniform method of employing them. However, the experiences gained promise success, and use of complex motions should be further expanded.

In sports, reactions arise in response to the stimuli of training and competition. The athlete develops great increases in motor abilities, strength, and endurance. Limits to this increase in performance are set by the individual's anatomic constitution and by learned or inherited neuromuscular reactions. If neuromuscular coordination has not been developed fully, the athlete is not able to respond adequately to the demands of training and competition. The stimuli for the athlete must be regulated by the technique of complex motions so that the desired reaction occurs. Weak points in the necessary motions for various athletic disciplines can be corrected and brought to optimal function through preventive or rehabilitative training. Patterns of motion (sensory engrams) weakened or disturbed by injury or lessened by specific stimuli are redeveloped through the application of complex motions; muscular strength is increased by the frequent repetition of the same motion, and the range of motion is increased. Only those combinations of motion that are purposeful treatments for the localized demands of a particular sport result in a successful "special training." Nonspecific, general exercises with and without apparatus do not produce the desired results, but rather hinder the development of optimal function.

The three-dimensional, diagonal-spiral shaped pattern of motion is most prevalent in all sports, particularly those requiring agility, coordination, and strength.

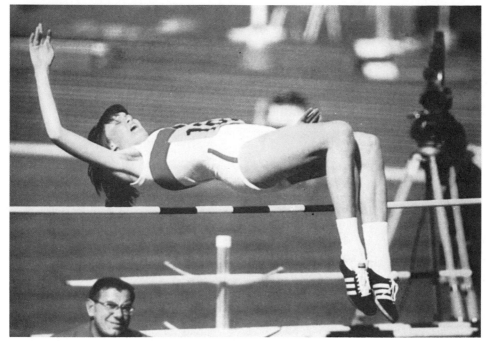

**Figure 7–3.**  Flop technique in high jump.

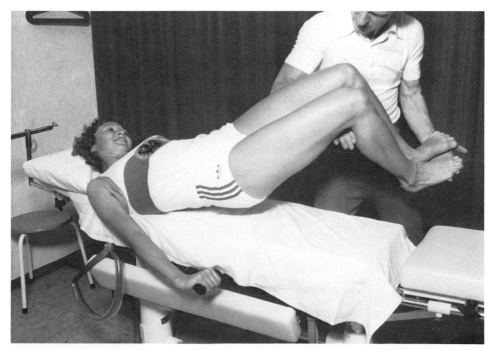

**Figure 7–4.**  PNF training for flop technique using hip extension.

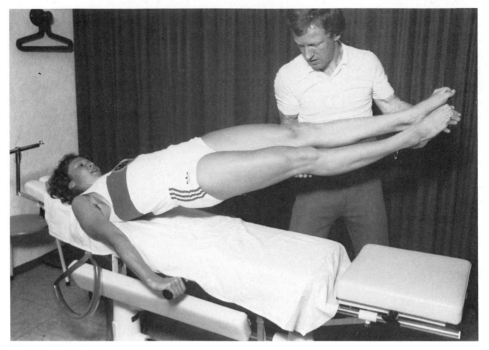

**Figure 7–5.** Hip, knee, and foot extension.

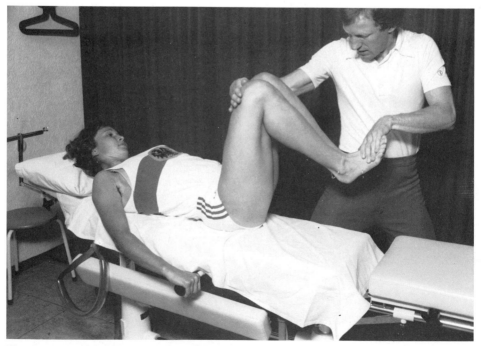

**Figure 7–6.** Hip, knee, and foot flexion.

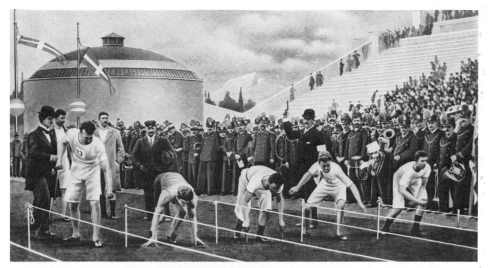

**Figure 7–7.** Start of the 100 m race at the first modern Olympic Games in Athens in 1896, showing the various starting positions taken by the runners.

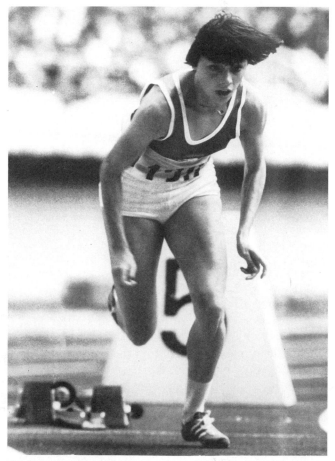

**Figure 7–8.** Sprinter shortly after start of race. Pattern of movement for supporting leg: the lower leg is rotated outward, and the foot is pronated.

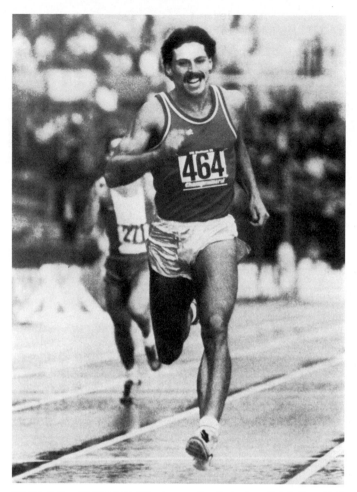

**Figure 7-9.** Runner of 400 m race shortly before finish line. Pattern of movement of swinging left leg: the lower leg is rotated inward, and the foot is supinated.

A 100 meter runner, who "only" runs straight ahead, actually demonstrates three-dimensional patterns of motion. The lower legs and feet are rotated outward and pronated shortly after the start. As the stride lengthens, the lower legs and feet are rotated more and more inward and supinated.

These diagonal-spiral patterns of motion exercised with the technique of complex motions are optimal preparations or training methods for the athlete because sports require similar patterns of motion. Furthermore, they correspond to the spiral, twisting motions that the body is capable of performing with bones, joints, muscles, and tendons. The human muscular system has a diagonal and spiral arrangement. Therefore, the direct path from a complete extension of a muscle to its complete contraction is also diagonal. This provides the basis for optimal muscular training for the athlete. This training can also correspond to the physiologic patterns of motion demanded by a particular sport, and thus it can have a preventive effect.

Complex patterns of motion in athletics that require a high degree of coordination are performed optimally when the antagonist and the agonist are completely synchronized. These patterns of motion can continue to occur as a result of reciprocal innervation. So-called minitraumas that take place during athletic events often go unnoticed, as they are not particularly painful. This is due to the poor correlation between the extent of the injury and the subjective sense of pain. Directed complex motions improve muscle sensation and control of motions. Free movements in antagonistic patterns during athletic training or as a preparation for competition have a stabilizing effect; at the same time, more demands are made on coordination. Special combinations of motion patterns act as an ongoing stimulation; thus, for example, complex motions of the extremities contribute to the development of the muscles of the torso.

Complex motions utilize stronger muscles in order to stimulate and strengthen weaker ones. In athletics the purpose is to prepare better for the

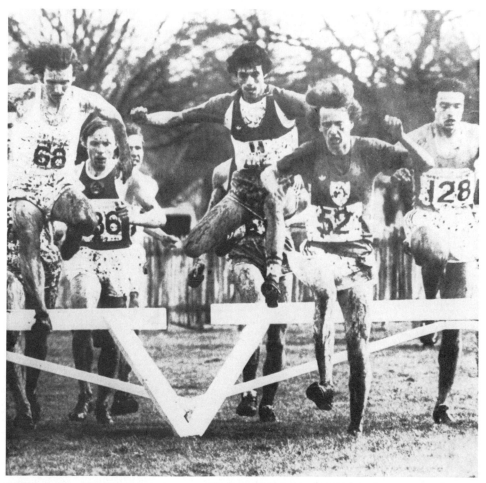

**Figure 7–10.** Cross-country runners with three-dimensional patterns of movement of the leg muscles.

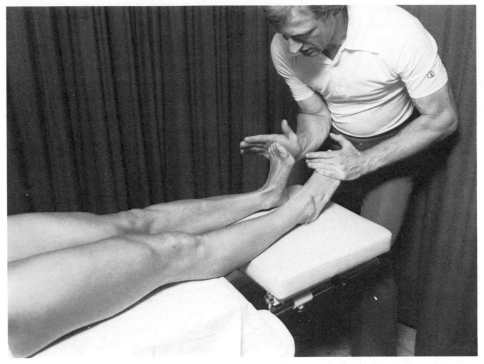

**Figure 7–11.** PNF training for running disciplines, using dynamic footwork: foot flexion with pronation alternates with foot extension with supination.

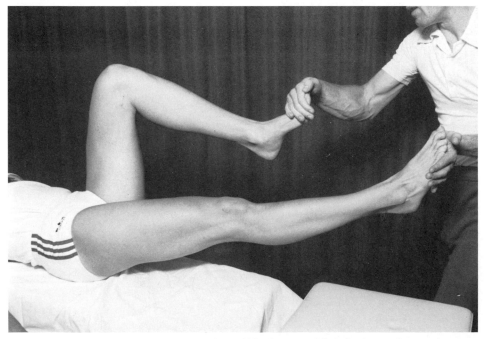

**Figure 7–12.** Dynamic legwork: alternation of hip, knee, and foot flexion and extension.

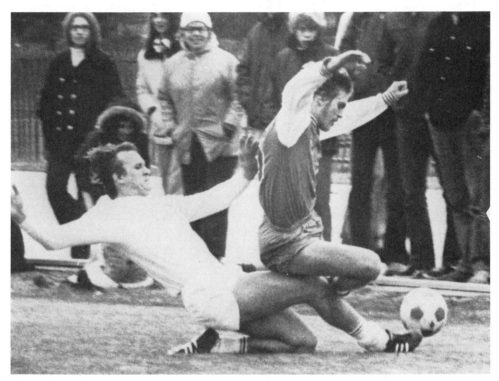

**Figure 7–13.**   Three-dimensional patterns of motion in soccer.

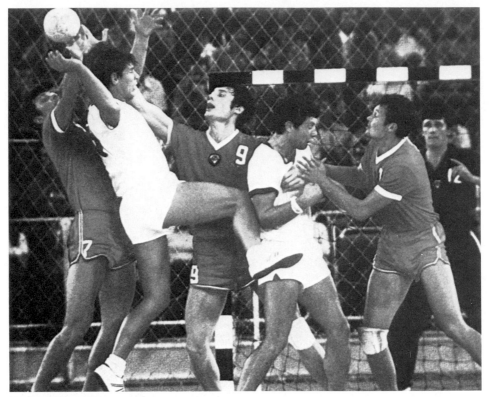

**Figure 7–14.** Three-dimensional patterns of motion in German handball.

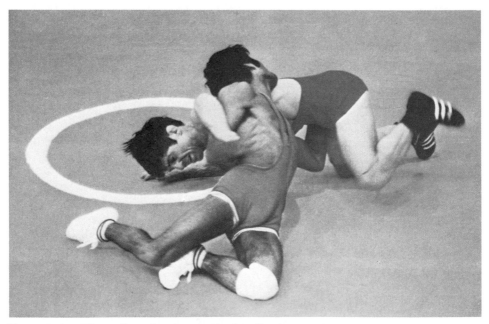

**Figure 7–15.** Three-dimensional patterns of motion in wrestling.

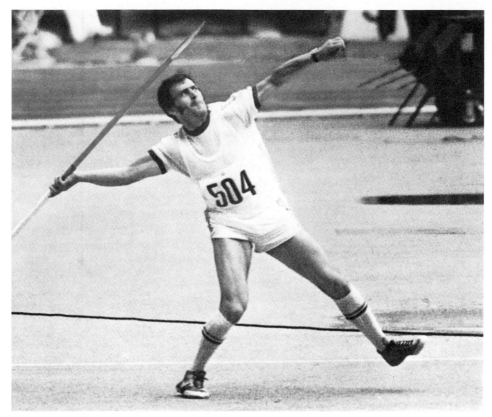

**Figure 7–16.** Three-dimensional patterns of motion in javelin throwing.

conditions of training and competition, to make use of those capabilities that exist or those that remain dormant, and to apply the motions in accordance with the demands of a particular sport. In this way the best training results are achieved — "optimal creation of function through function."

The athlete, healthy or injured, conforms to the demands of training and competition. Important requirements include a controlled pattern of motion for the particular sport and bodily condition that will permit this. Top performance requires the coordination among the series of motions required by a particular sport. This may involve balanced performance of the stressed muscle group, as in long distance running, or the increased performance of the muscles of only one side, as in javelin throwing.

All motion takes place in three-dimensional space and under the influence of the gravitational field of the earth. Complex motions in the various sports contain both lifting and supporting functions. This can involve an arm, a leg, and/or the torso, with the other extremity in free motion. Some sports involve lifting and supporting motions of both legs and arms at the same time, such as weight lifting, when the weight is held above the head, or skiing, in pushing off with both arms and legs together.

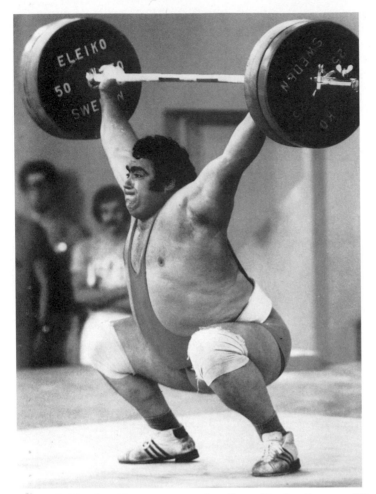

**Figure 7–17.** Complex sequence of motion with simultaneous lifting function of arms and supporting function of the legs in weight-lifting.

Limitations of the complex motion techniques in therapy depend on the specific sport of the athlete and type of injury.

## Limitations for Particular Sports

For some sports, the "pure" spiral-diagonal pattern of motion used in special training must be replaced with exercises aimed at developing muscles used in the particular sport. The demands of each particular sport determine which muscles of the muscle group to concentrate on, at the same time avoiding muscular imbalance.

Example: A shot putter requires optimal resilience in the upper arm extensors, particularly the triceps, for the final phase of the putting motion. The complex pattern of motion should benefit the athlete so that the upper arm extensors receive maximal preparation, whereas the opposing muscles are trained only to the extent that they can stretch optimally and thus prevent muscular imbalance. A biceps that is too thick and strong limits the maximal extension of the elbow and does not permit the athlete to hold the shot in the optimal position beside the neck. This would result in a restriction of the triceps.

In endurance training for the athlete, such as for long distance events, the complex motions required for training make use of many repetitions against a small amount of resistance. If the competition requires muscle strength training, as for events of short duration, the complex motion exercises utilize few repetitions against the greatest possible resistance.

Dynamic or static complex motions are thus carried out in accordance with the demands of the individual sports. If mobilization of individual components of the motion is desired, complex motions are combined with joint and muscle exercises to facilitate each action.

If stabilization is desired, the complex motions must be conducted with this stabilization in mind, stressing holding work in a variety of positions.

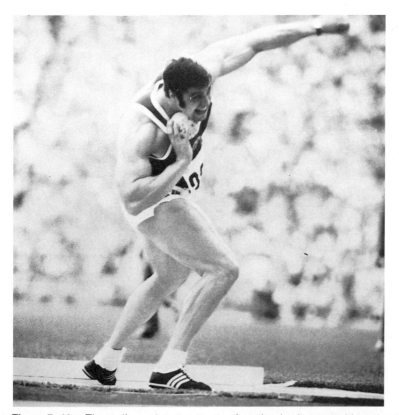

**Figure 7–18.**   Three-dimensional patterns of motion in shot-put with optimally positioned shot.

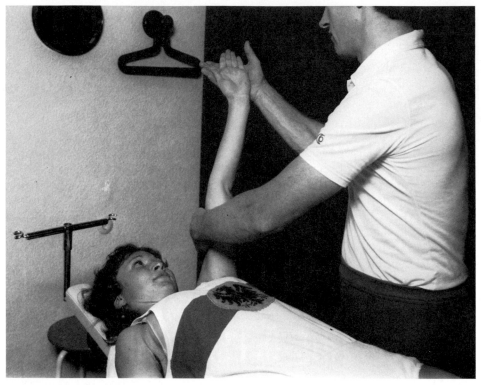

**Figure 7–19.** PNF training for arm muscles in supine position.

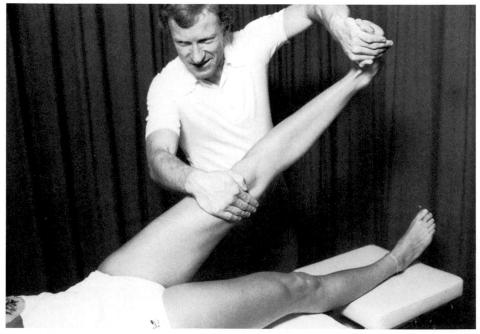

**Figure 7–20.** PNF training for leg muscles in supine position.

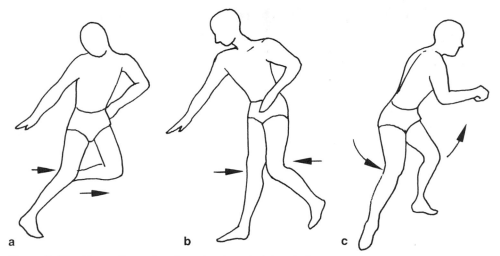

**Figure 7–21.**   Three-dimensional mechanisms in injury to knee.

# Limitations Determined by Injuries

Athletic injuries can frequently be explained by one-, two-, or three-dimensional causative mechanisms. Trauma from contact with opponents in competitive sports and games plays a role, as do external influences, such as the slalom poles in alpine skiing.

Injuries limit the execution of complex motions. As it is not always possible to carry out the complete motion, which may even be partially or completely forbidden by the limitations imposed by the injury, the therapist is forced to make do with slight extensions and contractions. The proper resistance is necessary in all the components of the motion pattern. Depending on the extent of the injury, only static complex motions may be used at first; in cases of slight injury, however, dynamic complex motions may be used as well.

Pain should be avoided during these exercises. Joints and muscles should be positioned without causing pain. This positioning begins the program of exercise. Pressure and traction are limited or are completely eliminated if they cause pain. The maximal resistance is reduced so that a painless complex motion is possible. The "pure" spiral-diagonal patterns of motions are changed so that the movements will not cause pain. Functional tests determine possible painful anatomic structures. The absence of pain permits an optimal training for the particular sport, with changes in the pattern of complex motions if they are necessary.

*Example:* A soccer player complains about pain during an outward rotation of his hip. Both components of the motion, abduction and outward rotation, are omitted in the complex motion exercises.

# Complex Motions in Rehabilitation

During the rehabilitative phase, the athlete is first made to sense the tension in his muscles. Patterns of motion are then taught, first without stress, then with stress.

Evasive motions, which develop from an acute protective position taken to avoid pain, are eliminated with the help of complex motions. Evasive motions are uneconomical for the athlete, serve little purpose, and generally are undesired. Repetitive faulty movements can be the result of trauma, muscular weakness, limitations of movement, and poor habits of motion.

The pain causes the injured athlete to search for alternative ways of getting the same results. If the athlete can be directed into the correct paths of movement, rehabilitation and recovery of capacity for stress are encouraged. Weak points in the pattern of motion required for specific sports are best corrected by practicing the entire sequence of motions. Prior to this, the pattern of movements is broken down into its component parts, and the painful segments are omitted or only exercised to the point of pain. The nonpainful motions are practiced.

Rehabilitation of athletic injuries and damages can be accomplished successfully by using the technique of complex motions. The technique of guiding the proprioceptive neuromuscular paths serves to facilitate movements. It favors and accelerates neuromuscular reactions. Particular stimuli can guide complex chains of motion through individual steps. Three-dimensional motions take place on three levels, sagittal, frontal, and transverse, around the corresponding axes. Advancing from isometric exercises to

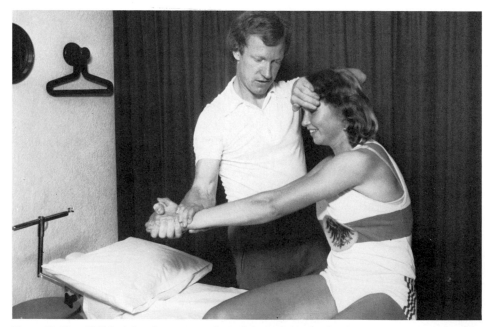

**Figure 7–22.**   PNF training for arm, neck, and throat muscles in sitting position.

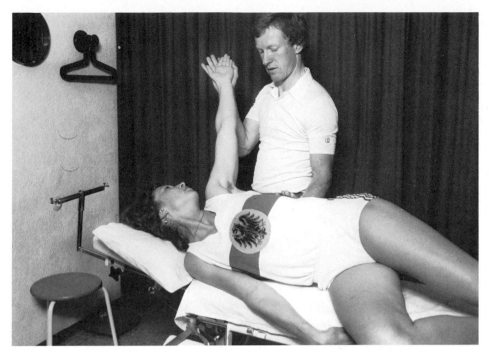

**Figure 7-23.**    PNF training for shoulder muscles in lateral position.

one-dimensional, two-dimensional, and finally three-dimensional motions has proved effective during the rehabilitative period.

## Positioning of the Athlete

The lateral position is suited for the start of the treatment with complex motions. This position favors the painless adjustment of joints and muscles of the extremities and the spinal column. The transition from the isometric exercises to one- and two-dimensional motions is possible in this position. Three-dimensional motions are done in a more supine position. The transition to movement involving the entire body depends on the individual sport of the athlete, and is carried out on a mat from all initial positions, such as lateral, prone, and supine. The complete sequence of movements gradually prepares the body for the maximal stress of individual sports. The use of complex motions is extended to include a variety of initial positions, such as sitting, kneeling, and standing.

## Summary

Complex motions represent an optimal method of "special training," with their three-dimensional, spiral-diagonal patterns of motion, and thus they are

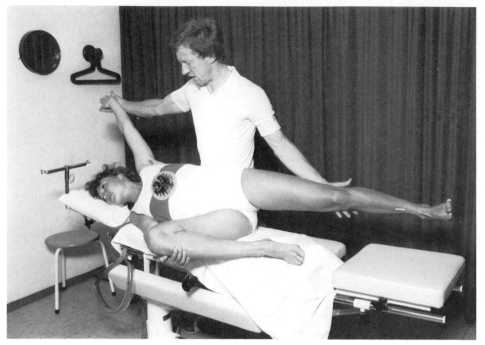

**Figure 7–24.** PNF training for torso muscles in lateral position.

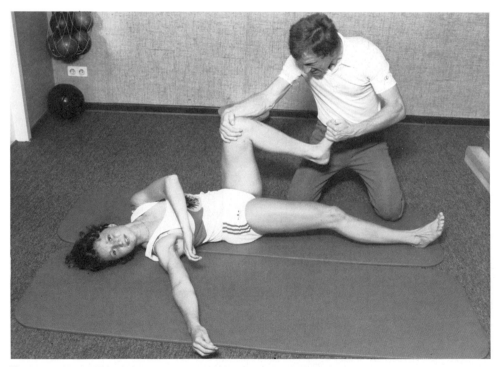

**Figure 7–25.** PNF training for torso muscles in supine position.

a splendid preventive measure against injuries, as well as an excellent tool for the rehabilitation of injured athletes and the training of healthy athletes. The limitless variability of the complex motions and the amount of stress used with them make them well suited for use in a large variety of sports. This method continually trains and prepares muscles and joints for stress. Limitations in use of this method due to the demands of individual sports and specific injuries should be observed. Complex motions are easily combined with other techniques of motion therapy. Applications of ice, special massage techniques, and other treatments of physical therapy can be included in the treatment with complex motions as necessary.

## CHAPTER 8

# Loosening

*DORIS EITNER*

Passive loosening is done by the therapist, whereas active loosening is done by the athlete himself. Maximal muscular tension results in greater subsequent relaxation. This alternation between stretching and relaxing makes the following passive and active loosening easier. The shaking motions should pass rhythmically into one another and should never be carried out jerkily.

## Passive Loosening

In passive loosening exercises changes in the volume of the muscle and in contractions are not the primary objectives; rather, only the length of the muscle is altered. This is accomplished by bringing the muscle origins and insertions closer together and then pulling them apart. In this way, muscle tension is reduced; this is why passive loosening is used for all spastic muscular conditions and for all muscle contractures.

### SHAKING

This treatment serves to loosen tense muscle groups. The shaking takes the form of small upward and downward motions or slight sideward rotations. During the shaking the position of the extremities or the torso can be altered. The therapist shakes with light traction and in a variety of positions.

### ARM SHAKING

The initial position is either lying on the side, sitting, or kneeling. The shaking loosens the arm muscles and the shoulders. If the shoulders and spinal area are to be loosened, the shoulder blades are alternately pulled away from the spinal column and then pushed back towards it with stiffly held arms. The muscles of the shoulder area are thus loosened, including the rhomboideus and subscapularis muscles. The therapist should make sure that the elbow is extended, as otherwise the shaking will not have the desired effect.

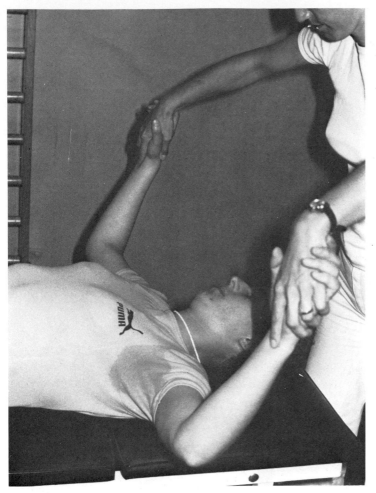

**Figure 8–1.** Passive loosening of arms by bringing muscle origins and insertions closer together.

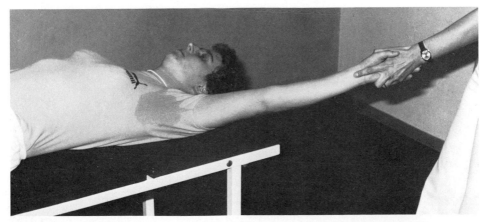

**Figure 8–2.** Passive loosening of arms by pulling muscle origins and insertions farther apart.

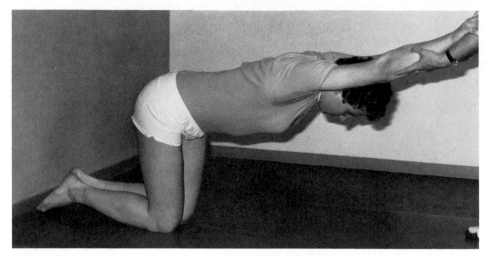

**Figure 8–3.** Arm shaking in kneeling position with elbows extended. This exercise affects the entire back.

## LEG SHAKING

Shaking is done with either bent or extended legs. Durng shaking with bent legs, the athlete lies on his or her back. The bent legs are shaken from side to side by the therapist, while the knees are clasped. The feet must be held in place, so that they don't slip out.

Shaking with extended legs can be done with both legs at one time or only one leg. The therapist shakes the legs from the feet, with the heels lying in the

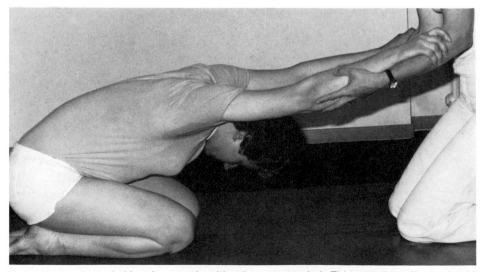

**Figure 8–4.** Arm shaking in crouch with elbows extended. This exercise affects shoulder muscles.

**Figure 8–5.** Leg shaking with extended knee.

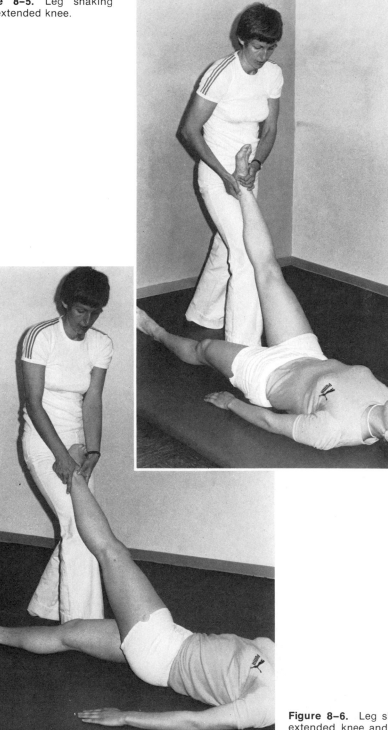

**Figure 8–6.** Leg shaking with extended knee and inward hip rotation.

palms of the hands. The athlete's knees are extended. In this treatment care must be taken to avoid an injured knee, particularly if the capsular ligament is damaged. In this case shaking would be contraindicated.

## HIP SHAKING

This shaking is carried out with the athlete lying on his or her side. Hips and knees are slightly bent. The therapist stands behind the athlete and places one hand on the ilium. He moves the upper thigh and pelvis rapidly back and forth with the other hand. This loosens the gluteus and hip muscles.

If only the hip muscles are to be loosened, the following procedure is used: The athlete lies on his back and draws up one leg at a time. He stabilizes the ankle joint with both hands. Then the leg is rotated slightly inward. This raises the pelvic side of the elevated leg slightly. Light pressure against the foot creates gentle vibrations in the hip area.

## TORSO SHAKING

Initial position is supine. Both legs are grasped above the ankles and then small lateral and turning motions of the legs are performed while they remain pressed together. If slower movements are carried out, the twisting motion of the torso can be precisely regulated and varied. Variations are possible for the

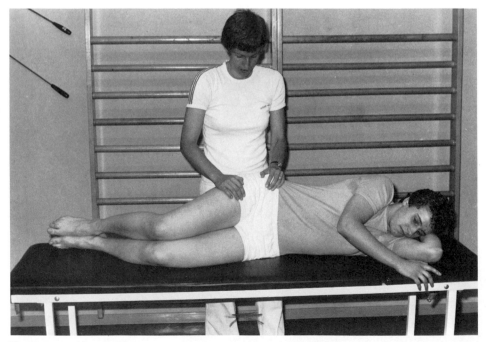

**Figure 8–7.** Hip shaking.

chest, groin, and abdominal areas. Vigorous small shaking motions against the knees of the bent legs allow a more precise treatment of the rectus abdominis muscles. A variety of effects can be obtained through shaking. For example, it is possible to beneficially influence the internal organs, such as the intestines, by shaking of the chest, torso, or pelvis. Variations of the shaking technique depend on positioning, type, and the goal of the treatment.

Shaking is used for athletes primarily as a preventive exercise. Athletes in particular are subject to limitations in the optimal flexibility of joints because of tensed and shortened muscles. Examples of affected areas include the shoulder for javelin throwers, the elbow for tennis players, and the hip for walkers and hurdlers. Shaking should always be used together with massage and other physical therapy exercises.

# Active Loosening Exercises

In contradistinction to passive loosening, which is administered by the therapist, the athlete himself performs the exercise in active loosening. Active loosening must be learned under supervision.

Its task is also to loosen overly tense tissue, to relax tight and shortened muscles, and to help in preventing athletic injuries. Active loosening exercises can be used both in the rehabilitative phase after injuries and as a preparation for training and competition.

The active loosening exercises are of the following types: (1) active rhythmic swinging of limbs, (2) active shaking of limbs, and (3) swinging and rotating of limbs and torso. During the active loosening exercises, the athlete either is in a prone, supine, or lateral position or is on his hands and knees, sitting, standing, or in motion. These initial positions vary according to the exercises. Objects such as Indian clubs, medicine balls, dumbbells, and jump ropes can be of great help. Rhythmic music can also aid swinging and therefore accelerate loosening.

## SWINGING EXERCISES

Swinging exercises should be conceived of as analogous to the motion of a pendulum around a focal point. They conserve energy, and have a loosening, stretching, and harmonizing effect on the pattern of motion.

A pendulum left to itself will eventually come to rest, but a new push will set it back into motion.

## ACTIVE SHAKING

Active shaking involves moving muscles against their supporting bones, causing loosening and relaxation. Active loosening exercises in the form of

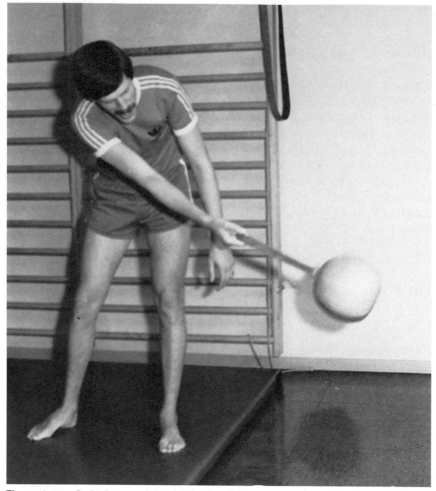

**Figure 8–8.**    Swinging exercises with sling ball.

shaking are an essential part of the athletic training program. We know from physiology that the relaxation of a muscle is just as important for its performance as its tension. Loosening exercises are always used during warm-up calisthenics and jogging, as well as between and after physical exertions. The muscles should be fully relaxed before each exertion.

Loosening detonicizes the muscle by changing its elastic structure. Loosening exercises facilitate more rapid recovery after stress. Athletes whose disciplines require great elasticity and endurance of the musculoskeletal system, such as participants in various games, will notice that when they are not sufficiently loosened up they will eventually experience a considerable loss of strength, tire early, and notice a slowing of movements. Physiologic experiments have shown that for two muscles of equal strength, the performance of the loosest muscle will always be superior. In all forms of sports, athletes are familiar with the effects of shaking the extremities for the loosening of the particular muscles. For example, a sprinter never gets into the starting blocks without having thoroughly loosened both legs and arms.

The legs are shaken while in a slight straddle position, as if one were trying to throw the leg away. Arms are shaken out while standing, with the upper body inclined forward and the arms hanging loosely. These two methods are the simplest forms of loosening.

The loosening of the arms and the shoulders is accomplished by moving the arms either in simple circles or in figure-eights. This can be done either with or without devices, such as a sling ball or Indian clubs. Shrugging the shoulders permits isolated loosening.

Another exercise is swinging the arms up high behind the back, both together and alternately.

The shoulders can be loosened with exercises while on hands and knees. These exercises are good not only for loosening but also for mobilization and strengthening.

*Text continued on page 141*

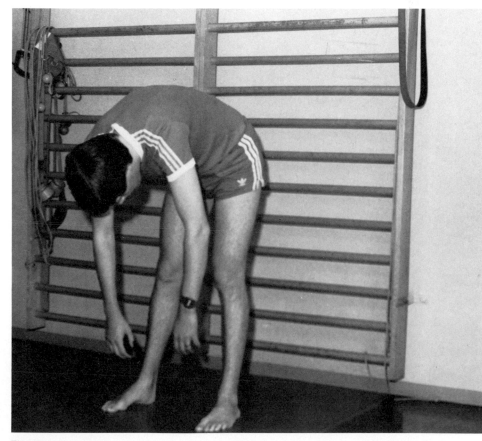

**Figure 8–9.** Active loosening exercise for arms.

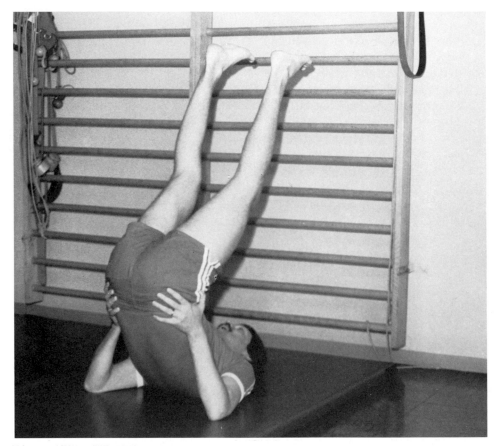

**Figure 8–10.** Active loosening exercise for legs.

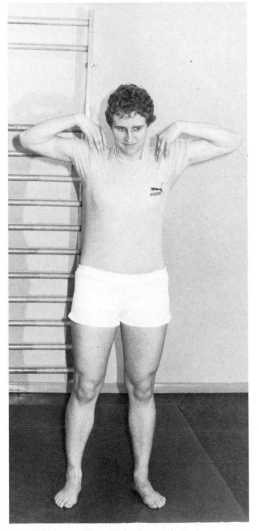

**Figure 8–11.**  Shoulder shrugs.

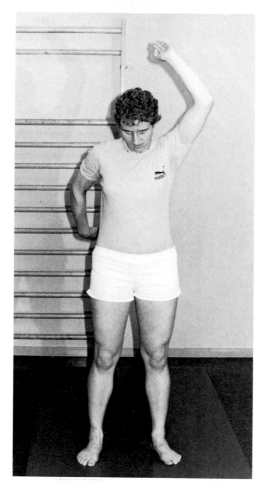

**Figure 8–12.** Alternating swinging of arms high behind back.

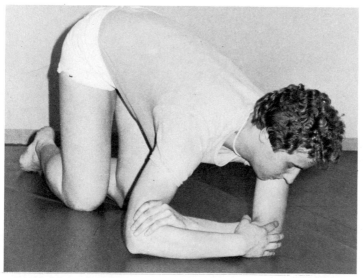

**Figure 8–13.** Shoulder loosening exercise.

**Figure 8–14.**  Trunk bending to the side.

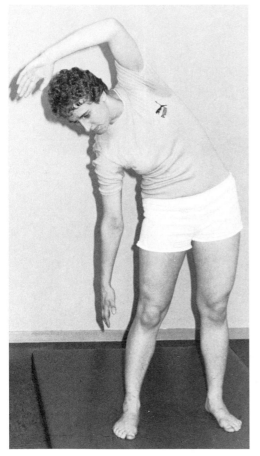

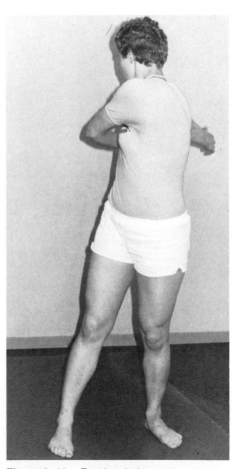

**Figure 8–15.**  Trunk twisting.

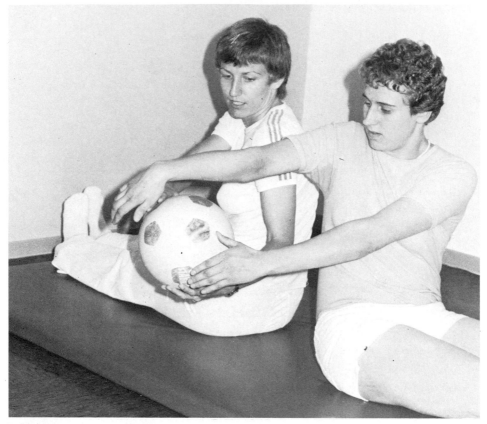

**Figure 8–16.** Trunk twisting as partner exercise with ball.

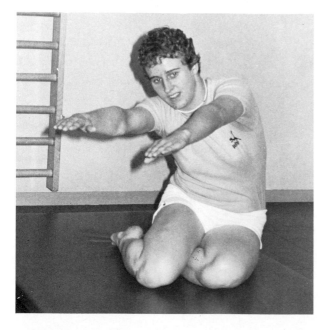

**Figure 8–17.** Hip loosening in kneeling position.

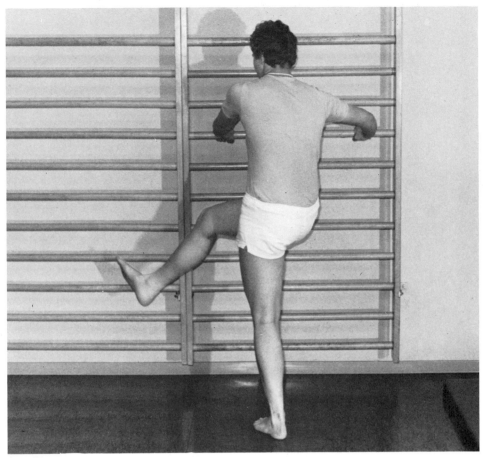

**Figure 8–18.**   Sidewards leg swinging.

Trunk twisting done with the athlete bending forwards, backwards, and sidewards loosens the torso. Trunk twisting to the right and left also serves to loosen. These trunk twisting exercises can be executed while standing, sitting, or kneeling.

The hips can be loosened by shifting the body to the right and the left of the feet while in a kneeling position. The arms should be held high. Pelvic circular movements are performed from the supine position with the support of the legs.

Wall bars can be used for the loosening of the legs and hips. The athlete stands facing the wall bars and supports himself by grasping the rungs at about chest height. From this position he can swing each leg back and forth for loosening.

Swinging legs in figure-eight patterns is more easily accomplished in a standing position.

As mentioned above, however, loosening exercises for the legs are primar-

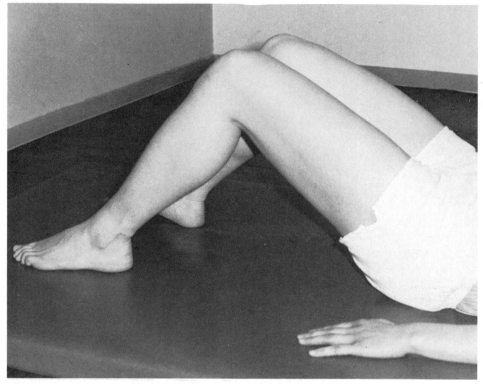

**Figure 8–19.** Loosening of calf muscles in supine position.

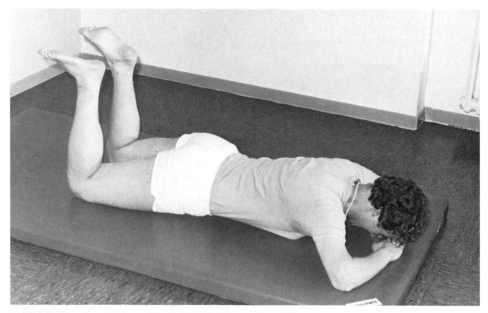

**Figure 8–20.** Loosening of calf muscles in prone position.

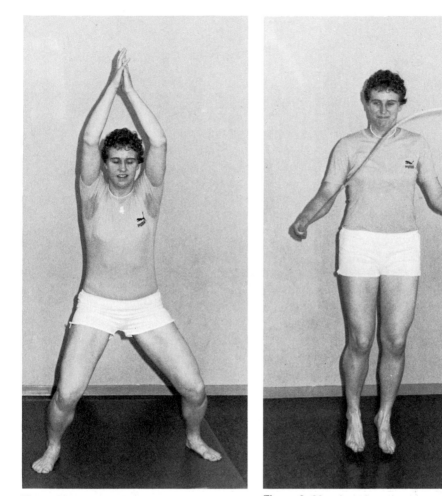

**Figure 8–21**   Jumping jacks.     **Figure 8–22.**   Jumping rope.

ily shaking ones. Positions taken for this activity include sitting, lying prone or supine, or standing. The lower legs in particular can be loosened well from a prone or supine position. The legs are bent and the lower calves shaken.

If the athlete wants to loosen the muscles of his entire body, jumping jacks are recommended. Another good method of loosening up the entire body is jumping rope in all its variations.

## CHAPTER 9

# Stretching

*HELMUT ORK*

## Introduction

Active and passive stretching of the ligaments and muscles permits increased motion in the most important joints. Stretching of muscles before an event is an extremely important factor in the achievement of optimal athletic performance. The requirement for performance of muscular work is an increased initial tension. If a weight is placed on an isolated muscle, it stretches. If the weight is increased, however, the flexibility decreases — that is, the muscle lengthens rapidly at first, but more slowly with increasing weight. After the weight is removed, the muscle returns to its initial state. Resting skeletal muscle is stretched to approximately half its maximal extension. Every time a muscle is contracted, antagonist muscle is stretched, thus increasing its readiness for work. For example, when the biceps is contracted, the elbow is bent and the extensor of the upper arm, the triceps, is stretched. This characteristic of muscles helps the athlete to increase his muscular capacity since these actions are performed repeatedly. Active, forced extensions of muscles cause an increase in their normal flexibility — for example, when the discus thrower swings his arms in the direction of flight or when a sprinter presses his feet against the starting blocks.

## Requirements for Stretching

The elasticity of a muscle prevents it from injury when a sudden high stress is placed on it. This elasticity is influenced by the temperature of the muscle, biomechanical considerations, and the mental state of the athlete.

*Temperature.* The elasticity of a muscle diminishes with cooling. As a result, the danger of muscle pulls is increased. Warm muscle, on the other hand, has an improved metabolism, contracts more rapidly, and is therefore in better condition for training and competition.

*Biomechanics and Mental State.* The exploitation of the optimal leverage of the body plays an important role in muscular activity. A disruption of coordination caused by momentary stresses during competition and need to change direction of motion quickly can often cause an injury of the muscle-ligament apparatus. This occurs, for example, during team contact sports.

Physiologic factors, such as relaxation or tiredness, and psychic components, such as one's feeling about the game and desire to compete, are also important in athletic performance.

# Passive Stretching

Passive and active stretching are indispensable for optimal competitive preparation. Both types of stretching should be undertaken only after the muscles are sufficiently warmed up. The mobility of the joints and the range of the motion in the phases of the active and passive stretching are important not only for the muscles specifically needed for the competition but for many other muscles as well. Therefore, stretching is carried out in a variety of directions for many different movements.

For example, a high jumper using the flop technique would not prepare by stretching out only the spinal column, but would also stretch the muscles of the torso with trunk twisting exercises. Thus, both motions — flexion and extension of the muscles — prepare the muscular system for the work to be performed.

Passive stretching exercises utilize the following: (1) constraining position, (2) support of partner, (3) traction, and (4) pressure.

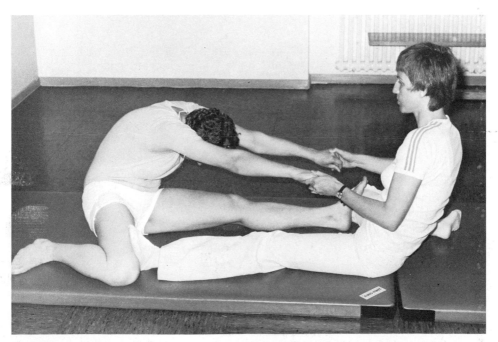

**Figure 9–1.** Passive stretching in hurdler's position with support of partner.

*Constraining Position.* This is a stretching exercise in which particular body positions are maintained for an extended period of time, such as a hurdler's position. These positions are maintained as the stretching is gradually increased.

*Partner Support.* With the support of a training partner, gentle stretching exercises of gradually increasing intensity are carried out. Use of both the hurdler's position and the aid of a partner can be valuable in eliminating and correcting improper stretching techniques and also in stretching particularly shortened muscles.

*Traction.* Sufficiently warmed muscles are brought into a very stretched position by traction. Traction should never be done jerkily or proceed beyond the point of pain. Gentle, repeated stretching can gradually bring the muscle to its maximum length.

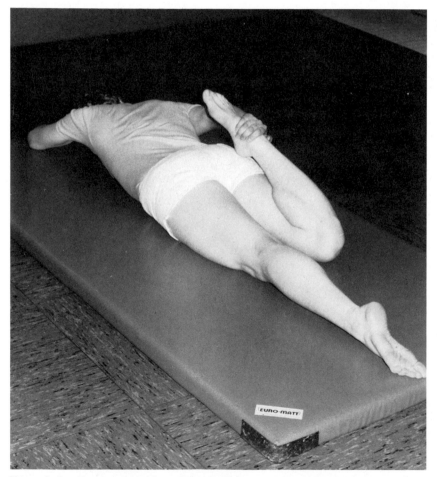

**Figure 9–2.** Passive stretching of the quadriceps of the right thigh with arm traction.

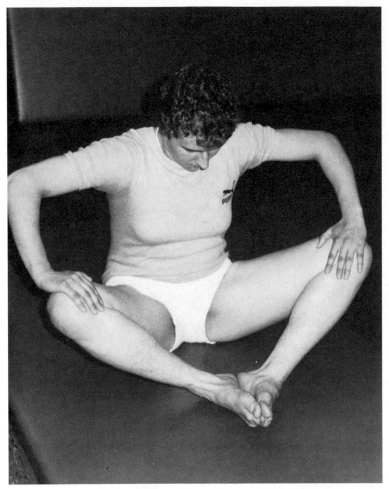

**Figure 9–3.** Passive stretching of the adductors with arm pressure.

***Pressure.*** Pressure can also be used to stretch muscles that were similarly warmed in advance. Maximal isometric tension must precede this stretching. After several repetitions, the gentle but increasingly stronger pressure brings the muscle to maximal tension, relaxation, and stretching, which increases the range of motion.

The exercises should be carried out gently and gradually increased in number, in order to avoid injuries. It is important to warm up before performing passive stretching exercises, because an increased tone within the muscle system aids the stretching. The extent of motion achieved through passive stretching is always greater than that achieved through active stretching. The threshold of pain should be approached carefully, slowly, and with the greatest possible sensitivity to the athlete's responses.

*Text continued on page 153*

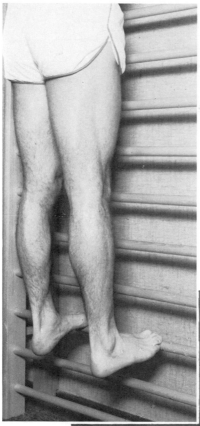

**Figure 9–4.** Stretching of both triceps surae of the legs.

**Figure 9–5.** Alternating stretching of triceps surae.

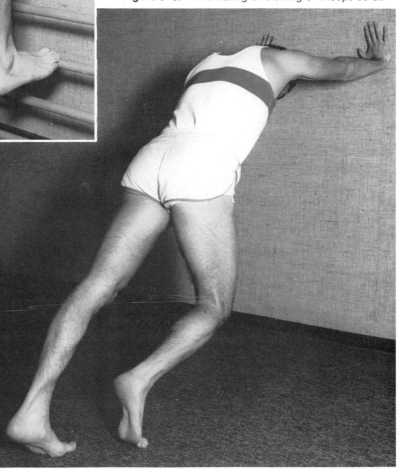

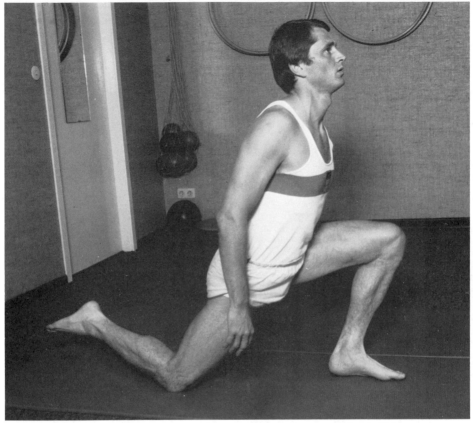

**Figure 9–6.** Active stretching of quadriceps and hip extensors of the right leg.

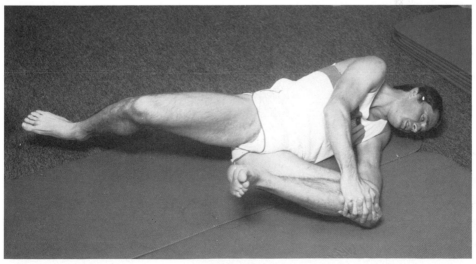

**Figure 9–7.** Active stretching of the quadriceps of the right leg and stretching of the hip extensors of the left leg in the lateral position.

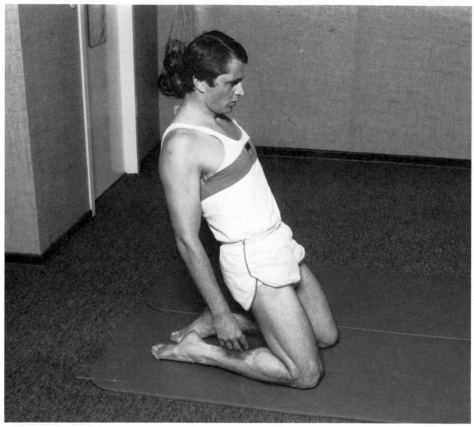

**Figure 9–8.** Active stretching of quadriceps.

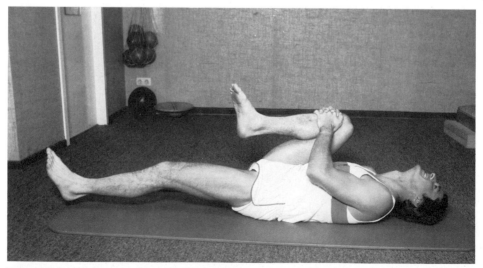

**Figure 9–9.** Active stretching of the hamstrings of the left leg and right hip extensor in the supine position.

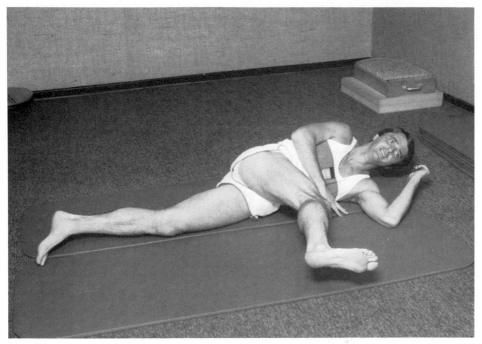

**Figure 9–10.**   Active stretching of the hamstrings of the left leg and the hip extensors of the right leg in the lateral position.

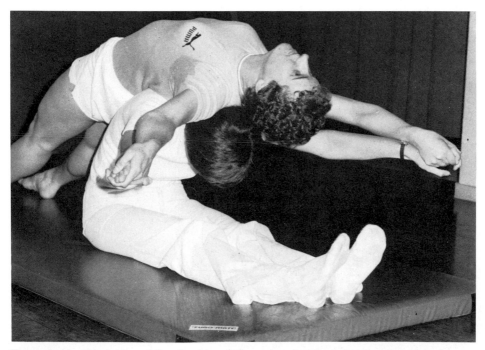

**Figure 9–11.**   Stretching of the shoulder girdle and pectoralis major as partner exercise.

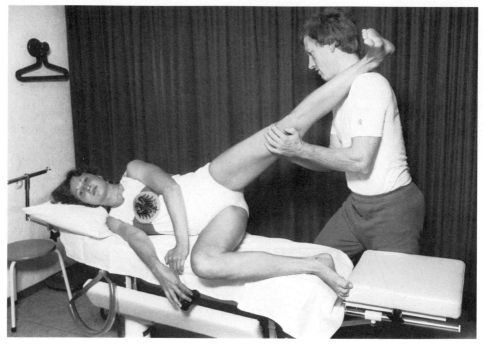

**Figure 9–12.**    Stretching of adductors in the lateral position with help of therapist.

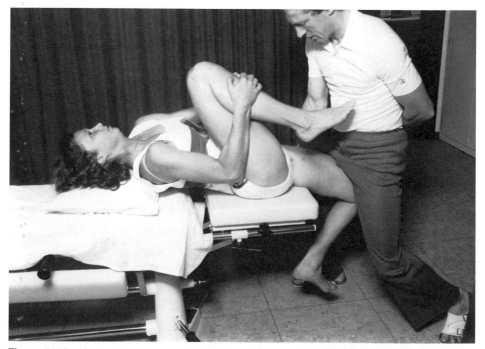

**Figure 9–13.**    Stretching of the hip extensors of left leg with support of therapist.

# Active Stretching

In active stretching the extent of movement is achieved by the appropriate active motions, that is, by means of a vigorous, quick extension to the limits of joint and muscular flexibility. The resulting stretching of the respective antagonist muscles and tendons is achieved by the intensity and rhythm of the exercise. At the same time, the resiliency of the muscular system is increased. At the start of training or during the competitive phase, active stretching should predominate at first. Jogging, trotting, light jumping, brief sprints, skipping, and practice starts serve as preparations for competition.

Passive stretching of the triceps-surae muscle group is achieved by placing the foot on an elevated surface. A landing or a step at the competition site or the wall bars in a gymnasium can be used.

The quadriceps and the hip extensors are stretched in a kneeling position. Moving the upper body in various directions achieves this active stretching.

The hamstrings and the hip extensor muscles are stretched optimally in a supine position. The right and left knees are alternately drawn as far as possible toward the head.

Further ways of stretching diverse muscle groups can be created with the support of the therapist by observing the various positions assumed by the athlete.

As flexibility of a muscle tends to be lower in the morning than in the afternoon, the athlete should limit morning stretching exercises when exercizing twice daily to avoid injury to the soft tissues. Concentration should be on the afternoon sessions.

# Conclusion

Optimal flexibility is based on physiologic, anatomic, and biomechanical considerations. One can assume that an increase in the range of motion results in increased mobility. The muscular work and the intensity of performance and endurance also depend on preparatory stretching. One must bear in mind when conducting special stretching exercises that one-sided strength training can result in a change of the muscle tone and therefore cause a permanent shortening of the muscle. The optimal contraction of the muscle is no longer possible, and a typical muscle dysfunction arises.

## CHAPTER 10

# Exercise in Water

*DORIS EITNER*

Exercise in water is not an individual branch of therapy, but rather a supportive treatment that is worked into the entire physical therapy program. Just being in the water acts as a psychologic stimulus to movement. Mechanical and thermal factors are important in this regard. Water displacement, water temperature, buoyancy, and frictional resistance of water all play an essential role in exercise in water. The therapist can make use of these properties as they relate to indications and goals for treating various disorders. The water temperature should not be higher than 32°C — that is, slightly below the neutral range. The patient's movements create energy, so that the water seems sufficiently warm. In this way neither overheating nor chilling develops. The form of the exercises is based primarily on the lowering of the force of gravity by immersion in water, yet buoyancy, frictional resistance, speed of performance, and water currents can also be used either to further facilitate these exercises or to increase their difficulty. Increased warmth in the water results in the relaxation of skeletal muscle. Maximal relaxation of the muscles can be reached when the temperature of the water exceeds the neutral point.

Buoyancy is explained by Archimedes' principle. Submersion in water reduces body weight by up to ninth tenths, depending on the extent of submersion. Motion thus becomes easier, which can be of great significance for the treatment. Remedial exercises can begin in the early stages of treatment, so that muscles can be loosened and the metabolism stimulated. As mentioned, frictional resistance, the surface area, speed of performance, and water currents can be used to increase the difficulty of the exercises. This is particularly important in the advanced stages of treatment of athletes getting back into shape. The frictional resistance is variable and depends on the size (surface area) of the body part in motion and the speed of the movements. The faster the patient moves, the larger the resistance of the water. This is ideal for permitting a precise gradation of exercises of increasing difficulty. The current produced by movements carried out in the water can be employed to reduce or increase the difficulty of the remedial exercises.

Running in ankle-deep water can be used as an initial exercise to increase the stress on the legs and feet. Gradually the running is performed in deeper water until it reaches hip level. Running in such "running trenches" is a good

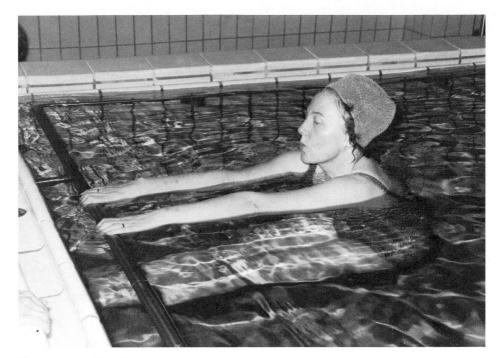

**Figure 10–1.**  Exercise in water.

means of rapidly developing strength following injuries to the feet, knees, or hips. Walking can begin in the water a long time before such treatment could otherwise be possible. Possible variations include stiff-legged walking, walking on the toes or heels, walking sideways or backward, walking in a slight or deep crouch, walking crabwise, and lunging. When these exercises have been mastered, they can be followed with step-climbing under water.

Remedial exercise in water for athletic injuries is particularly suited for fractures, pinned joints, the postoperative treatment of meniscal, Achilles tendon, and intervertebral disk injuries.

## Example: Postoperative Achilles Tendon Treatment

The following exercises are used:

Rising alternately on both toes and heels, and on toes of alternating legs; then standing on toes; walking on heels; running; lifting knees; and hopping, at first with both legs, then with one leg; and alternately opening and closing of legs while hopping and maintaining a straddling position. Jumping and stretching exercises follow in the later stages of recovery. A gradual increase is possible by increasing the number of repetitions, by using helping devices, and by carrying out the exercises in shallower water.

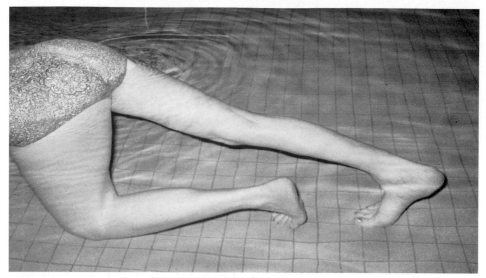

**Figure 10–2.**   Alternate stretching of triceps surae and Achilles tendon in exercise bath.

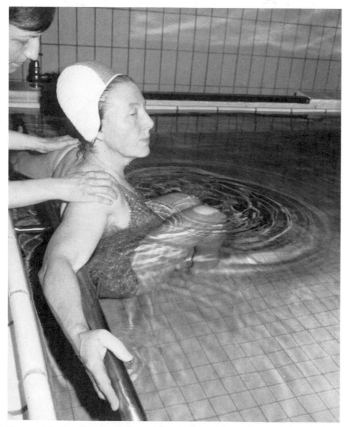

**Figure 10–3.**   Kyphosizing of lumbar vertebrae by drawing in legs.

Swimming is an additional possibility with remedial exercises in water. One should take particular care to ensure active motion of the ankles while performing particular strokes, such as the crawl or breaststroke. So that intensive stress is placed on the muscles of the lower legs, it is recommended that only the leg motions be carried out. If the kicking goes well, the athlete can proceed to swimming with flippers. This is a very effective means of increasing lower-leg strength. During the crawl stroke, whose movements begin in the hips, the knees should be bent only slightly. Propulsion must come primarily from the upward and downward motions of the ankles. Swimming with flippers should be part of the daily training program if possible.

Remedial therapy in warm water is also a good supplementary treatment to other remedial exercises for athletes with spinal deformities such as scoliosis, hunchback, lordosis, and kyphosis.

Back strains, such as those that occur in gymnastics, bicycling, and especially the track and field sports of javelin throwing and high jumping, can be eased or relieved with water exercises. These athletes should use the exercise bath as a preventive measure when not training and competing. Exercises are conducted in warm water that work against the motions required by the particular discipline as a type of balancing exercise. Thus, for example, back stroke is recommended for a gymnast along with balancing exercises in water, as the hyperlordosis which the discipline causes can be avoided by this treatment. This therapy is also recommended for such sports as javelin throwing and high jumping, which cause lordosis. On the other hand,

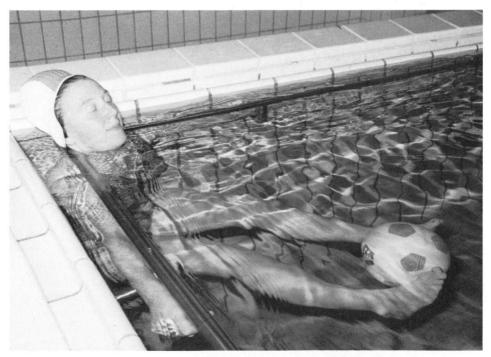

**Figure 10–4.**  Intensified stomach and leg muscle exercises with ball.

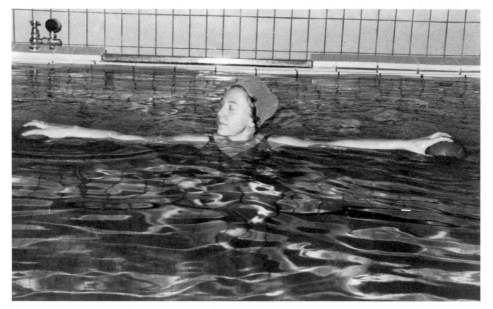

**Figure 10–5.**   Simultaneous downward pressure on two balls with arms.

breast stroke is recommended for a bicyclist along with other corrective exercises in water, as this balances out his kyphotic posture.

In summary, the exercise bath is a pleasant method of achieving relaxation and loosening of the entire body for the healthy athlete, as well as a means of affording relief from the stress of training and competition. Furthermore, there is an additional psychologic benefit. The injured athlete can be helped back to health and to recover mobility in his injured extremities, which is also beneficial to his state of mind.

Unfortunately, many competition and training areas lack suitable exercise or thermal baths.

## Cardiovascular Stress

The stress on the cardiovascular system that use of warm water for remedial exercises, rehabilitation, and retraining causes must be mentioned. Water at a temperature of 34°C stimulates and promotes peripheral arterial circulation. This circulation improves further during active remedial exercises. The stress on the heart and circulatory system is considerably greater in water than when remedial exercises are carried out on land. The hydrostatic pressure on the stomach and chest forces the heart to work harder and care must be taken by a person susceptible to heart trouble. Exercise in water can be viewed as a powerful stimulatory therapy for both muscles and circulation. Each individual's stress limit varies. In general, however, treatment should not extend beyond 20 minutes.

# Equipment

Basins of various sizes and specially shaped basins are used for exercise in water.

1. The exercise basin for adults is 1.25 m deep. The temperature is between 34 and 37°C, which is in the neutral range. Neither a buildup of warmth nor a loss of warmth should occur during an extended treatment in water.

Positions for the exercises include: along a bar that is underwater; sitting in water on a stool or on a broad, built-in stone step; standing; or at the rail on the edge of the basin, which permits exercises in prone or supine position. The therapist stands either outside the basin or in the water, which is the case for most resistance exercises. Sunken areas beside the basins, where the therapist can stand at the level of the water surface and direct and support the exercises, are also of great use.

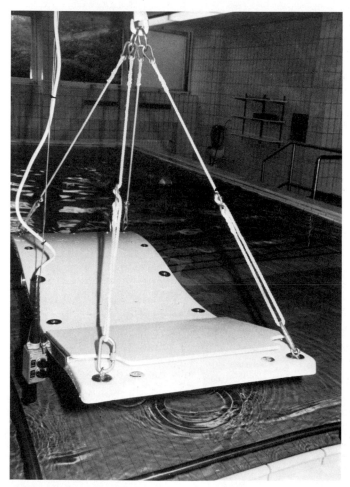

**Figure 10–6.**  Lifting platform for exercise bath.

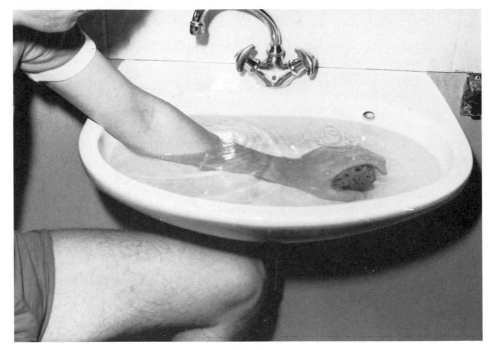

**Figure 10-7.** Exercise in water for hand and finger injuries.

2. The so-called butterfly tub permits localized treatment in water for the injured athlete. He or she lies comfortably in water about 30 cm deep with the head supported. Only the injured muscles are treated with localized exercises. They can be passive, active with the relief of body weight, active versus body weight, and active versus holding resistance. The therapist stands outside the basin.

The butterfly basin is suited for patients who should perform exercises in water despite open wounds.

3. The "walking trough" or "running trench" was invented for exercises for the lower extremities at the level of "learning to walk" — for example, for athletes recuperating from fractures of the lower extremities. The injured athlete runs in water, which can be up to shoulder depth. He or she is held on a harness, which is connected to a track above the basin. A lifting platform or stretcher brings the athlete comfortably in and out of the water.

4. Exercise in water is also possible for hand and finger joints. It is generally indispensable for the after-treatment of lower arm, hand, and finger fractures, as well as for existing contractures of the hand and finger joints. These exercises are carried out in armbaths and are particularly recommended in the early stages of the after-treatment.

CHAPTER **11**

# Manual Therapy

*LUTZ MEISSNER*

## History

Manual therapy, also known as chiropraxis, is as old as medicine. The art of "bone-setting" is mentioned as early as the times of Hippocrates, Galen, Avicenna, and Paracelsus.

The modern history of manual therapy begins with the American A. T. Still (1828–1919). Still termed his manual techniques for adjusting particular joints osteopathy. D. D. Palmer founded a school for manual therapy in America in 1895.

The techniques of manual therapy for the joints of extremities and the spinal column became better known in Europe through the work of the Swiss Naegeli, the Englishman Mennell (1877–1957), and the two Germans Schmorl and Junghanns.

The work of the Germans Zukschwerdt, Biedermann, and Zettel, as well as of the Englishmen Cyriax and Stoddard, the Czech Lewitt, and the Frenchman Maigne, to name a few, contributed to the further development of manual therapy.

In 1966 the German Society for Manual Medicine was founded in the Federal Republic of Germany. It arose out of the Research Institute for Arthrology and Chirotherapy, founded in 1953 in Hamm, and the Society for Manual Spinal and Extremity Treatment in Neutrauchburg. The German Society aims at eliminating dubious theories from manual therapy after critical examination and providing the physician with steadily improving techniques for treating and maintaining the well-being of patients.

Courses in manual therapy have also been given for physical therapists since 1975 in the Federal Republic of Germany. The course lasts seven weeks. They are conducted by the German Society for Manual Medicine together with the German Association of Physiotherapy–Central Organization of Physical Therapists. The book "Manual Therapy for the Extremity Joints" by the Norwegian F. M. Kaltenborn is the text used in this additional training course. It is also the text used today in many other countries.

# Introduction to Manual Therapy Techniques

Manual therapy includes all those diagnostic and therapeutic techniques that aid in treating injuries and functional disorders of the musculoskeletal system, particularly the reversible joint function disorders. Manual therapy is also a reflex therapy, because it creates reflex reactions through the mobilization of the joints, and thus acts on painful conditions and dysfunctions.

Chiropraxis is used to treat joints and the soft tissues. Thus, the treatments are divided into joint techniques and soft tissue techniques.

## Joint Techniques

Techniques for treating joints include the following: traction, gliding, stretching, and exercises.

## Traction

Traction mobilizes the joint by separating the two opposing joint components. Traction can be increased from one-dimensional to two- or three-dimensional exercises if the joints have been previously accustomed to one-, two-, or three-dimensional movements. Relief of pain is frequently possible with the use of this treatment alone.

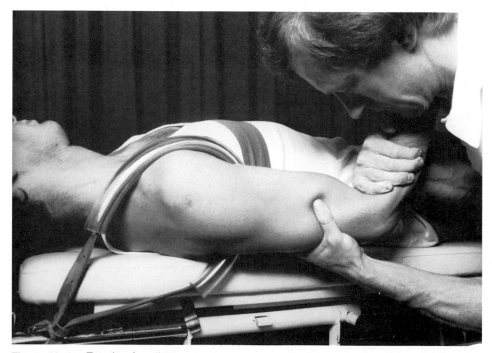

**Figure 11–1.** Traction for elbow.

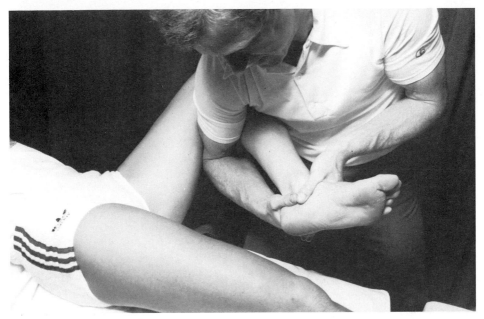

**Figure 11–2.**   Traction of ankle.

# Gliding

Parallel gliding in a medial, lateral, dorsal, or ventral direction mobilizes the joint. The proximal joint component is fixed in place, while the distal component is moved. Parallel gliding together with traction influences the

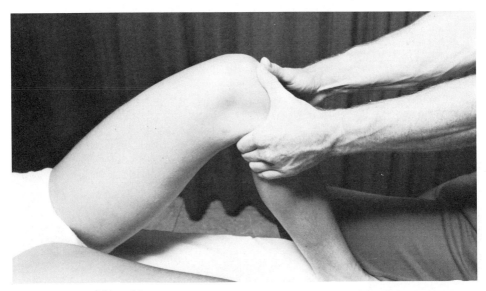

**Figure 11–3.**   Gliding of knee.

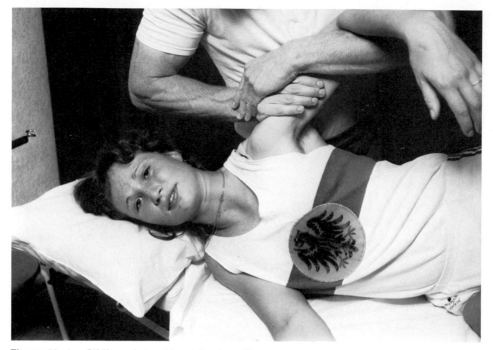

**Figure 11–4.** Gliding of shoulder, lateral position.

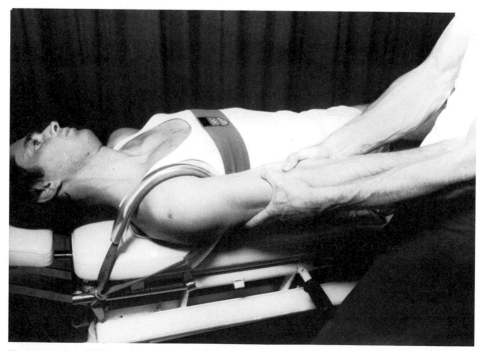

**Figure 11–5.** Gliding of shoulder, supine position.

"joint play." The free play of the joints should be reestablished through traction and gliding.

# Stretching

The connective tissue parts of the joints such as ligaments and joint capsules are stretched passively. This technique mobilizes the joint as well. Passive stretching should follow active muscular tension, as the muscle relaxes better after active tension.

# Exercises

The muscle sheath surrounding the joint also plays an important role in joint movement; shortened or inactive muscles hinder free joint play, for example. For this reason, active exercises together with traction, gliding, and stretching are extremely important. In this case pure joint techniques overlap with classic techniques of physical therapy. Complex motions and weight lifting, as recommended by Brunkow, together with isometric exercises for the mobilization or stabilization of joints, have proved to be particularly effective.

# Soft Tissue Techniques

Techniques for treating the soft tissues include the following: massage, muscle relaxation, stretching, and exercises.

## MASSAGE

Special massage techniques are used for mobilization of soft tissues. A method of treatment diagonal to the muscle or to the muscle insertion with its tendon is preferred. Frictions, vibrations, checks, and facilitations are to be used as techniques. They eliminate muscular dysfunctions, such as myogeloses and overly tense muscles.

## MUSCLE RELAXATION

Muscular function is improved by various techniques for improving muscle relaxation and muscle kinetics. After maximal stress has been placed on a shortened muscle, a rest period follows with stretching of the antagonist muscle. The dynamic tension of the antagonist muscle of a shortened muscle results in the reflex relaxation of this muscle. Sherrington's guidelines should be observed.

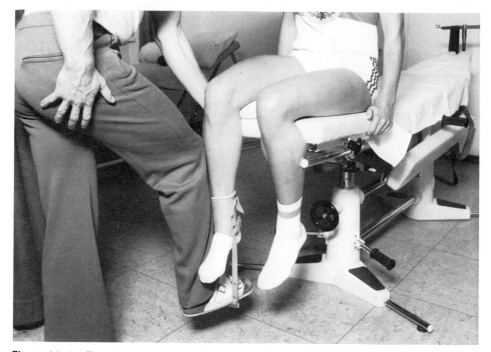

**Figure 11–6.** Traction of knee with stirrup.

## STRETCHING

Passive stretching of connective tissue structures in muscles and their tendinous insertions improves the flexibility of these tissues. Sherrington's instructions should be followed here as well.

## EXERCISES

Active exercises for the purpose of mobilization or stabilization improve, maintain, or lessen muscular tension and thus improve mobility as well. Complex motions and weight lifting (Brunkow) are suited for this purpose. Supportive techniques from thermo-, hydro-, or electrotherapy as well as immobilization with bandages can additionally improve the effect. The effectiveness of manual therapy can be increased with a variety of devices, such as specially constructed benches, apparatus, stabilizing and traction belts, stirrups, sandbags, and pillows.

# Manual Joint Therapy

Manual joint therapy is a passive treatment using gliding and traction of the joint. The bony components of the joint are the primary target of the treatment. This method forms the core of manual therapy; joint play is enhanced and the mobility of the joint is thus improved.

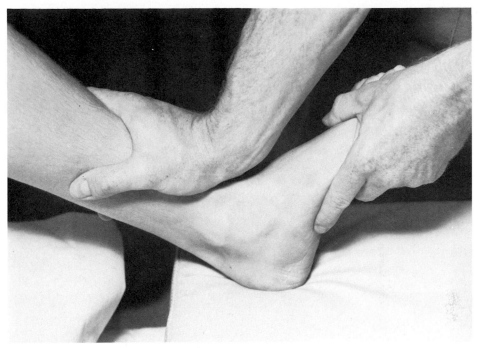

**Figure 11-7.**   Manual joint therapy after ankle sprain.

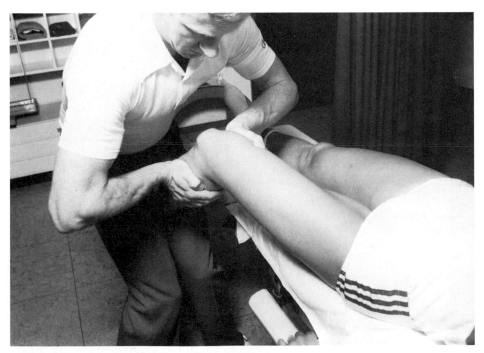

**Figure 11-8.**   Manual joint therapy after immobilization.

Physical therapy with manual therapy ameliorates disorders of the joint function, which manifest themselves as hypo- or hypermobility. Hypermobile joints are treated with manual joint therapy only if the joint is dislocated.

## MANUAL JOINT THERAPY FOR ATHLETIC INJURIES AND DAMAGE

This therapy is used in cases of improper stress, overloading, injuries, and immobilization.

Treatment with manual joint therapy restores proper joint function, which permits the painless, optimal motion in the joint, an essential requirement for good performance in most athletic disciplines.

Minor athletic injuries, in which there is no evidence of structural damage and no pain in the joint, but with displacement of the bone, can be treated directly with manual therapy.

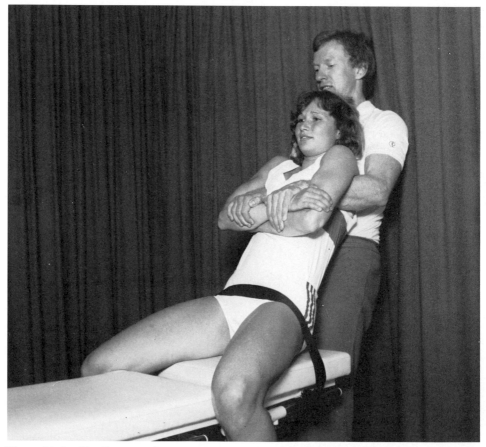

**Figure 11-9.** Traction on spine.

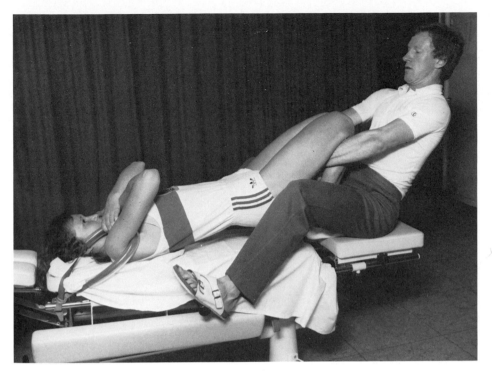

**Figure 11–10.**  Traction on spine in supine position.

Manual joint therapy is recommended for the subacute stages of athletic injuries, such as contusions, sprains, and dislocations, for fractures, and for reversible hypomobility of joints.

## INDICATIONS

Sprained fingers and wrists, such as occur in games like handball, volleyball, and basketball, benefit from manual therapy. It can also be used to treat improper stress on the hip, such as can occur in a bad landing after clearing a hurdle, in dismounting during gymnastics, or during walking or running. Other indications include spinal compressions, such as occur after falling on skis or from a horse, and bruises on the heel, such as take place in gymnastics, triple jump, broad jump, and cross-country running.

## CONTRAINDICATIONS

Manual joint therapy is always contraindicated when mobilization cannot occur painlessly.

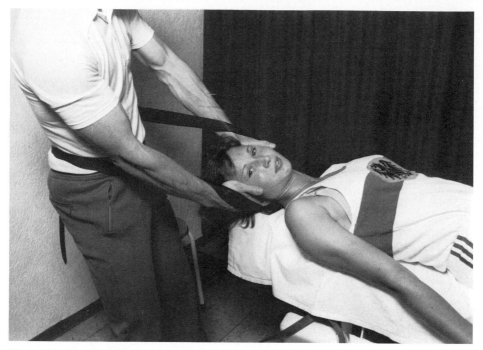

**Figure 11–11.** Traction on cervical vertebrae with traction belt in supine position; the focal point is the cervical vertebrae.

# Basic Principles

### PIVOTING AND GLIDING

Every joint motion begins with a gliding movement, which then becomes a pivoting. This alternation between pivoting and gliding results in the "pivotal glide," which is repeated several times during the motion of the joint. If either

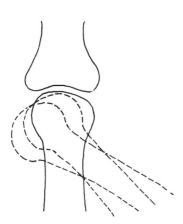
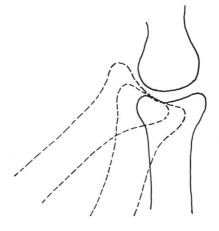

**Figure 11–12.** Pivotal glide.

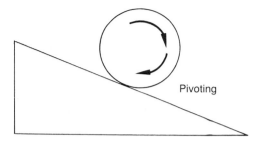

**Figure 11–13.**  Pivoting.

the pivoting or gliding cannot occur the motion of the joint is disturbed, as happens with contractures after immobilization. The free motion of the joint is thus made possible by the "pivotal glide." The two components will be discussed separately.

### Pivoting

Pivoting occurs around an axis. In this process, new points of contact are continually forming between the two components of the joint.

### Gliding

Gliding occurs along an axis. In this process one area of the same joint component makes contact with new points of the other component.

Gliding, which cannot be carried out actively by the patient himself, is also termed accessory motion; it is a necessary component of every joint motion.

Parallel gliding and traction are accessory motions.

## PARALLEL GLIDING

This is a gliding mobilization. The direction of the motion is tangential to the distal end of the fixed proximal joint component. The distal component is moved parallel in a medial, lateral, dorsal, or ventral direction.

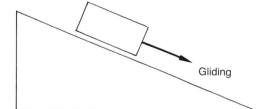

**Figure 11–14.**  Gliding.

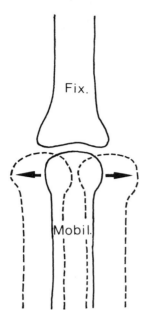

**Figure 11–15.** Parallel gliding. Fix, fixed joint component; mobil, mobilized joint component.

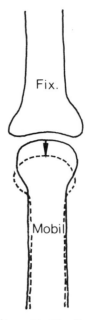

**Figure 11–16.** Traction.

## TRACTION

This is a traction mobilization. The proximal joint component is fixed and the distal component is moved in a distal direction by the traction.

The familiar levering, passive, and forced motions on hypomobilized joints create compression on one side and stretching on the other side of the joint.

In contrast, manual therapy, with its parallel gliding and traction movements, is a gentle treatment, particularly when active remedial exercises are not yet possible after an athletic injury, such as when there are effusions.

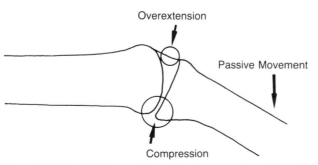

**Figure 11–17.** Effects on joint of leverage and passive and forced movements.

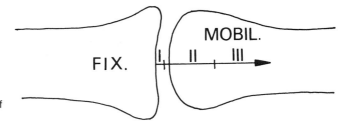

**Figure 11–18.** Traction of three grades.

# Administration of Traction and Gliding

Traction and gliding mobilization is administered in three stages:
Stage I. Joint loosening, in which the tension of adhesion is relieved.
Stage II. Joint tensing, in which contraction tension is relieved.
Stage III. Joint stretching, in which the residual tension is relieved.

# Rules of Treatment

The therapist moves the bone to be mobilized with the convex side of the joint opposed to and the concave side in agreement with the direction of the restricted bone movement.

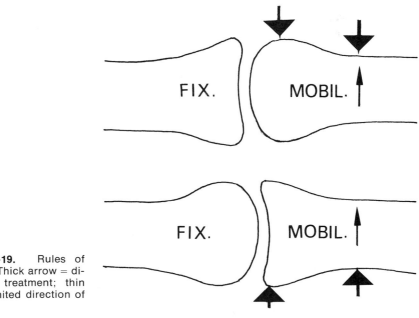

**Figure 11–19.** Rules of treatment: Thick arrow = direction of treatment; thin arrow = limited direction of movement.

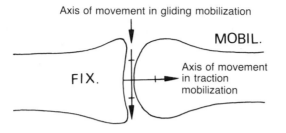

Axis of movement in gliding mobilization

MOBIL.

FIX.

Axis of movement
in traction
mobilization

**Figure 11–20.** Axis of movement in gliding and traction mobilization.

## Direction of Treatment

Traction is administered at a right angle to the tangential surface.

Gliding is administered parallel to the tangential surface.

When used for relieving pain, traction is placed on the joint entermittently for 10 seconds and then is slowly released. The intensity depends on the amount of pain. This is repeated several times.

Gliding can then be performed painlessly for further joint mobilization. Several repetitions in the same rhythm as the traction are administered.

Active "pivotal gliding" in the joint is achieved through accessory joint mobilization with traction and gliding. The extent of movement gained is preserved with active remedial exercises.

## Summary

Manual therapy is a method of treatment that is administered with localized techniques after diagnosis has been made. Its goal is to achieve normal free range of motion in the joints. This is absolutely necessary for their normal functioning, which permits the athlete to achieve optimal performance.

## CHAPTER 12

# Diagnosis

*LUTZ MEISSNER*

## Introduction

The foundation for all physical therapy treatments is always an individual diagnosis based on the results of a precise differential diagnosis by a sports physician. Before treatment by the physician or the physical therapist can begin it must be clear which structures of the soft tissues or bones are damaged. Only then can treatments that are unnecessary or even contraindicated be avoided.

Athletic injuries are almost always injuries to the soft tissues. The statistics of Herschfeld and Groh and Groh, of 75.3 per cent and 78.9 per cent, respectively, excluding open wounds, support this contention. X-rays are of little use in determining the nature of damage to soft tissues. For this reason, a clinical diagnosis with particular reference to the athlete's particular sport must first be undertaken. After the diagnosis has been made and any medical care which may be necessary has been given, the physical therapy treatment begins.

Before the therapist can begin treatment, he or she must also make a diagnosis, which forms the basis of the following physical therapy.

The plan of treatment is then created as the logical result of this diagnosis. The proper assessment and specific treatment of the injuries is important to the athlete and affects subsequent ability to resume training.

## Diagnostic Procedure

Name
Age
Sex
Athletic discipline
Diagnosis
Previous history
    Circumstances of the accident
    Initial injury
    Relapse
    Athletic injury

# Initial Situation

Complaints: Acute, chronic, sporadic
Pain: Localization, type, intensity
Functional limitations: Localization, type
    The following examinations facilitate the diagnosis:
Visual inspection
Function tests
Palpation

# Physical Examination

1. Inspection
2. Active and passive motions
3. Test joints
4. Test soft tissues
5. Palpation

# Inspection

Analyze the motions required by the athletic discipline.
Analyze the movements that caused the injury.
Motion, nature of stride, protective position.
General condition: Form, swelling, effusion, hypertrophy, atrophy, deformation, cavities, fissures.
Epidermis and subcutaneous tissues: Condition, color, wounds, swelling, edema, depressions, pressure points, calluses, scars, hair, appearance of nails.
Muscles: Profile, swellings, depressions.

# Active and Passive Motions

Active motions should be performed to check all anatomic structures and the patient's willingness or hesitancy to perform the motions.
Consider the following:
Extent of motion: Presence of evasive movements
Execution of motion: Local strength and endurance
Sounds/Noise: Crepitation
Pain: Course of pain
Anatomic motions are attempted in one-, two-, or three-dimensional configurations according to the structure of the joint.
Passive motions are performed to check all noncontractile structures, including the following:

Bones
Joint capsules
Ligaments
Bursas
Fasciae
Dura mater
Nerve roots

In the normal condition, the passive movements are identical to the actively executed anatomic movements.

A forced full extension gives information about joint stability and the so-called "end-feeling" of the joint. This end-feeling, an elastic checking of movement, can be soft if the joint ends on soft tissue; firm if it ends on capsule-ligament; or hard if it ends on bone. The extent of passive motion is somewhat greater than the active motion.

## Extent of Motion

0 = No mobility, ankylosis
1 = Very limited mobility.
2 = Slightly limited mobility.
3 = Normal mobility.
4 = Somewhat hypermobile without pain.
5 = Hypermobile with pain.
6 = Completely unstable.

Ascertain first whether the part treated is hypo- or hypermobile.

Active and passive movements in the affected areas can also be compared with the noninjured extremity or side of the body. The following should be noted:

Hypomobility
Hypermobility
Quality of motion
Pain
Shortened muscles
Capsular symptoms
End-feeling of joint

## Joint Measurements

Joint measurements determine the possible extent of motion — the angle of motion. In this book, we will use the neutral-zero method (Debrunner) of measurement. All measurements are taken from the neutral position. Examples: The extent of motion is measured on both sides of the neutral position. If there is flexion in a joint of 50 degrees and an extension of 15 degrees, it is recorded as 50-0-15. If there is a contracture and the flexion is limited by 20 degrees, it is recorded as 30-0-15. If a contracture makes extension completely impossible, leaving only flexion, both numbers are written to the left of the zero, 50-15-0.

There are two types of joint measurements:

Active measurement: Extent of motion is determined actively by the patient.

Passive measurement: Extent of motion is determined by the therapist.

Additional measurements: Measurement of circumference and length.

Equipment for measurements: Protractor, tape measure, supporting board, scale, holotopometer (universal measuring device).

## Differential Diagnosis by Means of Active and Passive Movements

1. If the active and passive movements are limited and/or painful in the same direction, the injury is in the noncontractile structures.

2. If the active and passive movements are limited and/or painful in an opposing direction, the injury is in the contractile structures.

3. If the passive movement is relatively limited in various directions, the injury is in the joint capsule. This so-called capsulary sign is for every joint the characteristic consequence of the limited motion.

## Resistance Test

The contractile structures are tested against maximal holding resistance, since the noncontractile structures remain uninvolved.

Contractile structures include the muscle fibers, connective tissue components, muscle-tendon transitions, and tendon insertions, known as the "muscle unit."

The muscles are tested for pain and strength with resistance tests. Results are interpreted as follows:

Pain and much strength: Small muscle-tendon injury.

Pain and little strength: Large muscle-tendon injury.

Painless and little strength: Neurologic defect.

Painless and much strength: Normal conditions.

*Text continued on page 185*

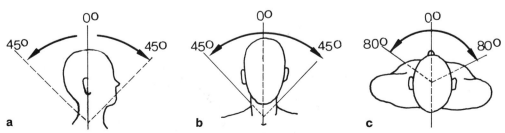

**Figure 12–1.** Range of motion of the cervical vertebrae. *a,* Extension and flexion 45 degrees; *b,* lateral inclination to 45 degrees; *c,* rotation to 80 degrees.

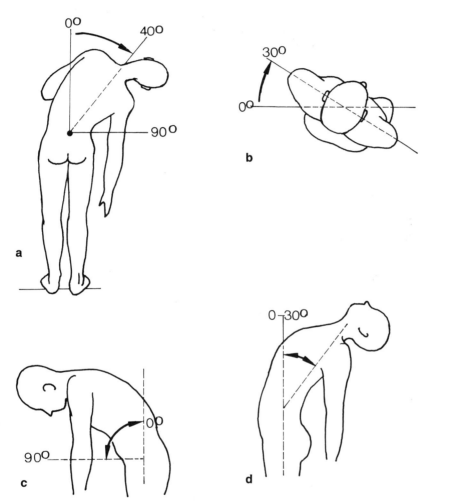

**Figure 12-2.** Range of motion of the lumbar vertebrae and torso. *a*, Lateral inclination to 40 degrees (from S1 through C7); *b*, rotation to 30 degrees; *c*, forward flexion to 90 degrees; *d*, backward extension to 30 degrees.

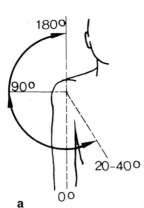
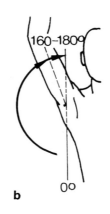
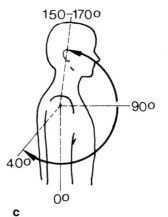
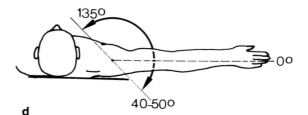

**Figure 12–3.** Range of motion of shoulder joint. *a,* Lateral lifting: abduction to 90 degrees, elevation to 180 degrees, towards head, 20 to 40 degrees; *b,* lifting up arm: elevation to 160 to 180 degrees; *c,* front lifting: elevation to 150 to 170 degrees, back lifting: extension to 40 degrees; *d,* horizontal motion: flexion to 135 degrees, extension to 40 to 50 degrees.

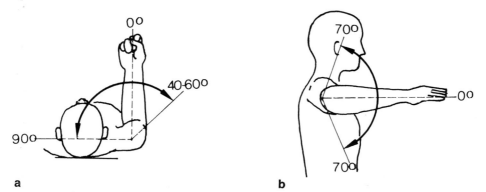

**Figure 12–4.** Rotation. *a,* In neutral position, inward rotation to 90 degrees, outward rotation to 40 to 60 degrees; *b,* in abduction position, inward rotation or outward rotation to 70 degrees.

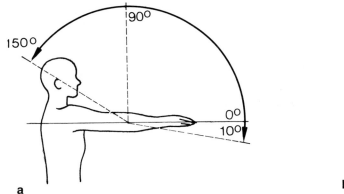

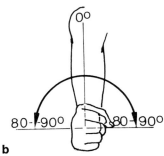

a

b

**Figure 12–5.**    Range of motion of elbow. *a,* Flexion to 150 degrees, hyperextension to 10 degrees; *b,* supination or pronation to 80 to 90 degrees.

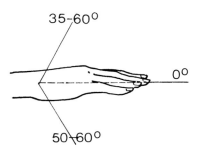

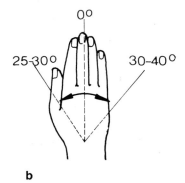

a

b

**Figure 12–6.**    Range of motion of wrist. *a,* Dorsal extension, 35 to 60 degrees, volar flexion, 50 to 60 degrees; *b,* ulnar abduction, 30 to 40 degrees.

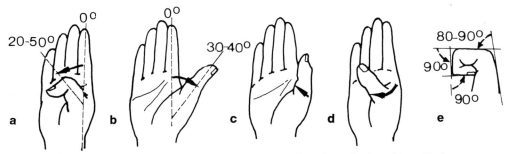

a        b        c        d        e

**Figure 12–7.**    Range of motion of thumb and finger. Thumb: *a,* flexion, 20 to 50 degrees; *b,* abduction, 30 to 40 degrees; *c,* adduction; *d,* opposition. Finger: *e,* flexion, proximal phalanges, 80 to 90 degrees, middle phalanges, to 90 degrees, distal phalanges, to 90 degrees.

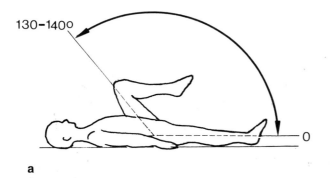

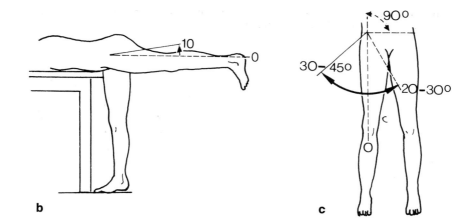

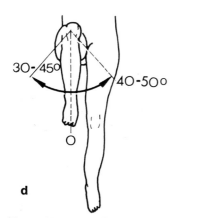

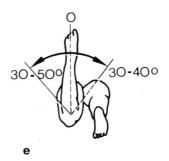

**Figure 12–8.**   Range of motion of hip. *a,* Flexion, 130 to 140 degrees; *b,* extension to 10 degrees with other hip at 90 degree flexion; *c,* abduction, 30 to 45 degrees, adduction, 20 to 30 degrees; *d,* inward rotation, 30 to 45 degrees in supine position, outward rotation 40 to 50 degrees in supine position; *e,* inward rotation, 30 to 50 degrees in prone position, outward rotation 30 to 40 degrees in prone position.

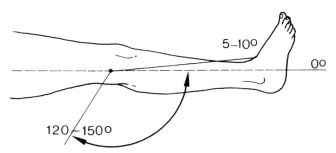

**Figure 12–9.** Range of motion of knee: Flexion, 120 to 150 degrees; hyperextension, 5 to 10 degrees; outward rotation, to 45 degrees with 90 degree knee flexion; inward rotation, to 15 degrees with 90 degree knee flexion.

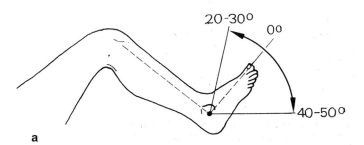

a

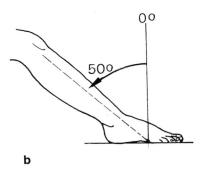

b

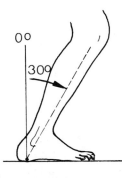

c

**Figure 12–10.** Range of motion of ankle. *a,* Extension (dorsiflexion), 20 to 30 degrees; plantar flexion, 40 to 50 degrees; *b,* plantar flexion, to 50 degrees while standing; *c,* dorsal extension, to 30 degrees while standing.

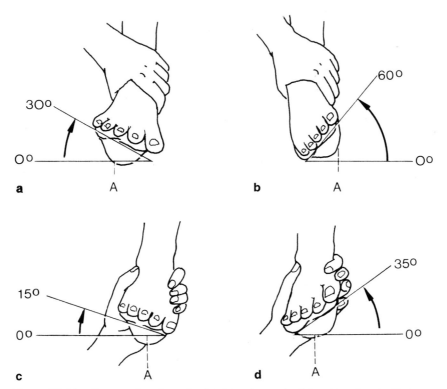

**Figure 12–11.** Range of motion of ankle (*A*, calcaneal axis). *a*, Eversion, to 30 degrees; *b*, inversion, to 60 degrees; *c*, pronation, to 15 degrees; *d*, supination, to 35 degrees.

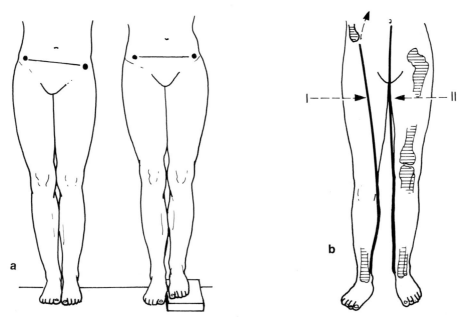

**Figure 12–12.** *a*, Measurement of difference in leg length with equalizing support; *b*, measurement of length of leg: *I*, true length of leg—measured from anterior superior iliac spine to medial malleolus: *II*, apparent length of leg.

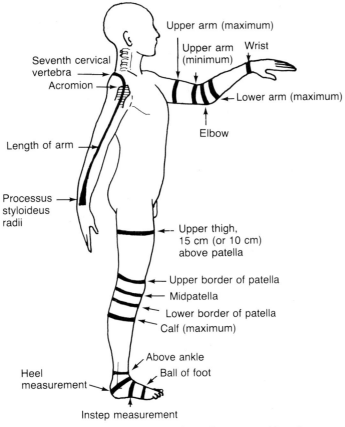

**Figure 12–13.**    Measurements of circumference and length.

# Joint Test

The joints and intraarticular structures are tested by accessory movements such as traction and gliding. A diagnosis of normal is made if joint movement is unrestricted (see Chapter 11).

# Soft Tissue Test

Muscles and connective tissues are tested for function, strength, endurance, flexibility, and coordination.

After the muscle function test, the muscle is evaluated. This evaluation is based on six grades of ability:

0   No muscle contraction                                    Paralyzed
1   Contraction is perceived but there is no movement        Trace
2   Movement with relief of body weight                      Poor
3   Movement against body weight                             Fair

| | |
|---|---|
| 4 Movement against slight resistance | Good |
| 5 Movement against maximal resistance | Very good/normal |

# Palpation

Epidermis and subcutaneous tissues:   Temperature, turgescence, surface sensitivity, mobility, adhesions, swelling, edema, depressions, lacerations, retractions

Muscle/tendon:   Tone, myogeloses, muscle-tendon transitions, muscle-bone transition, consistency, cavities, swelling, mobility, lacerations, crepitation, pain

Fasciae:   Thickening, swelling, mobility, adhesions, crepitations, pain, depressions, tears

Joints:   Effusions, form, improper position, pain

Capillaries/nerves: Swelling, inflammations, pressure points, bruises, tears.

Palpation zones are fixed anatomic areas with which every therapist should be familiar.

For a complete overview of the patient's circumstances, psychologic factors should also be taken into consideration; examples are general mood and difficulties at home, on the job, and on the playing field.

# Summary

Diagnosis may seem like a major undertaking, but experienced therapists only need a relatively short time. In this process the tests of inspection, function, and palpation produce a unified diagnosis. It must be reemphasized that a careful, individual diagnosis, which takes into consideration both the injury and the type of sport played is essential for an efficient program of physical therapy and remedial exercise.

# PART III  Possible Treatments with Physical Therapy and Remedial Exercise for Particular Athletic Injuries and Damage

## INDIVIDUAL DESCRIPTIONS

In this section typical athletic injuries and damages that are common in today's training and competitive events will be described. After a short introduction about the mechanisms of injuries and damages, the most important goals of a treatment with physical therapy and remedial exercises will be described. Purely medical treatments, which generally take place before the physical therapy, will either be sketched briefly or entirely dispensed with.

The goals of the treatment, the start of the treatment, and the diverse physical therapy and remedial procedures are depicted. The basic distinction between active and passive treatments is maintained. Passive treatments such as massages, positioning, cold, heat, electrotherapy, bandages, and so forth, are mentioned only briefly and are not described extensively. It is assumed that the therapist active in sports physical therapy will have mastered them. Moreover, these treatments have been described in the initial chapters of this work.

The active methods of remedial exercise are treated more thoroughly in discussions of individual disorders. Until recently they have remained insufficiently known and used in connection with athletic injuries and damages. Their application in particular sports has frequently been neglected. Whereas the passive treatment serves as preparation for active treatment and supplements it, the active methods are more important. They are the treatments that actually restore function. Only the active physical therapy treatments prepare the athlete for a resumption of training and therefore for full readiness for competition. Sperling once spoke of the "restoration of function through function" in this context. It is important to encourage the injured athlete to participate actively. This is a crucial requirement for the success of the treatment.

The schematic descriptions in the following chapters should be viewed as guidelines, not as a textbook. Their purpose is to inform sports physicians, physical therapists, trainers, students, and athletes themselves of the possibilities of treatment with physical therapy and remedial exercise for particular athletic injuries and damages.

The therapist must learn the techniques of treatment by actual practice, and practical experience is necessary before the techniques can be applied. In particular the selection of the proper treatments and their combination require many years of practical experience. The arrangement of the program of treatment, its modification, and if necessary, its correction in the course of the treatment must be individually tailored.

It is imperative that the team of attendants work closely together and communicate well. The treatment can be a success only if the trainer, doctor, and therapist work closely together to achieve complete recovery of the athlete, such as will permit him or her to withstand the full stress of competition. The trainer, physician, and therapist should consider themselves a team for the purpose of treating the athlete. On the one hand, they should work professionally toward the rapid recovery of the athlete to optimal strength after injuries, at the same time keeping the athlete's long-term health and freedom from injury in view. The individual needs of the athlete must be the primary consideration for each member of the team in each decision.

CHAPTER **13**

# General Considerations

*DORIS EITNER*

## Sprains

In a sprain the physiologic limit of a movement is surpassed. This generally involves a pull or even a tear of the capsule-ligament apparatus. In both cases there is bleeding. X-rays are necessary to determine the severity of the sprain and to make sure that the bone is not broken. In certain cases it is possible to determine if there is a ruptured ligament on x-rays.

Sprains occur frequently in the following sports: basketball, high jump and long jump — ankle sprains resulting from the foot being twisted during jumping motion; soccer and skiing — sprain of knee by overtwisting or wrenching; handball, volleyball, basketball — sprained fingers, resulting from sudden impact of ball.

### GOALS OF TREATMENT

Treatment aims at restoration of full function, strengthening of the muscle-ligament apparatus, and correction of improper stance.

### START OF TREATMENT

A period of immobilization is necessary, depending on the seriousness of the sprain. While the injured joint is immobilized, physical therapy of the other parts of the body can begin immediately. When immobilization is no longer necessary the injured joint is included in this treatment.

## PASSIVE TREATMENTS

*Positioning.*    Immobilization and elevation to stimulate venous and lymphatic return.

*Massage.*    The muscles of the adjacent extremity can be massaged immediately. After about 14 days, any adhesions that may have arisen can be relieved with localized friction, or in certain cases with stylus massage.

*Cold.*    Ice packs, cold baths, or application of cold towels can be used in the acute stages.

*Heat.*    Heat is applied by means of fango poultices and incandescent light in later stages. The applications of heat are important for the normalization of the metabolism in the joint.

*Electrotherapy.*    In the subacute phase, ultrasound, iontophoresis, and diadynamic currents are useful.

## ACTIVE TREATMENTS

*Physical Therapy and Remedial Exercise.*    Active remedial exercises, such as stabilization techniques, mobilization exercises, and resistance exercises in the form of complex motions are stressed. If these exercises are mastered, passive and active stretching begins. Exercises with devices such as balls, sponges, and jumpropes can be a part of the active exercise.

## SPECIAL NOTES

*Treatments Contraindicated.*    Passive exercise, overheating of the joint with hot baths in the acute phase, and massage of the injured joint are contraindicated. There is danger of causing myositis ossificans.

If the sprain is not completely healed, the joint is often left in an irritated condition. This is particularly true for the knee, where sprains usually take the form of injuries of rotation.

Several sprains on the same joint quickly cause an impairment of the metabolism in the joint. This can even lead to premature attrition (arthrosis deformans).

*First Aid at Competition Site.*    Measures include use of ice, compression bandage, with padding and a hollowing for the place of the injury; bandages treated with salves for the reabsorption of hematomas; and strengthening of the compression bandage with adhesive tape.

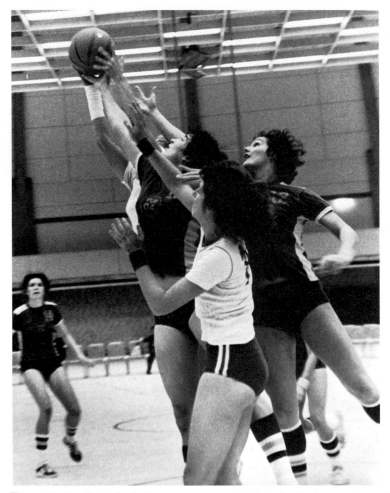

**Figure 13–1.**   Basketball players are at special risk of suffering sprained fingers.

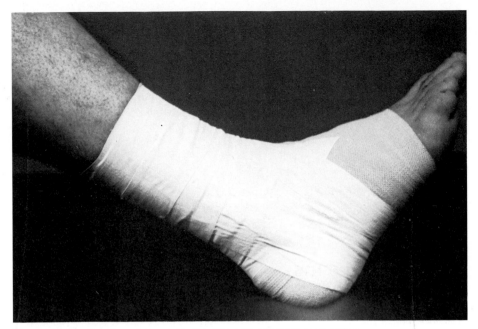

**Figure 13–2.**   Bandage for sprained ankle with adhesive tape strips.

*Prevention.*   Preventive measures are varied and include improvement of the strength and coordination of the muscle-ligament apparatus; preventive taping or bandaging; change of shoes (for example, to high-ankle basketball shoes); no cleats for young soccer players; improvement of motion techniques in the various sports.

# Contusions

A contusion is the result of a blunt impact on the body surface. This can lead to injury in the surface soft tissues, such as the muscles and the fasciae. The capsules and ligaments of joints can be damaged. The most common causes are falling, tripping, and collisions with another athlete, a piece of apparatus, or a natural obstacle.

The contusion is characterized by the immediate appearance of a hematoma, but most of all by the pain in the area of contact, which increases at first under pressure. The extent of bleeding varies, however. Sometimes the bruise is deep, making it difficult to ascertain how large it is. The impact results in damage to the surrounding areas as well. This can involve simply the compression of the muscles or a contusion of nerves or more deeply situated organs. In team sports, contusions usually result from direct collisions between opposing players. Soccer players speak of a "charleyhorse" when a player is hit in the thigh by the opponent's knee, resulting in a bruised upper thigh.

## GOALS OF TREATMENT

Goals of treatment are relieving of pain by the removal of the hematoma and restoration of complete motion.

Adhesions that have arisen should be removed, so that optimal function can be assured. Free motion and flexibility of the muscles, to reduce susceptibility to reinjury, such as strains, should also be achieved.

## START OF TREATMENT

Treatment of contusions of extremities can begin immediately. A patient with extensive bruising should rest for a day and elevate the extremity. Severe contusions on the torso are treated after a rest period of several days.

## PASSIVE TREATMENTS

*Positioning.* The injured extremity is elevated to increase the venous and lymphatic return. Serious contusions on the torso require temporary rest in bed. Additional alcohol-impregnated bandages aid in the reduction of hematomas.

*Massage.* Massage for the drainage of excess fluids can begin immediately, as can massage of the noninjured areas. Connective tissue massage is also recommended. Adhesions are treated with classic massage only after the irritation subsides, about 14 days.

*Cold.* In the acute stage, ice treatments are recommended. Bandages with alcohol or surgical spirits are also possible aids.

*Heat.* Heat is forbidden in any form during the acute period. After the pain has subsided, fango poultices, incandescent light, and other heat applications can be used.

*Electrotherapy.* In the acute phase, diadynamic currents, iontophoresis, and ultrasound can be used. After the period of irritation ends, high frequency waves in the form of short waves and microwaves are additional possible treatments.

## ACTIVE TREATMENTS

Physical therapy and remedial exercise. After 24 hours, isometric exercises can begin. After 2 days, active remedial isotonic exercises in an exercise bath can begin. Resistance exercises, including complex motions, begin on the third day. Active stretching exercises can also begin on the same day. On the fourth day, the patient exercises with devices such as dumbbells, sandbags, and medicine balls. Passive stretching exercises should be done only at the end of the physical therapy treatment. The threshold of pain must not be exceeded in either the active or the passive exercises. Exercises for the particular athletic discipline of the patient should begin before the start of training.

### SPECIAL NOTES

***Treatments Contraindicated.***    Heat and massage are contraindicated in the acute stage. Similarly, a vigorous massage in the area of injury can cause muscle ossification. All contusions require intensive physical therapy until full training can be resumed. If this is neglected, a painful irritated condition of the muscles or tendons often remains. This can easily lead to evasive motions, which affect the athlete's performance.

***First Aid at Competition Site.***    Ice treatment with cooling spray, or better, ice massage with icecubes for 3 to 5 minutes is helpful. Also useful is compression bandage treated with salve with foam-rubber cushioning. The compression bandage can be reinforced with additional adhesive tape to relieve pressure on muscle.

# Luxations

A luxation is a dislocation of the bony part of a joint, usually accompanied by a serious capsule-ligament lesion. This results in the displacement of the normal positions of the joint ends. Traumatic luxations occur frequently in athletic competition. Two forms may be seen — a complete, total luxation or a subluxation. In a subluxation, the two bones of the joint still remain in contact.

Clinically reliable symptoms include deformity, the empty joint socket, twisted head of the bone, and resilient fixation. The bone that is dislocated can be snapped back into the socket passively.

Doubtful symptoms include impaired function, pain from twisting, and bleeding.

Luxations frequently result in damage to soft tissues, particularly capsule and ligament tears, which results in bleeding in the interior of the joint and into the surrounding soft tissues.

The diagnosis is not always simple, particularly for deep-lying joints. X-rays are usually necessary to make the diagnosis certain.

Traumatic luxations can cause permanent damage in the torn capsule-ligament apparatus if the damage is severe enough or if it is improperly treated, and thus it can become a habitual luxation. This is characterized by repeated dislocations on performing the same motions; this can, however, be congenital. Habitual luxations occur most frequently in the shoulders and knees.

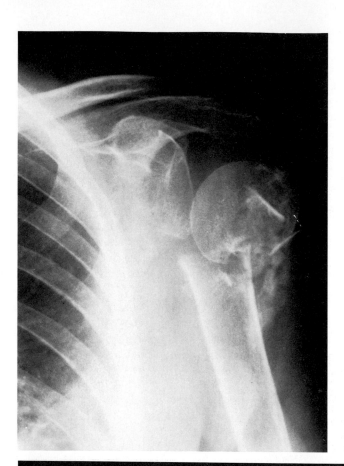

**Figure 13–3.** X-ray of a subcapital humerus fracture with concomitant shoulder dislocation.

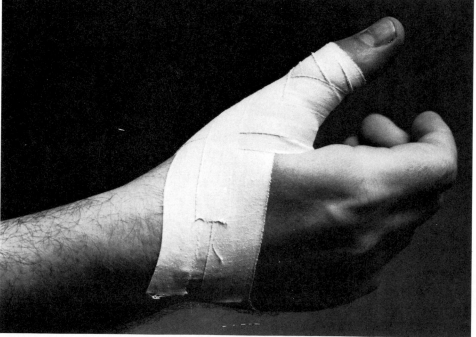

**Figure 13–4.** Adhesive tape bandage for the immobilization of a "skier's thumb."

The joint most frequently dislocated traumatically is the shoulder (about 50 per cent), followed by the elbow (20 per cent) (see Chapter 16, Shoulder Luxation). In sports such as handball, dislocation of an elbow of an outstretched arm can occur during a fall. A luxation of the thumb joint is known as skier's thumb. This involves a tear of the ulnar or radial ligament, which can range from a microscopic tear to complete severing. Tears that are only slight are treated conservatively. Complete severance requires an operation. Fingers can be dislocated by the unexpected impact of a ball, as in volleyball or basketball. Luxations of the kneecap occur frequently as a result of overextension or from lateral impact in soccer, jumping in ball sports, and dismounts from gymnastic apparatus. Luxations of the hip occur when jumping from great heights, such as in mountain climbing and parachute jumping.

Dislocations of the spine are rare, but do occur in gymnastics, riding, and ski-jumping.

Injuries to the blood vessels and nerves can also accompany traumatic luxations. Again, the shoulder and the knee are particularly at risk.

## GOALS OF TREATMENT

Goals of treatment include relief of painful hematomas, restoration of complete function, strengthening of the muscle-ligament apparatus, prevention of contractures, and prevention of capsule adhesions and connective tissue shrinkage.

## START OF TREATMENT

At the start of the immobilization period, the noninjured parts of the body can immediately be started on a physical therapy program. In this way, loss of strength and of conditioning is lessened. The active remedial treatment begins immediately after the period of immobilization ends. The extent of immobilization depends on the age of the patient, and the severity of the injury, and any additional injuries.

## PASSIVE TREATMENTS

*Positioning.*   The injured joint is elevated with the aid of splints. A frequent change of position is necessary for chronic dislocations in order to avoid contractures.

*Massage.*   Overly tense muscles are massaged after immobilization ends, with the exception of the injured joint in the early stages.

Connective tissue massage or brushing can be used for the general improvement of circulation. Adhesions of the capsules and fasciae are relieved in the later stages with massage, with use of a stylus if necessary.

*Cold.* If there is still joint effusion at the beginning of treatment, its reabsorption can be accelerated with ice.

*Heat.* Applications of heat, such as fango poultices and incandescent light, can be used in the late stages as a preparation for massage and remedial exercise.

*Electrotherapy.* On the second day, the ice treatments are alternated with a low dosage of ultrasonic therapy. Diadynamic currents can also be used to improve circulation.

*Hydrotherapy.* After the joint effusion has stopped, contrast baths and steam baths can be used as a preparation for active treatment.

## ACTIVE TREATMENTS

*Physical Therapy and Remedial Exercise.* Isometric exercises are used during the period of immobilization. After this period, exercises in the exercise bath begin. The movements should be slow and along the axis, up to the pain threshold. The muscles are strengthened while out of the water with isometric exercises. Movements not influenced by gravity follow, up to the pain threshold. The movement is increased with resistance against gravity and against the therapist. The joint play can be improved and normalized with manual joint therapy. The resistance exercises reinforce the newly restored range of motion. Devices such as medicine balls, sticks, Indian clubs, and jump ropes are aids to exercise.

During individual exercises, muscular tension must be greatest at the limits of movements, so that the range of motion is increased. During complex motions rotation must be only active and against carefully regulated resistance.

Exercise for shortened muscles consists of brief contractions followed by periods of relaxation.

Active and passive stretching of soft tissues as well as light swinging and pendulation exercises are added as soon as the contracture is free of irrigation and the joint play is largely possible without pain. The exercises must be used for both shortened and lengthened muscles, in order to achieve a functional improvement of the damaged locomotor unit.

## SPECIAL NOTES

*Treatments Contradicated.* Massage in the area of the injured joint in the acute phase, due to the danger of causing myositis ossificans; use of heat in the form of hot air or incandescent light because of the danger of causing Sudeck's dystrophy; pendulation exercises in the acute stage, passive motions, and motions which could lead to a redislocation are also contraindicated.

***First Aid at Competition Site.***    The dislocated joint is well padded and placed in a position that will permit transport with the least amount of pain. Dislocated joints should only be put back into place by professional medical personnel.

# Fractures

Fractures result from a violent impact on the bones. One can distinguish between simple fractures, i.e., closed, and compound fractures, i.e., those in which the skin is broken. In the latter case the broken ends of the bone are visible outside the body. Typical symptoms of broken bones include great pain, loss of function, considerable swelling from the hematoma, change of form, and a grating noise (crepitation).

Fractures usually involve torn capillaries and considerable damage to the tissues. This causes an increase in the metabolism and activity of the cells, which proceed from hyperemia and exudation to the reabsorption and reparation. The newly formed tissue is called callus. The formation of callus is increased and enables the fractured bones to rebind. The callus is later broken down. Excess callus can also be formed, known as a callus bridge, which blocks

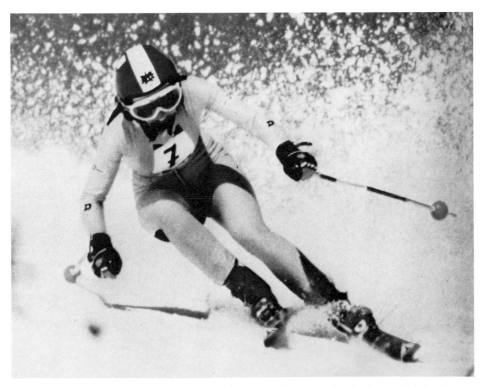

**Figure 13–5.**  The lower legs are particularly susceptible to fracture in downhill skiing (boot-top breaks).

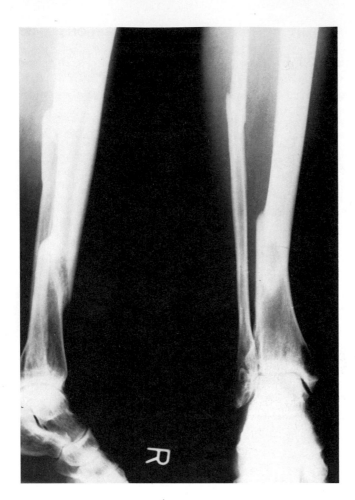

**Figure 13–6.** X-ray of a fracture of the lower leg.

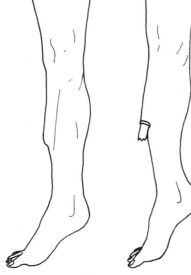

**Figure 13–7.** Simple closed fracture of the lower leg.

**Figure 13–8.** Compound fracture of the lower leg.

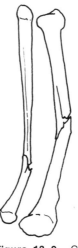

**Figure 13–9.** Complete fracture of the lower leg, a bending-break of tibia and fibula.

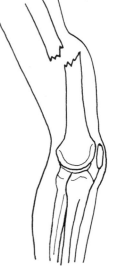

**Figure 13–10.** Complete bending fracture of the femur.

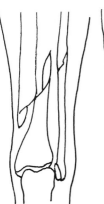 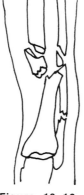 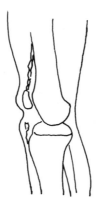 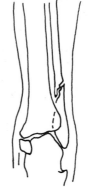

**Figure 13–11.** Twisting fracture of the tibia and fibula, with displacement of the broken ends.

**Figure 13–12.** Multiple fracture.

**Figure 13–13.** Torn fractured patella.

**Figure 13–14.** Cartilage fracture with triangular break (Volkmann's triangle).

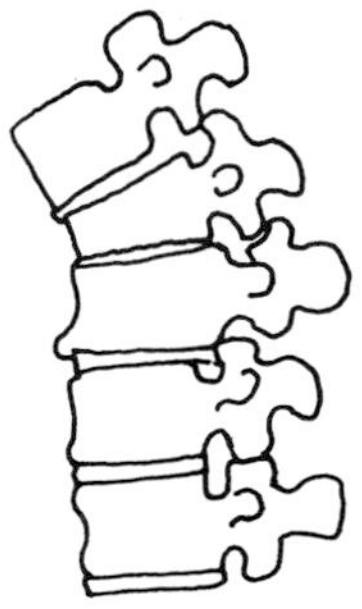

**Figure 13–15.** Stasis fracture of spine.

nerves and constricts vessels. As an example of this, the turning motion of the lower arm can be hindered after a fracture. According to the form of the fracture and the way the break occurred, diagonal, twisting, right-angle, spiral, fragmented, and joint breaks can be distinguished. Stress placed on the bones too early or a new accident can result in a callus fracture. These new fractures require renewed care and immobilization. It takes generally 8 weeks for fractures of the long bones of the upper extremity to heal, 12 weeks for fractures of the lower extremity, and 3 to 6 months for bones of the spinal column. Fractures occur in all types of sports.

Rapid treatment of the broken bone is important for the healing process. The bones of an athlete do not heal any more quickly than those of a non-athlete.

Fractures of the lower leg, which are the most common, occur primarily in soccer, downhill skiing, and track and field sports.

Fractures of the lower arm occur primarily in falls, as during games, downhill skiing, and gymnastics.

Fractures of the spine occur on the trampoline and in horse jumping, steeplechase, and gymnastics.

Broken collarbones and ribs occur in riding, boxing, bicycling, and ice hockey.

A broken pelvis may occur in serious motor accidents and in horse jumping.

## GOALS OF TREAMENT

Treatment goals are prevention of muscle atrophy, capsule shrinkage, and contractures. Additional goals include improvement of metabolism; prevention of thromboses and circulatory instability; and restoration of complete mobility, function, and muscle strength.

## START OF TREATMENT

The physical therapy begins on the first day, after both conservative and operative treatment.

## PASSIVE TREATMENTS

*Positioning.*   The fractured extremity is elevated with the aid of splints and sandbags.

*Massage.*   All parts of the body except the injured limb are massaged. The brush massage is a good way to stimulate general circulation. In the later stages, it is possible to loosen adhesions, which may have arisen with localized massage techniques.

*Hydrotherapy.*   This may be instituted after the cast has been removed or after the wounds have closed. After the immobilization period has ended, circulation-stimulating exercises are important. These can take the form of contrast baths, steam treatments, and warm baths.

*Cold.*   Contractures, if present, can be relaxed by laying an ice compress on the shortened muscles.

*Heat.*   Fango poultices and incandescent light are used in the later stages.

*Electrotherapy.*   If paralyses have arisen as a consequence of the fracture, they can be beneficially treated with electrogymnastic equipment. Iontophoresis and ultrasound can be used in the late phases if there is pain in the ligament origin and insertion. Diadynamic currents are used for joint capsule lesions.

## ACTIVE TREATMENTS

*Physical Therapy and Remedial Exercise.*   Starting on the first day, all joints that are not immobilized should be exercised actively several times daily throughout the immobilization period. Isometric exercises also begin on the first day for the immobilized limbs, along with exercises for the prevention of thromboses and embolisms. To prevent a lung infection in bedridden patients, intensive breathing exercises are needed. Manual therapy is later used to restore optimal joint function. Muscle strengthening exercises follow, which include isometric exercises, resistance exercises, complex motions, and light exercise with apparatus. Contractures are prevented through active muscle and mobilization training as well as through loosening and stretching exercises. If there is nerve damage the treatment consists of intensive muscle care, prevention of contractures, innervation training, and use of electrogymnastic equipment, during which the paralyzed muscle must be prevented from overstretching or overshortening by proper positioning. The final stage of the physical therapy exercise program includes both movements used in everyday activities and movements for the particular sport.

### SPECIAL NOTES

*Treatments Contraindicated.* Heat treatments in the acute phase and attempts to move the injured part after the injury has occurred are contraindicated.

*First Aid at the Competition Site.* For simple fractures, position the extremity comfortably and splint it. If there is no splint available, the undamaged extremity can serve as a stabilizer. For skiing accidents the boot should not be removed, as frostbite can easily occur; moreover, the foot is better stabilized in the boot. The primary danger in the case of a compound fracture is a secondary infection of the area of broken skin. The assistant should cover the wound with sterile material and splint the extremity well. Fractures must not be pushed back into place.

# Fatigue Fractures

Fatigue fractures arise from constantly repeated mechanical stresses that lie below the limit of the bone's strength. As Schmidt has argued, these should actually be considered exhaustion fractures rather than fatigue fractures, since fatigue is now believed to be a single reversible process.

The condition of the muscular system is of great importance, because exhausted muscles cannot perform fully their protective function, so that the traumas affect the skeleton directly. Fatigue fractures are aggravated by weaknesses in the connective and supportive tissues resulting from microtraumas. Microtraumas in sports usually result from repeated strong blows and shocks, maximal straining of muscles and tendons, and repeated rapid motions of the joints, such as in javelin throwing. Fatigue fractures do not occur suddenly, but are usually linked to painful previous stresses and radiologic changes.

Fatigue fractures occur in various types of sports. Runners and walkers show such fractures in the fibula, the os naviculare pedis, and the metatarsus; these are also known as march fractures. They can occur on the olecranon in participants in gymnastics and throwing sports.

## GOALS OF TREATMENT

Goals of Treatment include prevention of muscular atrophy, restoration of complete mobility and muscular strength, and prevention of a renewed fatigue fracture.

## START OF TREATMENT

The active physical therapy exercises begin immediately.

## PASSIVE TREATMENTS

*Positioning.*    The fractured limb is either splinted or put in a cast, depending on the severity of the injury. Rest in bed generally is not necessary.

*Massage.*    As with fractures, all noninjured body parts may be massaged.

*Hydrotherapy.*    Active exercises in water and contrast baths are recommended.

*Electrotherapy.*    Diadynamic currents and iontophoresis are an important part of the treatments and help to improve circulation.

## ACTIVE TREATMENTS

*Physical Therapy and Remedial Exercise.*    The functional treatment of fatigue fractures requires much experience on the part of the therapist. Isometric exercises are used for the prevention of muscular atrophy beginning on the first day of immobilization. In addition, active exercises for the noninjured joints are used, which progress from isometric exercises to complex motions. Training of all healthy parts of the body can begin immediately. When the period of immobilization is completed, mobilization exercises of the joints with manual therapy and active and passive stretching and loosening exercises for the soft tissues can begin. Various devices are also used to further increase the stress. The physical therapy program ends with exercises related to everyday movements and motion sequences required by the particular athletic discipline.

## SPECIAL NOTES

*Prevention.*    Intensive active warm-up of muscles, active and passive stretching, warming of the joints with warm sports clothing, and observance of rest periods between stress all help prevent fatigue fractures.

Early treatment is necessary for the fatigue fractures. The removal of stress is recommended as soon as strong pain sensations are noted in the lower extremities.

# Muscle Injuries

Muscles and their tendons have a particularly large task to fulfill, whether for everyday activities or for athletics. A trained muscle is considerably stronger than an untrained muscle. It gains in both mass and diameter. Normally a muscle does not operate at full strength, but instead adjusts to the demand made on it. Top competitive performances can only be achieved through harmonic neuromuscular cooperation.

The sudden loss of function in muscles or groups of muscles through damage during physical exercise is familiar to all active athletes and trainers. The causes include improper warm-up, resulting in muscles unprepared for the stress placed on them, such as take place in movements requiring flexibility and in uncoordinated motions, collisions, and falls. Microtraumas, degeneration or exhaustion of previously damaged tissue are further causes of this most common athletic injury. An incongruity between the muscle capacity and the stress can have the following effects on the locomotor system: (1) incomplete or complete muscle and tendon ruptures; (2) overextension or tearing of muscle constituents; (3) myogeloses as a result of local increase in muscle tone; (4) ruptures of the fascia with resulting muscle hernia; (5) tears of the origins and insertions of tendons with and without bony components, as in the head of the fibula; (6) tendonitis in the tendon insertions and origins that are free of periosteum.

# Torn Muscle

Muscle tears, which can occur during work or at rest, can be complete or incomplete, in the body of the muscle, at the transition to the tendon, in its tendinous part, or at its origin on the bone. Muscle tears usually result from violent overextension. A muscle that is not prepared for the amount of stress placed on it can also tear. Muscles tear more easily when they are unprepared and cold, as well as when they are exhausted or overtrained. A muscle can also tear spontaneously under direct force because it has lost elasticity and resistance strength.

Complete muscle tears are rare in athletics. Usually only muscle fibers tear, or a muscle tears at its tendon insertion. Bits of bone can also be torn in the process.

Tearing of the extensor and flexor muscles of the upper thigh in near spills while running occurs frequently.

Gymnasts and throwers often suffer tears of the biceps; wrestlers tear neck muscles.

Soccer players frequently tear the adductors.

Symptoms of torn muscles include sharp pain, which feels like a whiplash or a kick, swelling, and hematoma. A muscle depression can be seen and felt. Such depressions can, however, be covered with blood immediately after an accident and not be obvious.

Torn muscles are generally treated conservatively. Tears of smooth muscle require surgery.

## GOALS OF TREATMENT

Restoration of normal function, strengthening of muscle, and removal of adhesions are the goals of treatment.

## START OF TREATMENT

The physical therapy treatment begins immediately after the immobilization period ends. This is about 3 weeks for large injuries, a few days for smaller ones. The nonimmobilized body parts can be exercised during the period of immobilization.

## PASSIVE TREATMENT

*Positioning.*   The damaged extremity is elevated for the drainage of fluids. A lessening of the distance between the origin and the insertion of the muscle is also necessary for relaxation. This encourages the regrowth of muscle tissue.

*Massage.*   A classic massage is possible after the immobilization of the injured part. Adhesions are treated with local friction and stylus massages at the end of the healing process.

*Cold.*   Cold is applied immediately after the injury occurs.

*Heat.*   In the subacute stages, fango poultices or incandescent light can be used as a preparation for active remedial exercises.

*Hydrotherapy.*   Contrast baths or effervescent baths can increase the success of the treatment in the later stages.

*Electrotherapy.*   Diadynamic currents and ultrasound are used to improve circulation and to remove residues of the initial bleeding. Electrogymnastic equipment is used for severed nerves and for the care of a repaired nerve.

## ACTIVE TREATMENTS

*Physical Therapy and Remedial Exercise.*   Careful active exercises can begin after the period of immobilization. At first only isometric exercises are used. When the healing of the wound is complete, isotonic exercises can begin, followed by complex motions, loosening, and active and passive stretching.

The exercise bath is also eminently suited for the after-treatment.

The individual strengthening exercises, which are gradually increased, must be continued until the end of therapy, because the injured muscle must regain full use, including athletic function.

## SPECIAL NOTES

*Treatments Contraindicated.*   Massages, hot air, and incandescent light are contraindicated in the acute phases because of the danger of causing myositis ossificans; premature use of injured muscle is also forbidden.

If scars and adhesions are not completely loosened, there is danger of renewed injury. If the muscle is completely restored, competitive athletics can be resumed.

*Prevention.*   Muscle care in the form of intensive stretching exercises, muscle preparation through warm-ups, loosening techniques, and massage are helpful. In addition, active exercise with complex motions or with a Universal Gym may be used.

*First Aid at Competition Site.*   The torn muscles are wrapped in ice with a compression bandage. Additional strips of adhesive material increase the compression by bringing the origin and the insertion of the muscle closer together.

# Muscle Pulls and Torn Muscle Fibers

A muscle pull involves the overextension of individual muscle fibers. The web of muscle remains intact, however.

The muscle pull manifests itself as a needle-like, jabbing pain. Pressure on the affected area causes this sharp pain, and the pain subsides when the pressure is relieved. Muscle pulls are further evidenced by a loss of function, a guarding position, and later development of a hematoma. A muscle fiber tear is a more serious injury to several bundles of muscles; the symptoms are more severe than for a muscle pull. The most common causes of muscle pulls are the following: coordination mistakes; neuromotor disorders in the muscle; insufficient flexibility of the muscle and tendons, as in an abrupt braking after a

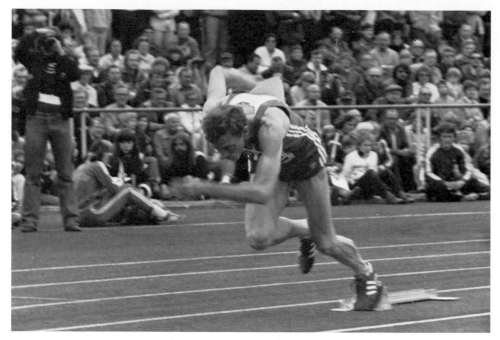

**Figure 13-16.** The starting phase of a race: the muscles on the back of the thigh and the calf are particularly vulnerable to tearing.

sprint or during a high jump, which can cause pulled adductors and hernias; insufficient elasticity because of hypertonia; myogeloses and insufficient blood supply in the muscles; and insufficient warm-up and local exhaustion. In addition, other causes, such as sudden pressure or a blow from another competitor, overloading with weights, a rough playing surface, and cold and wetness, can cause muscle pulls or torn fibers.

## GOALS OF TREATMENT

Treatment goals are relief of pain and hematoma and regaining of full training stress with guided remedial exercises.

## START OF TREATMENT

The treatment starts immediately after the injury.

## PASSIVE TREATMENTS

*Positioning, Immobilization, and Bandages.* The affected body area should be immobilized immediately with a compression bandage and ice. In addition, the part should be elevated to encourage reabsorption. Supportive bandages should be put on after the swelling goes down.

*Massage.*    The noninjured muscles can be massaged. In the area of the pulled muscle, massage should, however, be avoided until the pain from pressure is completely removed. Adhesions and scars are removed with gentle kneading, friction, and stylus massage if necessary. Underwater massage and the suction-wave massage are recommended later for general muscle loosening.

*Cold and Heat.*    Ice and other cooling agents are needed immediately after the accident to combat exudations and as an analgesic. Heat treatments can follow when the pain is gone. Fango poultices, which act as preparation for the active treatments, are useful. Warm baths are also recommended.

*Electrotherapy.*    Diadynamic currents, ultrasound, and iontophoresis can begin immediately. Short wave treatments can begin 14 days after the accident.

## ACTIVE TREATMENTS

*Physical Therapy and Remedial Exercise.*    The active physical therapy treatments begin after the second day. They begin with isometric exercises and light isotonic exercises with resistance. If these exercises are painless, resistance exercises up to complex motions can follow. Active stretching and loosening exercises are also recommended for this period. The pain threshold should not be crossed upon resumption of training.

## SPECIAL NOTES

*Treatment Contraindicated.*    Premature heat and massage treatments on the injured muscle should be avoided, as should premature active and passive motions.

*First Aid at the Competition Site.*    Apply cold in the form of ice; apply a compression bandage, if necessary with a salve to aid the reabsorption of hematomas; completely immobilize the muscle.

*Prevention.*    Preventive measures include increased coordination exercises, special strength-endurance training of the stressed muscle group, and increased loosening and stretching exercises during training. Muscles can be kept warm with proper clothing, blankets, and so forth. Warm-up and stretching of the muscles that are particularly stressed in the particular sport and use of preventive bandages are optional measures.

# Muscle Cramps

A muscle cramp is a local increase in tension in a muscle. An extremely painful muscle contraction is the result. The cramped muscle can be loosened only by a stretch reflex arc.

Muscle cramping is primarily due to excessive or improper stress; lack of salt and circulatory disturbances; or blockage of blood vessels by tight shoes, elastic bands in socks, bandages, and so forth. Psychologic factors, such as those found in a stressful situation, can also influence development of cramps.

## GOALS OF TREATMENT

Treatment goals are relief of muscle cramps and restoration of function.

## START OF TREATMENT

Treatment should begin immediately after the cramp sets in.

## PASSIVE TREATMENTS

*Positioning.*   The affected extremity is extended and left in the protective position taken as a result of pain. Severe cramps require a stretcher.

*Massage.*   Gentle massage in the acute stage should alternate with stretching of the affected muscle. Shaking is particularly good.

*Heat.*   Heat is extremely important for reduction of susceptibility to cramps. Damp warm towels, warm partial baths, and incandescent light can prepare the muscle for subsequent physical therapy.

## ACTIVE TREATMENTS

*Physical Therapy and Remedial Exercise.*   Active dynamic exercises are used to tense and relax the muscle. Avoid causing renewed cramps while doing this. The relaxing phase of the dynamic exercises should be stressed.

Rhythmic swinging exercises and exercises in an exercise bath are particularly good. These also prepare the muscles for resumption of training.

## SPECIAL NOTES

*Treatments Contraindicated.*   Violent stretching of the cramped muscle and vigorous massage should be avoided.

Resume training or competition only after complete and lasting relief of cramp has been achieved.

**Prevention.**   Keep muscles warm during training and competition; perform extensive warm-up exercises, including loosening and stretching exercises; combine loosening exercises with the suitable massage techniques; take salt tablets or balanced electrolyte solutions.

***First Aid at Competition Site.***   Assume relaxing, extending position; remove tight clothing; use cold applications; stretch muscle carefully against the cramp. Afterwards move cramped muscle against manual resistance.

# Sore Muscles

Scientific opinion is divided on the causes of muscle soreness. Surplus lactic acid, lowered pH, and the buildup of heat are thought to be important factors. The muscle tissue becomes overly acidic due to accumulation of lactic acid, pyruvic acid, carbonic acid, and other acidic metabolic products. Excessive or incorrect stress and insufficient training can also play a role. More recent opinion holds that muscle soreness results from microtrauma in the connective tissue — that is, in the tiny fibers of structural protein that surround the muscle fibers. According to this view, muscle soreness is an early stage leading to muscle pulls and tears. It differs primarily in a quantitative way from these traumas; the boundaries are not rigid.

## GOALS OF TREATMENT

Goals of therapy are removal of the muscle soreness and restoration of normal function.

## START OF TREATMENT

Treatment begins immediately after the muscle soreness sets in.

## PASSIVE TREATMENTS

***Positioning.***   The athlete is positioned so that the muscles are in a position of optimal relaxation.

***Massage.***   Careful massage is performed after muscular exertion to break down the residual acidic metabolic wastes. The effects of this relaxing massage can be improved with the help of alcohol preparations and fluids.

*Heat and Hydrotherapy.*  Warm showers, steam showers, baths, partial baths and dry applications of heat, such as incandescent light, are also good preparations for the massage. Sauna baths can likewise be good for the relief of muscle soreness.

## ACTIVE TREATMENTS

*Physical Therapy and Remedial Exercise.*  In the beginning exercises are carried out only in an exercise bath at 28°C. Afterwards, shaking, active and passive stretching, and loosening exercises can be used to restore the normal condition of the muscle.

## SPECIAL NOTES

Painful active and passive stretching exercises and further intensive training and competitive stress should be avoided. A light continuation of training with the emphasis on loosening should be used; this accelerates the breakdown of metabolic wastes. Warm showers and light, loosening exercise in a relaxing bath are simple and effective treatments for muscle soreness.

# Myogeloses and Difficulty in Stretching

Myogeloses are localized hardenings of the muscles which are painful when pressed against.

There are two types of myogeloses: One can be called thread-like and the other round-oval.

The entire muscle may also be hardened because of a surplus of metabolic wastes. Neurophysiological experiments have confirmed the connection between emotion and muscular tension. Nervous tension can also contribute to muscle contractions and cause pain. Generalized hardening is relieved by narcotics, whereas the myogeloses remain unaffected.

The epidermis and dermis overlying the tense muscles generally are capable of moving. Myogeloses can be felt and have a very specific point of pain which can be probed with the finger.

The causes are not always simple. Usually they result from an overloading of the muscle, however. Muscles that perform the same task for an entire day are inclined to be affected such as the shoulder and neck muscles of weight lifters, gymnasts, and also stenotypists and drivers; and the upper and lower arm muscles of tennis players. Deformities of the spine and degenerative changes in the joints are likewise frequent causes of painful muscular hypertension.

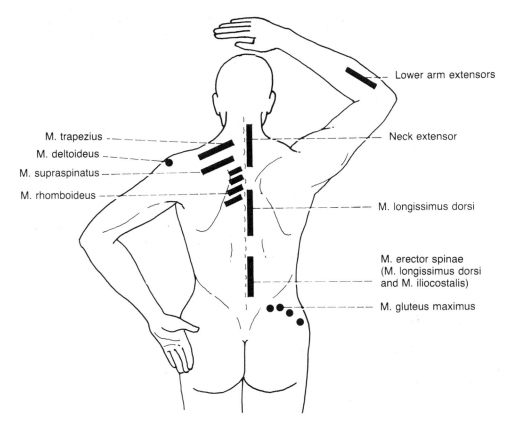

**Figure 13–17.**   Primary areas at which myogeloses occur.

## GOALS OF TREATMENT

Treatment aims at relief of myogeloses and of hardened muscles, as otherwise the flexibility of the muscle is decreased.

## START OF TREATMENT

Immediately upon feeling the hardened muscle, or as soon as the pain is felt, treatment is begun.

## PASSIVE TREATMENTS

*Position.*   The athlete should be in the optimal relaxing position during massage.

*Massage.*   The primary treatment of myogeloses is a localized massage. Local kneading, friction, circling, and stylus massage if necessary are to be used. Too vigorous massage can result in reflex pain in tensing the muscle, however. This must be avoided. The hardening that generally forms as a reflex zone around a myogelosis can be treated with a relaxing massage on the lightly stretched muscle. The blood supply is in this case particularly intensive. Underwater massages can also be used.

**Heat.**   The massage must be preceded by a warming of the muscles. This can be done with incandescent light, fango poultices, hot rolled towels, and so forth.

**Hydrotherapy.**   Showers and steam baths can be used as a preparation for massage. Sauna baths are also recommended.

**Electrotherapy.**   Circulation can be stimulated with diadynamic currents. Short-wave radiation, ultrasound, and histamine iontophoresis together with suction electrodes are often used. Treatment with interference currents is also recommended.

## ACTIVE TREATMENTS

**Physical Therapy and Remedial Exercise.**   Active and passive stretching of the muscle affected by myogelosis is important at first. All of the fibers of the muscle group which are hardened must be well mobilized. This can be achieved through minimal changes in the axis and plane of movement. If the stretching exercises are painless, loosening exercises can begin. These must be very gentle and smooth.

Strength is then improved with resistance and tension exercises. The relaxing phase must always be stressed during resistance exercises, however, with gentle massage techniques or repeated shaking to prepare the muscle optimally for a renewed tension. Active techniques for relaxing muscles are also to be used.

Psychologic factors are also of importance in the treatment of muscular tension.

## SPECIAL NOTES

Rapid muscle contraction and jerky motions during stretching are contraindicated.

Myogeloses should be noticed and taken seriously in competitive sports, as they can lead to further damage to the soft tissues.

**Prevention.**   Muscle care with massage, self-massage, sauna, and stretching and loosening exercises are helpful in preventing myogeloses. The athlete should see to it that muscles are always warm, supple, and well vascularized.

# Inflamed Muscles

The symptoms of muscle inflammation include redness, swelling, warmth, and pain. In addition to these symptoms there is dysfunction of the muscle tissue.

The most common causes of muscle inflammation are mechanical, chemical, climatic, or nervous, or attributable to the presence of foreign bodies. The primary causes from participation in sports include overexertion, muscle pulls, cramps, and insufficient flexibility of the muscles. The athlete feels a persistent pain in the inflamed area. Moreover, there is an enduring tension in the muscles. Pressure on the painful area causes an increase in pain, which lasts for an extended period of time.

## GOALS OF TREATMENT

Treatment goals are removal of the inflammation, pain, and restoration of the disturbed function.

## START OF TREATMENT

Begin treatment immediately upon appearance of symptoms of inflammation.

## PASSIVE TREATMENTS

***Positioning, Immobilization, Bandages, and Massage.***  The affected region is immobilized and elevated. Extremities are placed under additional immobilization with an immobilizing bandage.

Draining massage and connective tissue massage in the nonaffected regions of the body, carefully avoiding the inflamed area, are helpful.

***Hydrotherapy.***  During the first days, damp, cold towels are alternated with medicated ointment towel compresses and salve bandages, such as zinc, ichthammol, and similar compounds.

***Electrotherapy.***  A well-regulated ultrasound treatment with histamine iontophoresis has proved effective; also, treatment with diadynamic and interference currents are helpful.

## ACTIVE TREATMENTS

***Physical Therapy and Remedial Exercise.***  The primary task is the immobilization of the inflamed area. Active physical therapy treatment begins in the form of isometric exercises only after the inflammation has subsided. Dynamic exercises and resistance exercises follow, along with complex motions for the affected muscle group. In this way, possible coordination loss is prevented. Exercises in an exercise bath are a good transition and preparation for the stress of training.

### SPECIAL NOTES

Training should resume only after the subsidence of the inflammation. Sufficient diuresis must be encouraged with liquids such as tea and fruit juices, which also supply important vitamins. This is beneficial to the healing process.

*Treatment Contraindicated.*   Local muscle massage and applications of heat and premature resumption of training are to be avoided absolutely.

# Periostitis

Symptoms of periostitis include warmth, swelling, pain, and dysfunctioning of the affected limb, as occurs in every inflammation. The causes can be overloading of the joints on an uneven surface or hard floor, incorrect stress, such as on the take-off leg for high jumpers, local circulatory problems, insufficient flexibility of the respective tendons and muscles, and inflammation of the joints of the affected limb.

Periostitis causes stabbing pain, which is triggered by muscle contraction or stress. The pain extends into the surrounding inflamed area and can also be provoked and increased through pressure. Large periostitic inflammations are characterized by persistent pain while resting.

### GOALS OF TREATMENT

Treatment eliminates both the inflammation and the pain.

### START OF TREATMENT

Begin therapy immediately after the symptoms of inflammation arise.

### PASSIVE TREATMENTS

*Positioning, Immobilization, and Bandages.*   The extremity is relieved of stress and elevated. Immobilizing bandages are indicated.

*Massage.* Drainage massage can be carried out, avoiding the inflamed area. Connective tissue massage is helpful, particularly in the affected segment.

*Cold.* Cold poultices with arnica, heparin, ichthammol, and other anti-inflammatory materials can be applied.

*Heat.* Damp, warm poultices in the later stages, hot rolled towels, and fango poultices are indicated.

*Electrotherapy.* Iontophoresis and ultrasound have proved effective in the acute stage. Diadynamic currents and later microwave and short-wave irradiation are good electrotherapeutic treatments.

## ACTIVE TREATMENT

*Physical Therapy and Remedial Exercise.* Remedial exercises begin in the later phase, after the acute inflammation has subsided. Isometric exercises enhance circulation and help bring the muscle back to its normal strength. The periosteum must not be reinjured in this process. If there is no pain, treatment can progress through resistance and coordination exercises to complex motions. Exercises in the exercise bath prepare the muscles and tissues for the resumption of training stresses. Training should resume only when these movements can be performed painlessly; it should begin slowly at first and gradually progress to the normal extent and intensity.

## SPECIAL NOTES

*Treatments Contraindicated.* Direct massage of the inflamed periosteum and use of heat in acute stages are contraindicated.

*Prevention.* Well-regulated training, improvement of coordination, training on soft ground, use of better athletic shoes, regular muscle massage, and treatment of focal infection, if necessary, are good preventive measures.

# Injured Tendons

A healthy tendon is extremely resistant to most stresses. A sudden, unexpected blow can cause the tendon to be detached from the bone. The condyles may tear in the area of tendon insertions or apophyses in young people. These apophyses have their own growth lines. For this reason, complete healing is necessary to avoid permanent damage.

Tendons which have degenerated owing to lack of exercise, inflammation, or even overweight can be subject to pulling at relatively slight tension.

The following types of injuries may occur: torn tendon, pulled tendon, or strained tendon.

# Torn Tendon

A torn tendon involves the complete severance of the entire tendon insertion of a muscle. The best known are the torn Achilles tendon and the tearing of the tendon of the long head of the biceps on the upper arm where it attaches to the socket of the shoulder joint. These generally are not the result of traumatic injuries, but rather stem from uncoordinated motions. Volleyball, basketball, and handball players experience torn extensor tendons on the distal phalanges; soccer players may tear the quadriceps tendons.

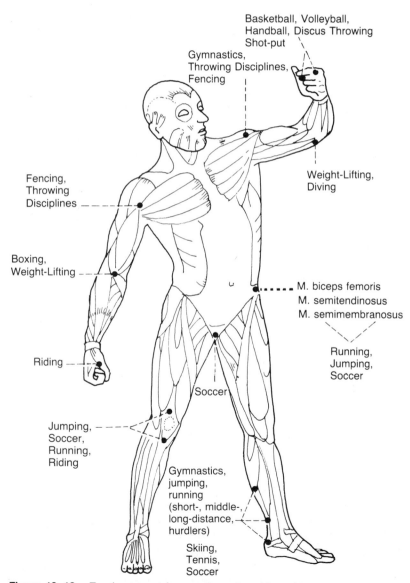

**Figure 13–18.**   Tendons most frequently ruptured in sports.

In contradistinction to torn muscles, ruptured tendons often give indication of previous injury. This previous injury cannot be more specifically defined, however, as ruptures occur in both trained athletes and nonathletes. Histologically intact tendons can also tear; this is known as spontaneous rupture. The tearing of a tendon feels like a sudden blow, and the affected tendon can no longer be tensed. Even when held in a protective position there is throbbing pain. Pressure on the point of injury reveals a hollow, collapsed region. Causes include maximal tension of the muscle, as in jumping or releasing a throw, abrupt stopping of an active motion, passive overextension of a working muscle, and direct, blunt trauma.

Ruptured tendons should be operated on as soon as possible, by the third day at the latest.

## GOALS OF TREATMENT

Goals of treatment include restoration of normal function, prevention of muscle atrophy, and prevention or removal of adhesions.

## START OF TREATMENT

Treatment should begin immediately after the period of immobilization.

## PASSIVE TREATMENTS

***Positioning.***   The sutured tendon is relaxed and the extremity is elevated to encourage venous and lymphatic return.

***Massage.***   Massage of the noninjured body parts is performed. Drainage massage of the injured extremity is helfpul, with strict avoidance of the affected region. Later, massage of the scar will help prevent adhesions.

***Cold.***   Ice treatment, particularly before remedial exercises, can be done.

***Hydrotherapy.***   Lukewarm partial and contrast baths are used before and during the exercises.

***Electrotherapy.***   Galvanization, faradization, and diadynamic currents can be used for the improvement of circulation; use of electrogymnastics equipment is helpful for damaged nerves or innervation disorders.

## ACTIVE TREATMENTS

***Physical Therapy and Remedial Exercise.***   Active exercise begins with isometric tension, then isotonic exercises after a few days. Functional and resistance exercises follow. Careful active stretching and loosening exercises are alternated with the resistance exercises. The threshold of pain should not be exceeded. Exercise baths are a good way to prepare for full stress.

Strengthening exercises in the form of complex motions and training of movement sequences for the athlete's particular sport make up the final phase of treatment.

### SPECIAL NOTES

The active exercises are the most important. These exercises should be painless because of the danger of causing Sudeck's dystrophy.

*Treatments Contraindicated.* Overheating or damp heat; premature massage near the area operated on; and all passive movements are contraindicated.

*First Aid at Competition Site.* Apply cold, elevate extremity, and use immobilizing bandages.

# Strained and Pulled Tendons

A strained tendon results from a sudden, violent overextension of the tendinous tissue, which involves the tearing of the smallest vessels. The athlete feels a stabbing pain, which increases with pressure on the tendon.

Unlike the ruptured tendon, the pulled tendon is usually treated conservatively with immobilization.

A pulled tendon constitutes a more serious injury to the tendinous tissue, in which individual parts of the tendon are torn.

### GOALS OF TREATMENT

Relief of pain, restoration of normal function, prevention of muscular atrophy, and prevention or removal of adhesions are the goals of treatment.

### START OF TREATMENT

Treatment should begin immediately after the immobilization period.

### PASSIVE TREATMENTS

*Positioning, Immobilization, and Bandages.* The injured extremity is elevated and wrapped in an immobilizing bandage, which brings and holds together the insertion and origin of the tendon and its muscle.

*Massage.* Massage of the unaffected body parts and drainage massage of the affected extremity, with strict avoidance of the injured area, are helpful. Later, after the healing, gentle massage can be done for the improvement of circulation. Follow this with deep-reaching massage techniques to loosen adhesions.

*Hydrotherapy.* Fango poultices, contrasting affusions, and contrast baths are recommended.

*Cold and Heat.* Cold applications in the form of ice compresses or ice massage are given in the acute stage. Both cold and heat can be used in the late stages as a preparation for massage and remedial exercises.

*Electrotherapy.* Galvanization, faradization, and diadynamic currents are useful for improvement of circulation. Electrogymnastics aid in treatment of damaged nerves or disorders of innervation.

## ACTIVE TREATMENTS

*Physical Therapy and Remedial Exercise.* Physical therapy is introduced immediately after the immobilization period. This begins with isometric exercises for restoring tone and strength to the affected muscle. Afterward light isotonic exercises are used; the injured tendon must not be overextended in this process. Exercises against manual resistance with the help of devices and in the exercise bath follow. Complex motions can begin when there is no pain. Coordination exercises and exercises for the particular sport conclude the treatment.

## SPECIAL NOTES

*Treatments Contraindicated.* Premature massage and dry heat treatments are contraindicated, as are premature stress on tendon.

*Prevention.* Pulled and strained tendons can be prevented by increased stretching, loosening, and coordination exercises in the endangered area; observance of regular muscle care; and taping of areas at risk before training.

*First Aid at Competition Site.* The pulled tendon and the area surrounding it are treated immediately with ice. Afterward, the tendon is immobilized by fixing the appropriate joint in a protective position with tape or a nonelastic bandage.

# Tendinoses and Tendopathies

The insertion zone of the tendon is the area that receives maximum stress and has the poorest circulation. The tendinous fibers at the transition to the rigid bone are particularly subject to sudden pulls. Overloading this insertion zone can even lead to ossification of the cartilage and to the development of bone spurs. This occurs frequently in the heel. Improper training, prolonged stress, poor coordination, hard running or vaulting surfaces, and other equipment problems frequently are responsible for the development of tendinoses. Incompletely healed traumas can also cause tendinoses. Tendinoses can arise wherever muscle-tendon insertions are found. The muscle-tendon insertions most frequently affected by tendinoses in the particular sports listed are the following:

*Running:* Achilles tendon insertion; insertion of the tibialis anterior and posterior

*Jumping:* Achilles tendon insertion; back extensor insertions

*Throwing, Putting:* Back extensor insertions; insertions on the epicondylus lateralis and epicondylus medialis; insertion of the triceps tendon

*Soccer:* Insertions of the adductors and the iliopsoas, the gracilis, and the rectus abdominis muscles

*Ball games:* Achilles tendon insertion, insertion of the tibialis anterior, insertion of biceps

*Weight lifting:* Triceps tendon insertion

*Tennis:* Insertion of the lower arm extensors

*Fencing:* Insertions on the epicondylus medialis and lateralis; pubic insertion

*Rowing:* Insertion on the spinal processes of the thoracic and lumbar vertebrae.

Tendinoses are characterized by pain at the tendon insertion whenever the muscle is activated. If the muscle, nevertheless, continues to be exercised, pain soon persists when the muscle is at rest, and function ceases completely.

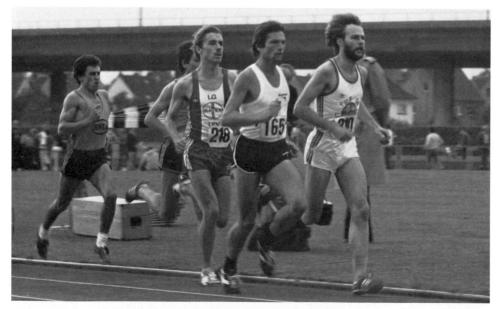

**Figure 13–19.**  Tendinosis and tendopathies of the lower leg in runners, particularly long-distance runners, occur more frequently on artificial surfaces.

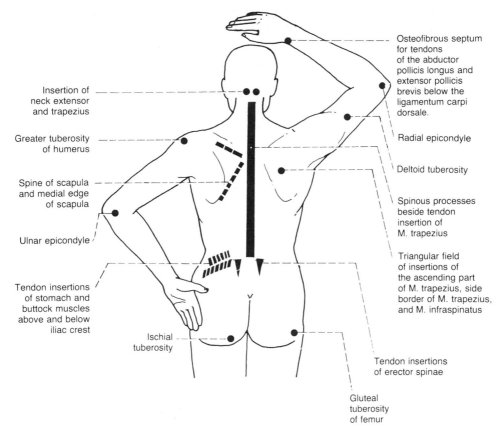

Osteofibrous septum
for tendons
of the abductor
pollicis longus and
extensor pollicis
brevis below the
ligamentum carpi
dorsale.

Insertion of
neck extensor
and trapezius

Greater tuberosity
of humerus

Radial epicondyle

Deltoid tuberosity

Spine of scapula
and medial edge
of scapula

Spinous processes
beside tendon
insertion of
M. trapezius

Ulnar epicondyle

Triangular field
of insertions of
the ascending part
of M. trapezius, side
border of M. trapezius,
and M. infraspinatus

Tendon insertions
of stomach and
buttock muscles
above and below
iliac crest

Ischial
tuberosity

Tendon insertions
of erector spinae

Gluteal
tuberosity
of femur

**Figure 13–20.**    Major areas at which tendopathies and periostitis occur.

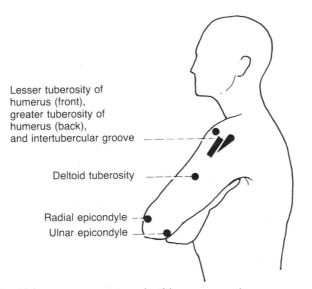

Lesser tuberosity of
humerus (front),
greater tuberosity of
humerus (back),
and intertubercular groove

Deltoid tuberosity

Radial epicondyle

Ulnar epicondyle

**Figure 13–21.**    Major areas at which periostitis occurs on the upper arm and shoulder.

Usually participation in sports is then forbidden for 3 weeks. The rest period and athletic prohibition can last several months in serious cases.

Tendopathies are degenerative changes in the tendon itself or inflammatory processes in the tendon sheath (tenosynonitis). Insufficient circulation in the tissues under maximal one-sided stress causes these changes to occur frequently in athletics. Audible friction noise in the injured tendon is known as paratenonitis crepitans. These injuries arising from faulty stress often require a lengthy recovery period for complete healing.

## GOALS OF TREATMENT

Removal of the irritation and therefore of the pain, restoration of normal function, and strengthening of the muscles are the goals of therapy.

## START OF TREATMENT

Begin treatment immediately after the pain begins.

## PASSIVE TREATMENTS

*Positioning, Immobilization, and Bandages.*    Maintain the protective position. Use immobilizing bandages in the acute condition and supportive bandages to guide motion and limit painful movements.

*Massage.*    Massage can be used for the improvement of circulation exception in the injured area. Connective tissue massage and underwater massage are also recommended.

*Cold.*    Icepacks are helpful in the acute condition; ice massage or other application of cold may also be used.

*Hydrotherapy.*    Contrast baths, Kneipp affusions, later fango poultices, to shorten the recovery period.

*Electrotherapy.*    Electrotherapy plays an important role in the entire treatment of tendinoses and tendopathies. Histamine iontophoresis is particularly effective. These medicines can also be given along with ultrasound.

## ACTIVE TREATMENTS

*Physical Therapy and Remedial Exercises.*    Improvement of the blood supply in the tissues during work periods and in the rest period is of fundamental importance for a successful treatment. Active exercise is at first restricted to isometric exercises, which cause hypertrophy of the muscle fibers.

Furthermore, local, slow isometric muscle contraction to the point of maximal tension permits full relaxation in the muscles. This maximal muscle relaxation prepares for the maximal flexibility of the tendons necessary in athletics. When these isometric exercises are mastered, resistance exercises in the form of complex motions follow. These are primarily for the improvement of coordination. After a week, light active stretching exercises are included in the treatment. Exercises can also be carried out in the exercise bath. Light training on soft ground is possible after 14 days.

## SPECIAL NOTES

*Treatments Contraindicated.*   Massage in the area of the tendon, heat treatment, and intensive exercise before the inflammation has subsided are contraindicated.

*Prevention.*   Training on soft ground; increased coordination exercises to improve the flexibility of the muscle; enhancement of circulation; and regular muscle and body care with massage and sauna are good preventive measures.

*First Aid at Competition Site.*   Cool the area around the tendon and immobilize with bandages in a position that relieves stress.

## CHAPTER 14

# Foot and Leg

*LUTZ MEISSNER, HELMUT ORK,
AND WERNER KUPRIAN*

## Toe Injuries

Toe injuries, such as contusions and sprains, result from sudden impact or kicking of the ground in soccer or in handball and track and field events. Deformities such as hallux valgus or hammer toes encourage such injuries.

### GOALS OF TREATMENT

Goals of treatment include relief of swelling and pain, and restoration to normal stride and to complete readiness for participation in sports.

### START OF TREATMENT

Treatment should begin immediately after the injury.

### PASSIVE TREATMENTS

*Positioning, Immobilization, and Bandages.* Elevate the extremity and apply compression bandages. Tape after the swelling has gone down to permit static stress. Improve the position of the injured toes with foam rubber, felt rings, or tape.

*Cold.* Ice massage may be used, and a cold towel bath for the entire foot may be given.

*Electrotherapy.* Ultrasound and diadynamic currents are helpful.

### ACTIVE TREATMENTS

*Physical Therapy and Remedial Exercise.* Manual therapy is used to put the joint back into place. Traction for the relief of pain is the primary

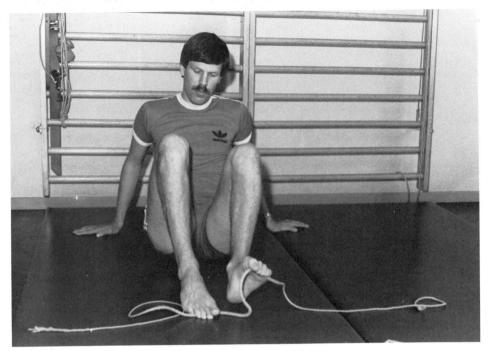

**Figure 14–1.** Foot exercises with rope to strengthen muscles in sole of foot.

consideration. Supportive remedial exercises with and without helping devices reinforce the range of motion gained. The entire mobility of the foot can be improved with exercises, such as tracing shapes in a piece of rope, balling paper together and then flattening it out again with the feet; and picking up pencils with the toes. Six to eight treatments two to three times per week are necessary.

## SPECIAL NOTES

Improvement of strength and stability of the entire foot should be achieved with a program of special exercises (see *Fallen Arches* and *Bruised Heels*). Athletic shoes with protective toepieces are preferred.

*First Aid at the Competition Site.* Apply cold and compression bandage.

# Fallen Arches

Fallen arches develop from stress on the foot that is either too great or lasts too long. Both the soft tissues, particularly the tendons and muscles joined by the plantar aponeurosis, and the bony parts of the foot are affected.

Displacements in the metatarsals and the tarsus called "step formation" can arise. Periostitis or inflammation follows frequently. Deformities of the foot, such as flatfoot, splayfoot, pes valgus, and weak foot muscles contribute to the development of fallen arches. This injury can occur to long distance runners, particularly road and cross-country runners, from stepping into a pothole or on a root; tennis players who play on hard surfaces, soccer players, and gymnasts are also at risk.

## GOALS OF TREATMENT

Relief of pain, reduction of irritation in soft tissue, repositioning of the displaced bones, and resumption of competition are the goals of treatment.

## START OF TREATMENT

Treatment is begun immediately after the injury occurs.

## PASSIVE TREATMENTS

*Positioning, Immobilization, and Bandages.*   Elevate the foot until pain is relieved, then put on supporting tape bandages.

*Massage.*   Massage the foot and leg muscles with exception of the acutely painful area. Relieve adhesions on the sole of the foot and the plantar aponeurosis with friction and stylus massage if necessary.

*Cold.*   Ice massage and ice bath of the entire foot are helpful.

*Electrotherapy.*   Ultrasound and diadynamic currents can be used.

## ACTIVE TREATMENTS

*Physical Therapy and Remedial Exercise.*   Manual therapy is initiated to achieve normal joint function and position, if it is a case of a blocked joint and there is no structural damage to the soft tissues. Remedial exercises are used after relief of pain for strengthening of the entire foot and lower leg to stabilize the arch. Exercises with rope, pencils, paper, towels, balls, and sticks also train the foot muscles. These exercises correct foot statics. Eight to twelve treatments, every other day, generally are necessary.

## SPECIAL NOTES

The athlete should wear shoes with arch supports if necessary. Support the deformity of the foot with tape and foam rubber during training. Running

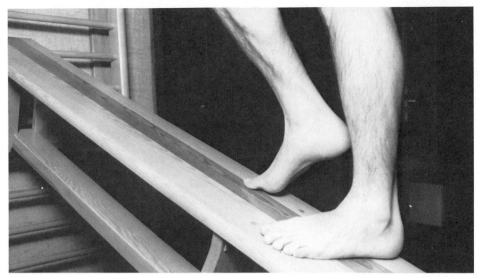

**Figure 14–2.**    Special exercises on a slanted surface: Walking uphill with twisting motion.

barefoot is a good exercise for strengthening in all direction of stress; walking on toes, on heels, and with stiff legs, and running sidewards or backwards strengthen the various running muscles. Also helpful are slow running over uneven terrain, running on sand in large S-curves from dry sand into wet sand, and running in shallow water to water up to the knees and then back again. Repeat the running in water exercise several times, at a quicker tempo; in this exercise, mechanical and thermal qualities of the water are both utilized. Running on stones, up and down hills, diagonally to a slope, and on beams and

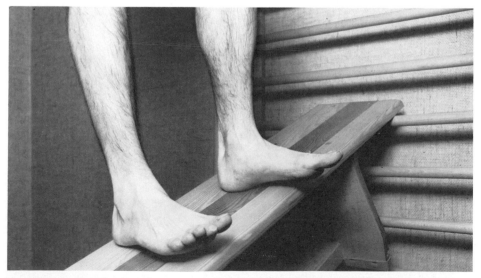

**Figure 14–3.**    Special exercises on a slanted surface: Walking uphill sideways on heels.

fallen tree trunks improves the stability of the foot. Further possibilities for training the muscles of running include special exercises on an incline, with devices for practicing balance, or with a medicine ball.

**First Aid at Competition Site.**    Apply cold and supportive bandages.

# Deformities of the Foot

Deformities such as hammer toes, flatfoot, splayfoot, pes valgus and so forth, should be supported with shoe inserts and tape even if there is no pain during the stress of the sport. If the pain is serious, the athlete must be advised to take up a sport less taxing to the feet.

## GOALS OF TREATMENT

Stabilize and improve the muscles and statics of the foot with active and passive physical therapy treatments and in this way prepare the foot for stresses encountered in sports.

## START OF TREATMENT

Preventive care, if possible, should be taken before the damage occurs; treatment should begin as early as possible.

## PASSIVE TREATMENTS

**Bandages and Inserts.**    Correct and equalize the deformity of the foot with bandages and inserts, thereby relieving stress on the foot.

**Massage.**    Massage the soft tissues of the foot intensively with stylus massage if necessary; remove adhesions and relieve contracted muscles.

**Cold and Heat.**    Stimulate circulation with affusions, rising temperature footbaths, and contrast foot baths.

## ACTIVE TREATMENTS

**Physical Therapy and Remedial Exercise.**    Prevent worsening of the deformity with manual therapy. Reinforce the range of motion achieved with remedial exercise. Improve foot statics. Prevent damage from excessive stress with a correctly adjusted training program, with or without helping devices. (For exercises, see *Injured Toes* and *Fallen Arches*.) Several series of treatments must be conducted with rest pauses.

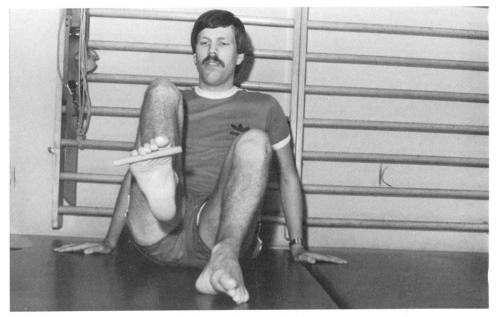

**Figure 14-4.**   Foot exercises with stick for flatfoot and splayfoot.

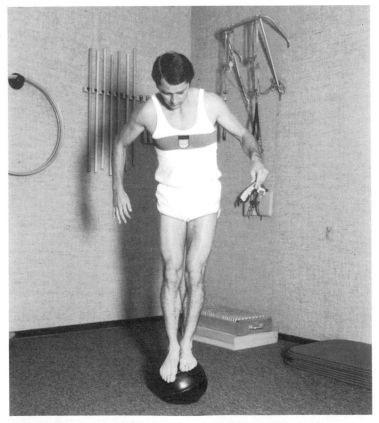

**Figure 14-5.**   Foot and leg exercise with medicine ball.

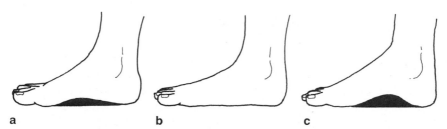

a                          b                        c

**Figure 14–6.** Medial arch of the foot: *a*, normal arch; *b*, flatfoot; *c*, pes cavus.

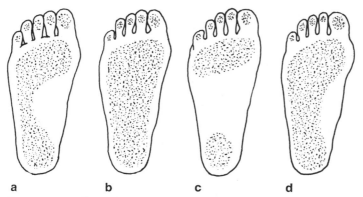

a               b              c              d

**Figure 14–7.** Footprints: *a*, normal; *b*, flatfoot; *c*, hollow-foot; *d*, splayfoot.

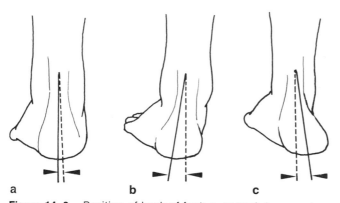

a                         b                        c

**Figure 14–8.** Position of back of foot: *a*, normal; *b*, pes valgus; *c*, pes varus.

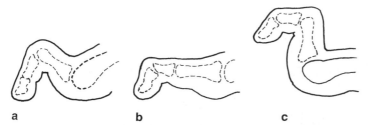

a                         b                        c

**Figure 14–9.** Toe deformities: *a, b,* hammer toe; *c,* cock-up toe.

# Bruised Heels

Bruised heels result from coming down violently on the heel onto a hard surface. The soft tissues of the heel are bruised; additional displacement of the calcaneus occurs only when there is massive bruising. This blockage can reduce the motion of the ankle in both pronation and supination. Periostitis can follow. These injuries occur in jumping events in field sports, hurdling, steeplechase, handball, volleyball, basketball, and gymnastics. The heel swells and is painful when weight is put on it.

## GOALS OF TREATMENT

Treatment goals are relief of swelling and pain, restoration to normal stride and ability to withstand stress, and from there to complete readiness for sports.

## START OF TREATMENT

Immediately after the bruise occurs treatment should begin.

## PASSIVE TREATMENTS

*Positioning, Immobilization, and Bandages.*  Relieve weight and elevate the limb for 24 hours, or longer if the pain continues. Foam rubber compression bandage may be used for the reabsorption of effusion; tape is used later for support.

*Cold.*  Ice therapy and brief submersion of the entire foot in an ice bath are helpful.

*Electrotherapy.*  Ultrasound and diadynamic currents are sometimes used.

## ACTIVE TREATMENTS

*Physical Therapy and Remedial Exercise.*  Manual therapy is used to correct joint blockages. While the leg is elevated, general remedial exercises are suggested for strengthening foot and leg muscles. Afterwards careful stress is placed on the leg in remedial walking, and also in the exercise bath. For remedial walking, the heel should be elevated with a foam rubber insert. The heel can also be covered with a nylon heelpiece for protection. Daily treatment for 8 to 12 days is generally necessary.

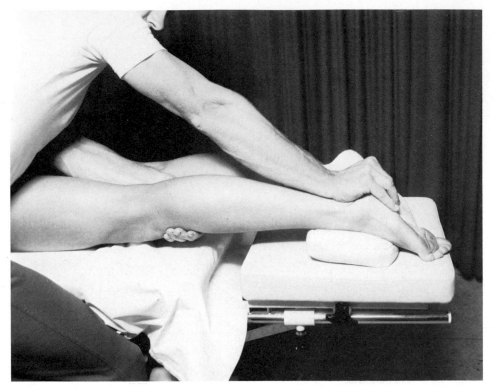

**Figure 14–10.** Manual joint therapy for bruised heel.

## SPECIAL NOTES

Resume training when the pain subsides; avoid hard ground and use a tape bandage for support at first. Use athletic shoes with raised heels. Put additional foam rubber heel pads in the shoes.

*First Aid at Competition Site.* Apply cold and elevate the leg with bandages.

# Sprained Ankle

Sprained ankles are among the most frequent and most typical athletic injuries to the lower leg. The susceptibility to this type of injury is due to anatomic structure and functional stress. Over 15 per cent of all athletic injuries are to the ankle.

Sprained ankles occur frequently in games such as basketball, volleyball, handball, and soccer. They can be precipitated by uneven ground, edges of mats, and cracks in the floor in gymnastics and jumping sports, as well as in combative sports such as judo and wrestling. They can result in both strained ligaments and ruptures and tears of the origin on the malleolus or the insertion on the tarsus. The tight connection needed for proper functioning is

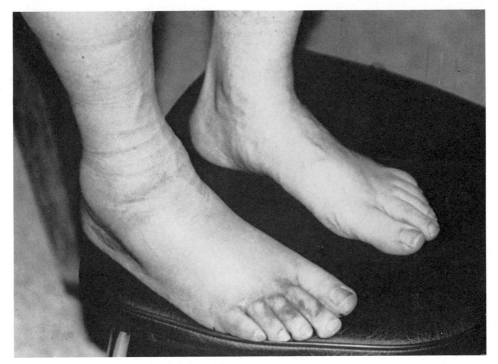

**Figure 14–11.** Badly sprained right ankle.

performed by a complex system of ligaments. If the functional limits of the ligament system are overextended, ligamentous or ankle injury can occur.

## GOALS OF TREATMENT

Goals of treatment are avoidance of swelling and stases in ankle region; reabsorption of hematoma; restoration of normal function; and avoidance of muscular atrophy.

## START OF TREATMENT

Immediately after the athletic injury occurs, treatment should begin to prevent the development or expansion of a hematoma.

## PASSIVE TREATMENTS

***Positioning, Immobilization, and Bandages.*** Elevation to encourage venous and lymphatic return and drainage. Compression bandages are used in the acute stage, then supportive elastic bandages, tape, and zinc ointment bandages.

**Cold.**  Ice treatment is helpful for the reabsorption of effusion; immersion in partial ice bath, ice bag, and ice massage are additional measures.

**Heat.**  In the late stages, after the complete reabsorption of the effusion, use heat to prepare for massage.

**Massage.**  In the acute stages, perform drainage massage of the entire lower and upper leg muscles of the noninjured leg. Relieve adhesions and deposits in the area of the moving joint in the late phases.

**Electrotherapy.**  Ultrasound, iontophoresis, ionomodulator, and diadynamic currents are useful.

## ACTIVE TREATMENTS

**Physical Therapy and Remedial Exercise.**  Isometric exercises begin while the leg is elevated. Then dynamic exercises begin, with and without resistance, with emphasis on dorsal flexion and pronation, as sprains generally involve supination of the foot. Complex motions for the entire leg are introduced for further stabilization of all the leg muscles. Training for partial stress on balances and seesaws, with remedial walking in the exercise bath follow. Manual therapy is used to achieve free joint play. The joint is placed under increasing stress in walking and running motions and limited jogging on soft ground. Eight to twelve treatments are necessary.

## SPECIAL NOTES

Most sprained ankles require an interruption in the training schedule for those sports that place particular stress on the legs and feet. Well-fitted shoes and supportive bandages are important upon resumption of training. The soles of the shoes must be constructed so that they prevent the foot from twisting. Further considerations include the good physiologic pattern of motion, coordination training, and further strengthening of the muscle-ligament apparatus of the foot and leg.

**First Aid at the Competition Site.**  Apply cold and use cool spray, which can be sprayed on through sock; elevate the leg and relieve stress on the injured ankle; use compression bandages and salves to aid reabsorption.

# Ruptured Achilles Tendon
# (Postoperative Treatment)

Ruptured Achilles tendon is a classic athletic injury. It has become considerably more frequent in various athletic disciplines in recent years. The reasons for this increase are still uncertain. Schoberth reports that he encounters ruptured Achilles tendons more frequently in athletes who perform indoors than in those who perform outdoors such as soccer players. A connection between the injuries and the widespread use of artificial track surfaces and floors is suspected. This injury affects track and field athletes, long and high jumpers, triple jumpers, gymnasts, soccer players, and tennis players.

The Achilles tendon usually ruptures suddenly. The injured person says that he felt a strong blow in the area of the Achilles tendon, as if he had been hit with a stone. This typical "whiplash" is frequently reported. The rupture generally occurs without having received a blow from either an opposing player or a foreign object, however. Causes include previously damaged tendinous tissues, degenerative changes, persistent overloading of the joint, peritonitis achillea, and traumatic damage. Excessive cortisone injections and sudden cold have also been considered causes of the injury.

## GOALS OF TREATMENT

Among the goals of treatment are prevention of muscle atrophy, particularly of the triceps surae, but also of the rest of the upper and lower operated leg; prevention of adhesions; removal of trophic disorders; restoration of normal function to complete athletic ability; and prevention of training loss in the healthy areas of the body and in general condition.

## START OF TREATMENT

For the healthy parts of the body, treatment can begin on the first postoperative day, and on the injured leg 2 to 6 weeks after the operation and immobilization in cast.

## PASSIVE TREATMENT

*Positioning.*   Place the extremity in a comfortable position for both the sutured tendon and the entire leg, with slight elevation to encourage venous and lymphatic return and drainage.

*Massage.*   Massage the healthy leg, buttocks, and the lower back as well as the upper thigh of the injured leg; later perform scar massage.

*Cold.*   Ice treatment should be done before the remedial exercises.

*Hydrotherapy.*   Contrast foot baths or lukewarm partial baths are helpful after the scar from operation has healed, and before or during the therapy with remedial exercises.

*Electrotherapy.*   Galvanization, faradization, diadynamic currents, and electrogymnastic equipment are used for innervation damage and accompanying nerve damage.

## ACTIVE TREATMENTS

*Physical Therapy and Remedial Exercise.*   Remedial exercises begin on the healthy leg with active motions of all joints, at first without resistance, but soon against strong manual resistance. Also included are general circulatory, breathing, and conditioning exercises. Back and stomach muscles and arms must be exercised to limit the loss in strength.

Isometric exercises are recommended first for the muscles of the injured leg and foot. Afterward one- and two-dimensional exercises with bending in the knee and ankle are advised. These are performed first without resistance, then with manual resistance. Careful and complete active stretching exercises

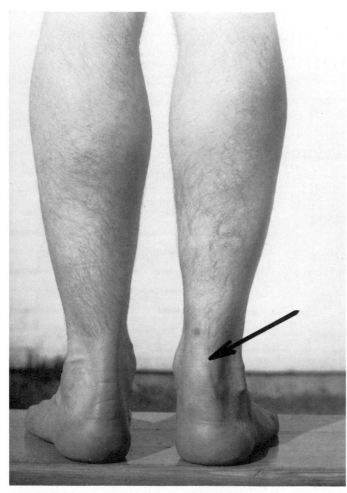

**Figure 14–12.**   Healed scar from operation.

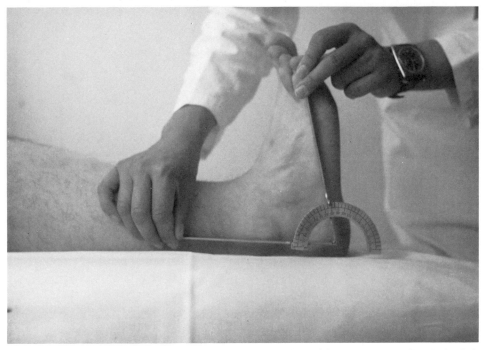

**Figure 14–13.**  Measurement of the mobility of the ankle with protractor at the start of the treatment.

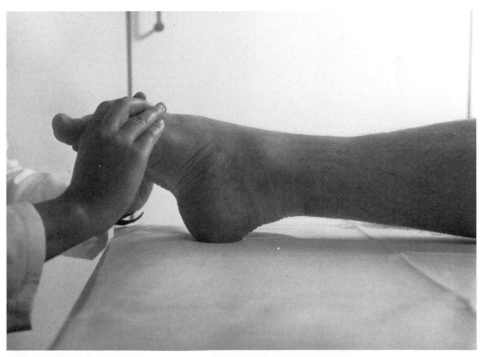

**Figure 14–14.**  Exercise of plantar flexion against manual resistance.

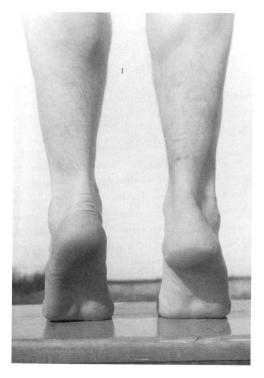

**Figure 14–15.** Exercise of plantar flexion under stress.

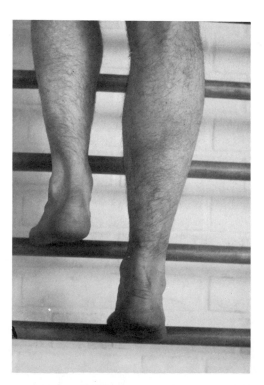

**Figure 14–16.** Stretching exercises on the wall bars.

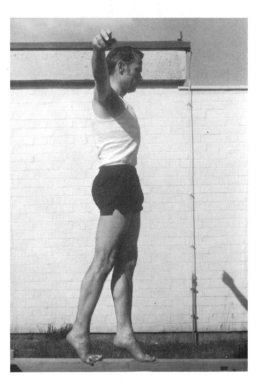

**Figure 14–17.** Walking on toes on the balance beam.

can be recommended for limited dorsal and plantar flexion. The pain threshold should not be exceeded. Active supination and pronation exercises follow; grasping with toes and plantar flexion against strong resistance follow. All exercises should be carried out in a position that encourages venous and lymphatic return. Three-dimensional complex motions for further strengthening of the muscle groups are recommended. After eight to ten treatments, exercises in the sitting position and partial stress in standing and walking — also in the exercise bath — can begin. Functional exercises follow, such as walking and climbing steps, use of slanted surfaces and wall bars, standing and walking on toes; later exercises include running, hopping, and jumping, at first extremely carefully, on mats and soft grass. The final stage of physical therapy includes cross-country running, skipping and jumping rope, running on uneven ground, kicking a medicine ball, exercises for the athlete's particular sport, and exercises for coarse and fine motor skills. Concentration must be on the restoration of strong plantar flexion and thus the restrengthening of the gastrocnemius and the soleus muscles.

Twenty treatments are needed daily at first; later treatments are scheduled two to three times per week.

## SPECIAL NOTES

All overheating and hyperemia-causing passive treatments, such as hot air, incandescent light, hot baths, and so forth, should be avoided because of

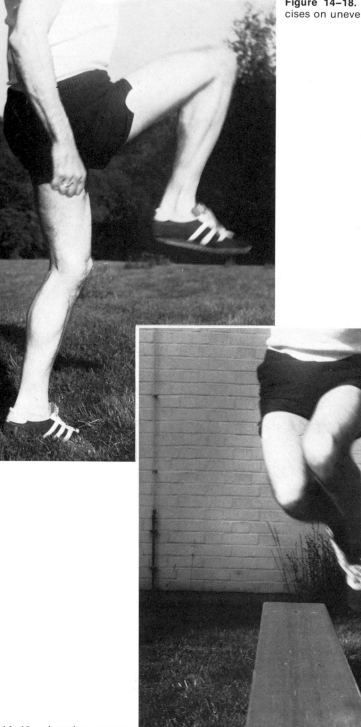

**Figure 14–18.** Skipping exercises on uneven surface.

**Figure 14–19.** Jumping over a bench. Function is normal.

the danger of causing Sudeck's dystrophy. Massage techniques other than massage of scar tissue are contraindicated on the operated leg (lower leg). The emphasis should be on a well-regulated active physical therapy program of exercise. The pain threshold should be observed during all exercise. Passive exercises, other than light stretching after active dorsal and plantar flexion, are not necessary. The use of athletic shoes that are "kind to the Achilles tendon," having a good insole and a slightly raised and padded heel, is recommended.

Bandages, tape, and socks for the protection of the sensitive scar are also recommended. Excessive stress should be avoided upon resumption of training. Exercising on soft ground is important. The trainer's supervision and advice are necessary.

# Achillodynia

Achillodynia is an irritation of the insertion of the Achilles tendon. It is one of the most commonly encountered tendon disorders in athletics. It affects runners, sprinters, tennis and soccer players, hockey players, speed skaters, and skiers. Symptoms include pain in the tendon during and after the athletic performance, and pain from pressure, particularly on the tuber calcanei, the tendon, and the surrounding area. Pain usually builds gradually; it seldom occurs suddenly. Excess stress is usually the cause. Additional causes of this irritation include improper statics of the feet, splayfoot, pes valgus, flatfoot, deep-lying calcaneus, false running technique, poor shoes, hard ski slopes, and artificial running surfaces, as well as strained tendons, which can finally make running impossible.

## GOALS OF TREATMENT

Treatment goals are reduction of irritation, relief of pain, and restoration of normal running function.

## START OF TREATMENT

Immediately after the injury occurs, immobilize the leg and apply bandages. After about an 8 day rest, ice treatments, diadynamic currents, remedial exercises, and massage are offered.

## PASSIVE TREATMENTS

***Positioning, Immobilization, and Bandages.***    Immobilize the leg for 8 to 10 days in either a plaster cast, a supportive Elastoplast, or a tape bandage with additional elevation. A stirrup made out of Leuko-Tape with foam rubber cushioning for the Achilles tendon is recommended. The discomfort is usually relieved simply by elevating the heel with an insert, or better, by placing a wedge between the welt and the sole of the shoe.

*Massage.*   Stylus massage in the area of the tendon and manual massage of the upper and lower leg can be done.

*Cold.*   Ice therapy is used before the massage and remedial exercise.

*Electrotherapy.*   Ultrasound, microwaves, and diadynamic currents are helpful treatments.

## ACTIVE TREATMENTS

*Physical Therapy and Remedial Exercise.*   Physical therapy begins with isometric exercises for the entire leg while it is elevated. These are followed by dynamic exercises for dorsal and plantar flexion, supination and pronation, and adduction and abduction in the ankles, after the acute condition has receded. Light, complete active and passive stretching of the Achilles tendon and the triceps surae is recommended. Foot statics should be corrected with active exercises, and the muscles of the foot and lower leg should be strengthened. Complex motions for the entire leg and remedial walking and running complete the program of physical therapy. Afterward a guided transition is made to exercises for the athlete's particular sport and finally to the resumption of normal training. Eight to twelve treatments, two to three times per week, are necessary.

## SPECIAL NOTES

The use of heat is not recommended. Particularly good athletic shoes with slightly raised heels are very important. It may be necessary to fit an insert

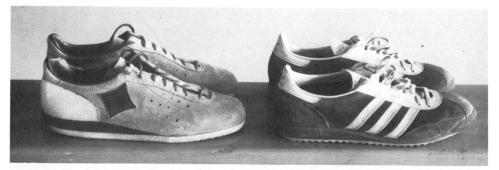

**Figure 14–20.**   Athletic shoes with slightly raised heels to relieve stress on Achilles tendon.

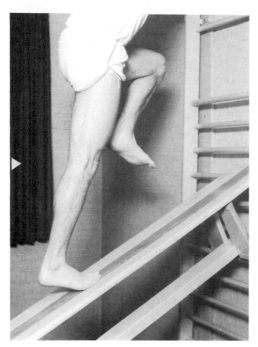 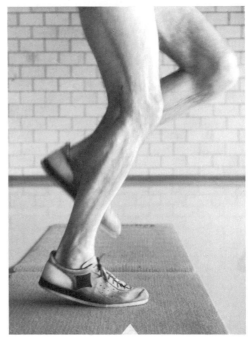

**Figure 14–21.** Stretching exercises for the Achilles tendon and calf muscles on a slanted surface.

**Figure 14–22.** Running in place.

into the shoe to correct the foot statics. The athlete should avoid hard surfaces and train on soft ground. Use of a supportive bandage is recommended upon resumption of training and in competition. Active stretching of the calves is valuable after a good warm-up; the actual training should begin only then. Persistent discomfort may indicate focal infection, which must be eradicated.

# Meniscus Injury (Postoperative Treatment)

The traumatic tearing of the meniscus results from a sudden twisting of the knee. If the tibia is locked in position and stress is placed on the knee on the inner side when the upper body is rotated, the result can be an injury to the inner meniscus. This motion occurs in skiing, track and field sports, wrestling, soccer, handball, basketball, and ballet. Trauma to the inner meniscus is always connected with damage to the transverse ligament of the knee. The larger medial meniscus surrounds the small circular lateral meniscus in the shape of a half moon. The medial meniscus is tightly connected to the broad transverse ligament. Injury to the outer meniscus is considerably less common.

Degenerative damage to the meniscus results from recurrent stress in a kneeling or squatting position. It is a chronic disorder for miners and gardeners. The traumatic damage is frequently preceded by degenerative changes. It is characterized by frequent relapses, pinching, instability of the knee and a feeling of unsteadiness under stress and in particular movements. Associated symptoms include joint effusions, pain, and atrophy of the quadriceps.

Typical signs of recent meniscus damage include strong pain in an overextension of the knee, spontaneous pain during the rotation of the bent lower leg at the hinge of the joint, pinching, and joint effusions. The surgical removal of the torn meniscus cannot be avoided by such conservative treatments as immobilization, and so forth. The results in a properly diagnosed case are generally good, if remedial exercise and other physical therapy treatments follow.

## GOALS OF TREATMENT

Goals of treatment include removal of joint effusions; restoration of normal joint function; reinforcement of the knee by strengthening the muscle-ligament apparatus of the entire leg, particularly of the quadriceps and the muscle group of the pes anserinus; prevention of training loss in the healthy body parts; prevention of loss of general conditioning; and restoration and resumption of training to achieve complete athletic ability.

## START OF TREATMENT

On the healthy leg, torso, and arms treatment should begin on the first postoperative day; conditioning also begins on the first postoperative day.

Joint effusion treatment and isometric exercises should begin on the operated leg on the second postoperative day, after the acute pain has receded, while the leg is still in a splint or cast, if necessary.

## PASSIVE TREATMENTS

*Positioning.* Elevate the leg by propping up the bed or the leg supports of the training table to encourage venous and lymphatic return and drainage. Use light hip and knee flexion, as well as neutral rotation position. Strive for 90 degree dorsal extension in the ankle.

*Massage.* Drainage massage of the upper and lower thigh and feet is helpful. Later, vigorous massage is given in preparation for remedial exercise.

*Cold and Bandages.* Ice treatment with compression bandage aids reabsorption of the joint effusion and swelling. Cold towels, ice compresses, or icebags are applied for 10 to 15 minutes. Afterward a pressure bandage, which has foam rubber padding, is applied. The bandage is worn for 2 to 3 days and is removed only for renewed ice treatments during this time.

***Electrotherapy.*** Ultrasound and diadynamic currents are good therapeutic modalities.

## ACTIVE TREATMENTS

***Physical Therapy and Remedial Exercise.*** Active physical therapy begins on the healthy body parts while the affected knee is still immobilized after surgery. This is done to maintain their function and general conditioning.

The stitches are removed from the knee after about 14 days. A joint effusion treatment during this time is valuable. Daily isometric exercises can also be carried out while the leg is being treated with the previously described ice compression bandage. The strengthening of the muscle-ligament apparatus, the achievement of complete extension, and the stabilization of the knee with isometric exercises are the most important goals. Once the patient is introduced to these exercises, he should carry them out himself several times daily.

When the wound has closed and the stitches are removed, exercise can also begin in the exercise bath. The stability of the knee is more important than its flexibility, however. The ligaments, which are usually also damaged, as well as all the muscles of the upper thigh (primarily the quadriceps, vastus medius, sartorius, gracilis, and the semitendinosus), must be strengthened.

After the cast or splint has been removed, isometric and then dynamic exercises are added for the foot, knee, and hip muscles, at first without and later with manual resistance. The flexion of the knee should be practiced only actively and at first without resistance. It plays a less important role in stabilization and walking movements. Flexion must not be passively forced. The movements originally exercised in insolation are soon combined in prone, supine, and side positions while the weight on the leg is relieved. Sitting on the edge of the treatment bench or bed is a good initial position for the exercise. The lower leg hangs down under its own weight, in so far as the contracture permits. Stretching can be practiced against the weight of the lower leg. The patient can easily see progress in this motion. A sandbag or weighted shoe (2 to 4 kg) can accelerate this process. Manual therapy is possible also in cases where free joint play is limited.

Complex motions serve to increase strength. The leg is under maximal tension. The tension is built up from the distal to proximal regions. The patient should move his leg smoothly over the full range of its motion. The exercise can be increased with holding work. The athlete must exercise until tiring to train muscular strength and endurance. Only when the knee is stabilized can resistance be given distally from the knee joint.

Sling supports can also be used for valuable stretching and bending

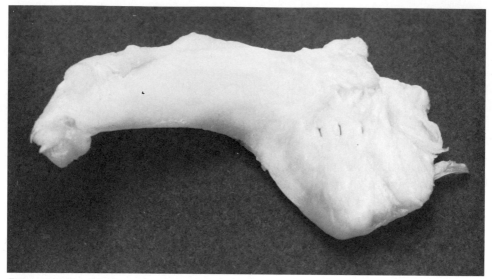

**Figure 14–23.** Meniscus specimen.

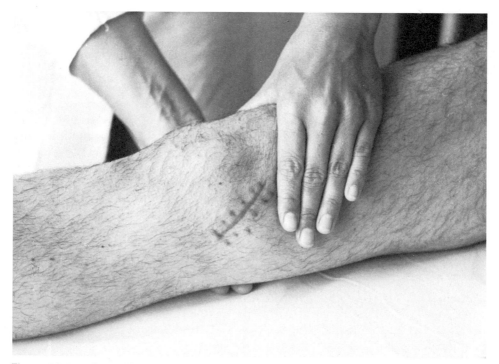

**Figure 14–24.** Isometric exercises after meniscus operation.

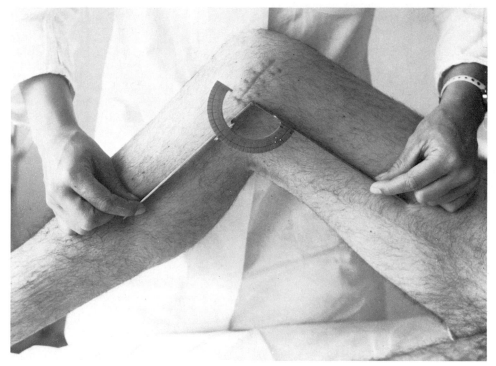

**Figure 14–25.**  Measurement of mobility of knee.

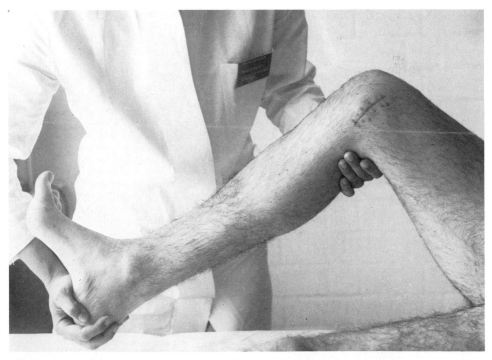

**Figure 14–26.**  Extensor exercises against manual resistance.

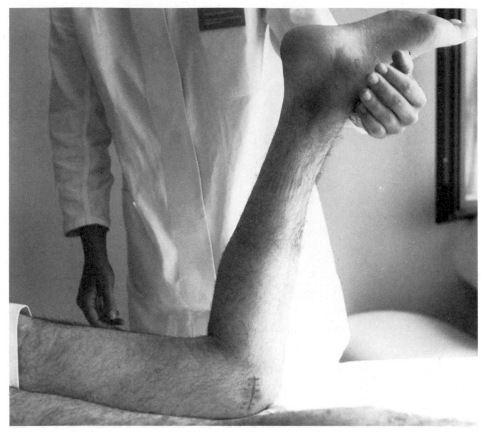

**Figure 14–27.** Flexor exercises for knee. Overcoming force of gravity with manual guidance.

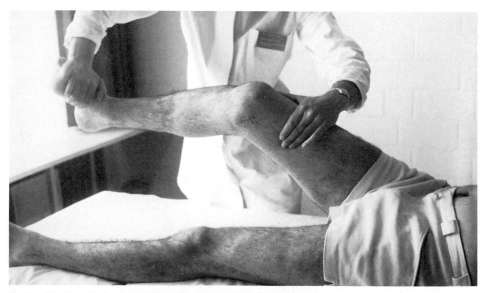

**Figure 14–28.** Complex motions for the leg after surgery.

exercises for the knee and for adduction and abduction of the hip with resistance with spring pulls and weights.

The first partial stress should be carried out in water, at first in deep water, later in shallow. Climbing steps in water should also be practiced. The patient walks with the aid of lower arm supports. Later, partial stress while standing follows. The patient supports himself on wall bars or a rail. Shifting weight in a straddle and split position follows, and then the first walking exercises without support. Use forward, backward, and sideways walking; climbing stairs; and devices such as medicine balls, dumbbells, exercise bicycles, rowing machines, and Universal Gym. The Deuser belt can be used for individual exercises.

Gradually the remedial exercises merge into training exercises for the particular sport. Knee bends, with dumbbells, small jumps, running, dribbling a soccer ball, jumping rope, and exercises suited to his or her particular sport bring the athlete to the goal of ability to withstand complete stress in training and competition after about 6 to 10 weeks. Twenty to 30 treatments are necessary for this, daily at first, then two to three times per week.

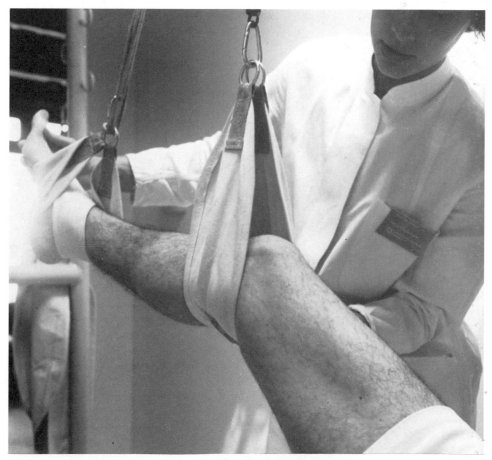

**Figure 14–29.** Flexor and extensor exercises in supporting sling.

**Figure 14–30.** Flexor exercises with small sandbag.

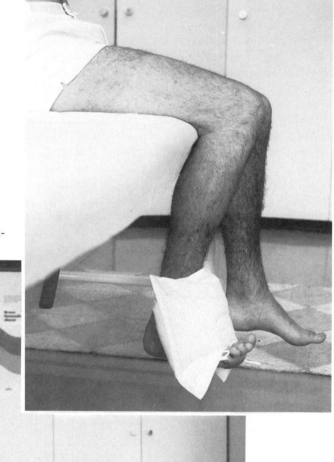

**Figure 14–31.** Extensor exercises with small sandbag.

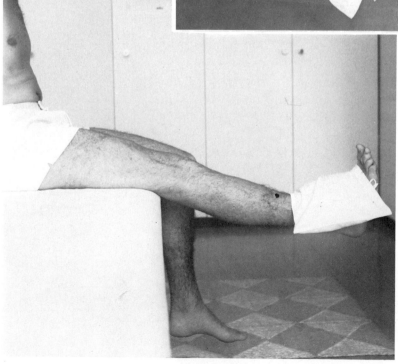

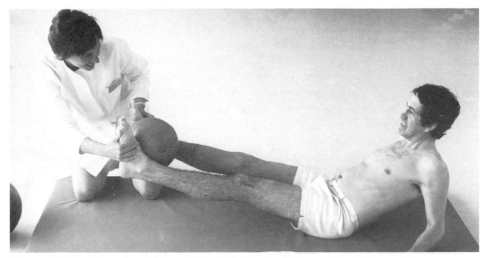

**Figure 14–32.**   Strengthening exercises for both legs with medicine ball.

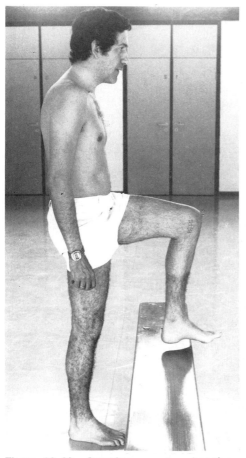

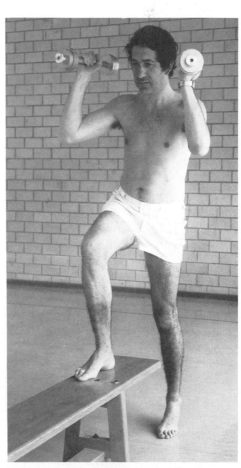

**Figure 14–33.**  Stepping up onto a bench —
strengthening of knee extension.

**Figure 14–34.**  Strengthening of extension
with additional weight.

## SPECIAL NOTES

All uses of heat, such as hot air, incandescent light, fango, and so forth, are contraindicated; so is massage of the joint and surrounding areas.

Passive and jerky movements of the knee are to be avoided. Treatment in water should begin only after the scar has completely closed.

Only isometric exercises should be used if renewed effusion occurs, and there should be no further motion of the knee; renew ice treatments.

At the start of the normal athletic training, bandages and tape can be used to protect the knee. The muscles should be kept warm with the proper training gear. Supervision and advice by the trainer are recommended.

*First Aid at the Competition Site.* Use of ice compression bandage, removal of stress, and elevation of the leg are advised.

*Prevention.* Avoidance of extreme torsion motions in the knee joint, strengthening of the muscle-ligament apparatus of the knee, and use of tape bandages are good preventive measures.

# Ligament Injury to the Knee

The knee is the most frequently injured joint in athletics. This is due to the specific demands of the various sports and the knee's special susceptibility to injury, owing to its specific anatomic and mechanical structure. Capsule ligament injuries usually occur in connection with flexion, rotation, abduction, and adduction mechanisms of the knee. Both collateral ligaments, both cruciate ligaments, and the joint capsule can be injured. The tibial collateral ligament is most frequently injured. An additional injury to the meniscus and bones is also possible. A conservative immobilization using an upper thigh cast with the knee bent at an angle of about 20 degrees is usually sufficient for capsule ligament injuries resulting from stretching or very minor injuries. An operation is required for capsule ligament ruptures and more serious instabilities. This type of injury occurs primarily in soccer, handball, downhill skiing, and combative sports such as judo and wrestling.

## GOALS OF TREATMENT

After conservative or operative treatment and immobilization, restoration of the normal joint function, stabilization of the knee, and strengthening of the muscle-ligament apparatus are the primary treatment objectives; other goals include prevention of losses of training and conditioning in the healthy body parts; renewed stress on the injured leg; and training to bring the athlete to complete athletic ability.

## START OF TREATMENT

All noninjured body parts are exercised during immobilization to avoid unnecessary training loss. Isometric exercises are also possible for the injured leg during immobilization. After the cast is removed, isometric stretching exercises begin.

## PASSIVE TREATMENTS

*Positioning.*   Keep the knee elevated at an angle of approximately 20 degrees between treatments. Higher elevation encourages venous and lymphatic return and drainage. The hips are slightly bent and the ankle placed in 90 degrees dorsal extension.

*Massage.*   Drainage massage of the entire leg, with exception of injured area, is performed. Vigorous massage of the other body areas prepares the athlete for remedial exercise. Transverse friction on the injured area in the late stages will break down adhesions and deposits.

*Cold and Bandages.*   A compression bandage with icebags or ice compresses is used for about 15 minutes if swelling develops after the cast is removed or if effusions develop during initial stress. After the remedial exercise, put on a new compression bandage with foam rubber padding. This continues until the swelling dies down.

*Electrotherapy.*   Ultrasound and diadynamic currents are helpful treatments.

## ACTIVE TREATMENTS

*Physical Therapy and Remedial Exercise.*   The noninjured parts of the body are intensively exercised while the injured knee is immobilized to maintain the function of joints and muscles and the body's overall condition. Medicine balls and other apparatus aid in this treatment. Cardiovascular exercises can take the form of one-legged or two-legged work on an exercise bicycle or use of a rowing machine.

After the cast is removed, a series of isometric exercises for the injured knee begin, every 2 to 3 hours. The primary concern in treatment is developing the stability of the knee and its full flexibility. The joint play and also the movement of the patella are improved with gentle manual therapy without endangering the recently healed tendons. The extent of motion achieved is reinforced with active exercises. Only then does training for strength, muscular endurance, and flexibility begin. The active exercises must improve the condition of all the muscles of the leg and thus provide for muscular stability.

Active one- and two-dimensional motions begin after the isometric exercises, first without and then with resistance. The following three-dimensional complex motions represent a further increase. The athlete initially lies on his or her side; prone and supine positions follow. The exercises are in accordance with the extent of the newly developed strength. The legs are first exercised in water. Remedial walking in water is practiced along with relaxing exercises, such as swimming crawl stroke and later swimming with fins. The stress is increased as the water becomes shallower. This so-called "minus training" permits a gradual increase of stress on the injured area. Bicycling with both legs, then with one, and bicycling forward and backward with the injured leg represent further increases in training. These are followed by remedial walking together with stair climbing and walking on various surfaces. Running without full weight is a transition to the stresses found in sports; this is possible by having the athlete support himself partially with the arms in a Universal Gym or by running in a supporting harness. Running on soft mats and soft ground permits a further increase in strength. Athletic training begins only when stability, muscular strength, and endurance have become normal. (See also *Meniscus Injury.*) Twenty to 30 treatments, three times per week are required.

## SPECIAL NOTES

*Treatments Contraindicated.*   Heat and passive motions should be avoided, as should overextension of the capsule-ligament apparatus.

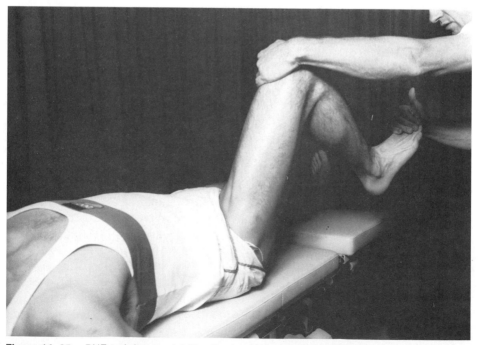

**Figure 14–35.**   PNF training to stabilize the knee after damage to cartilage.

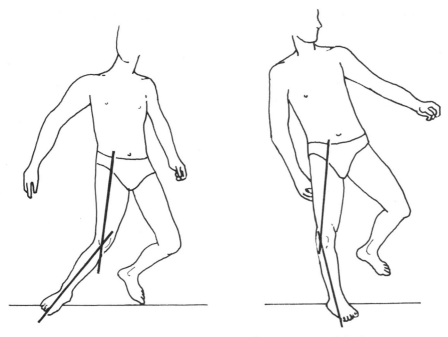

**Figure 14-36.**   Mechanism of injury in capsule-ligament tears of the knee.

**Prevention.**   Participants in sports with heavy stress on capsule liga-ments of the knee, such as soccer, handball, and downhill skiing, should take care to develop strength, muscular endurance, and stability in the knees.

**First Aid at Competition Site.**   Apply cold and compression bandages, relieve stress, and elevate the injured leg.

# Irritated Knee

Irritation to the knee can result from a variety of causes. It is usually coupled with vague complaints, and symptoms frequently include irregular swelling and fluctuating joint effusions with a "floating patella," particularly after heavy athletic stress. In most cases the irritated knee results from an unphysiologic stress. The extent and frequency of the occurrence depends on the amount of stress, conditioning, tiredness, age, and type of running surface. Incompletely healed athletic injuries of the knee and premature stress after recent injury can also lead to chronic inflammations and irritation. A diagnosis of the cause and its elimination are important.

## GOALS OF TREATMENT

Relief of irritation, freedom from pain, and restoration to normal running function are the goals of treatment.

### START OF TREATMENT

Begin treatment immediately after the irritation develops.

### PASSIVE TREATMENTS

*Positioning, Immobilization, and Bandages.*   Use immobilizing bandages at first, or a plaster cast, if necessary; elevation of the leg while relaxing is recommended for 8 to 14 days.

*Massage.*   A drainage massage of all leg muscles should be performed.

*Cold.*   Apply cold in form of ice packs, cold towels, and ice massage to relieve swelling and to prepare for remedial exercise.

*Electrotherapy.*   Diadynamic currents and ultrasound are useful.

### ACTIVE TREATMENT

*Physical Therapy and Remedial Exercise.*   Isometric and later isotonic exercises are begun with active resistance until maximal flexion in the knee is achieved while the leg is elevated horizontally. Isometric and isotonic exercises

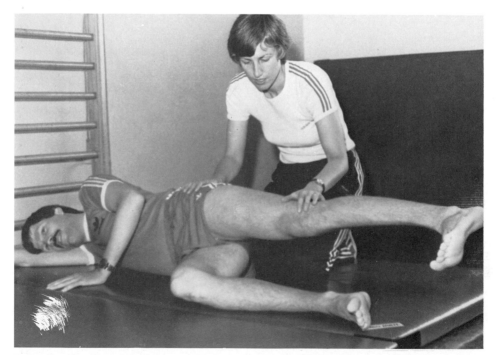

**Figure 14–37.**   Exercise of leg muscles in the lateral position with relief of stress on knee.

are also used for the preservation of muscular strength in the entire leg and foot and for attaining normal knee function. These are followed by complex motions. Begin all exercises with the leg elevated and horizontal. Make slow transition to exercise with partial and later full stress only when there is no more pain. Follow this with remedial walking and running of increasing duration and intensity. The exercise bicycle may be used for supplementary training. About 12 to 20 treatments are necessary.

### SPECIAL NOTES

All uses of heat are contraindicated in the acute stages. Check the ground condition and movement sequences. If a relapse occurs, relieve stress immediately and cool the knee again.

# Chondromalacia Patellae

Chondromalacia patellae is a prearthritic condition observed even in early years of life. It is most common between the second and fourth decades of life in participants in sports like soccer, judo, volleyball, basketball, and downhill skiing. Its symptoms include pain from pressure and motion, crepitation, and possible swelling in the knee.

The degenerative symptoms in the knee are caused by biomechanical processes, which begin with poor blood supply in the synovial capsule or improper nourishment of the cartilage. For example, these symptoms may result from enzymatic and compressive damage to the synovial vessels through irritation and blood effusions; fibrosis of the synovial capsule through inflammation; and hypertrophy of the cartilage in young top competitive performers.

An understanding of the biomechanics and the pathophysiology of the knee is therefore required for a correct interpretation of the symptoms of chondromalacia patellae, which can also include the following endogenous and exogenous disorders: form variations and deformities of the knee, improper position of the patella, dysplasia of the femoral condyles, local or general infection, physiologic change, disrupted joint mechanics, meniscus and capsule-ligament lesions, repeated or excessive stress, and trauma.

Chondromalacia patellae can also arise secondarily from other damage to the knee, such as meniscal injuries.

Both conservative and surgical treatment may be required, depending on the indications. Operative treatment permits early dynamic exercise, whereas conservative therapy can require a cast for 6 to 10 weeks.

### GOALS OF TREATMENT

Treatment aims at removal of effusion, restoration of the muscular strength to the entire leg, and achievement of normal running function.

### START OF TREATMENT

Treatment begins after immobilization or following surgery.

### PASSIVE TREATMENT WITH CONSERVATIVE CARE

*Positioning.*    Elevate the extremity and relieve stress while the leg is slightly bent, at an angle of approximately 20 degrees.

*Massage.*    Perform drainage massage of the entire leg and vigorous massage of the other body parts as a preparation for the remedial exercises.

*Cold and Bandages.*    Apply cold together with compression bandages for swelling and irritation, while the leg remains elevated.

*Heat.*    In the chronic state, incandescent light, hot towels, and fango poultices are helpful.

*Electrotherapy.*    Diadynamic currents, ultrasound, and iontophoresis can be used.

### PASSIVE TREATMENT WITH SURGERY

*Positioning.*    Elevate the leg and relieve stress while the knee is bent to approximately 20 degrees.

*Massage.*    Perform drainage massage of the upper thigh with the exception of the area that was operated on. Vigorous massage of the other leg and other parts of body may also be done as a preparation for remedial exercises.

*Cold and Bandages.*    Apply cold together with compression bandages for swelling and irritation during elevation.

### ACTIVE TREATMENT AFTER CONSERVATIVE AND SURGICAL CARE

*Physical Therapy and Remedial Exercise.*    Strengthen entire leg with isometric exercises after immobilization or on the first postoperative day, with emphasis on the quadriceps. Follow with transition to dynamic motions, first without and then with resistance in lateral, prone, and supine positions. Increase exercises with complex motions, beginning on the edge of the training table or bed. Stress exercises begin in the exercise bath and are continued with remedial walking.

After normal walking movements are achieved, light running on soft ground begins. About 12 to 20 treatments are necessary. Since the regeneration time of cartilage varies, full athletic stress should not begin until a full three months have passed. Gradually training increases under constant observation of the motion sequences, in order to prevent a relapse. A supportive bandage is recommended for relief of stress upon resumption of training.

## SPECIAL NOTES

***Treatments Contraindicated.***    Use of heat in acute stage and postoperatively; massage on the joint; movements which cause compression; jumping; and lifting weights while standing are to be avoided. Correct foot and leg statics with proper athletic shoes and inserts.

# Dislocated Kneecap

Dislocated kneecaps occur in various games, particularly soccer. They also occur frequently in wrestling, judo, and other combative sports.

Dislocated knees are caused by a pathologic change of the axis of the leg, among other factors. The knee cap (patella) usually slides laterally, very rarely medially. A blow or kick against the medial or lateral side of the kneecap or the knee is a characteristic cause of traumatic dislocation of the kneecap. Repositioning is necessary. In the case of chronic dislocations, the kneecap slides laterally across the lateral condyle of the femur when the knee is bent. This occurs during weightlifting, for example. When the knee is extended, the kneecap usually slides back into place. Repeated dislocations must be operated on, as otherwise they result in osteochondrotic changes in the gliding path of the kneecap, which causes athletic disability.

## GOALS OF TREATMENT

Goals of treatment are intensive training of all leg muscles for stabilization of the knee joint, removal of joint effusions, and prevention of training loss in the healthy areas of the body.

## START OF TRAINING

Training continues through immobilization.

## PASSIVE TREATMENTS

*Positioning, Immobilization, and Bandages.* Immobilization in a cast or splint follows the repositioning. Slight elevation is used to encourage venous and lymphatic return. After the hematoma has subsided, a circular cast or, depending on the seriousness of the injury, a tight elastic bandage is put into place.

*Massage.* Perform drainage massage to enhance venous and lymphatic return in the lower and upper leg muscles. Massage of the knee itself is to be avoided in acute stages. Loosening of adhesions in late stages will improve the gliding of the kneecap.

*Cold.* Cold is applied to combat tendency of the knee to swell during immobilization and as a preparation for remedial exercises.

*Electrotherapy.* Diadynamic currents and ultrasound are useful.

## ACTIVE TREATMENTS

*Physical Therapy and Remedial Exercise.* Physical therapy begins after immobilization with isometric exercises for the entire leg while it remains

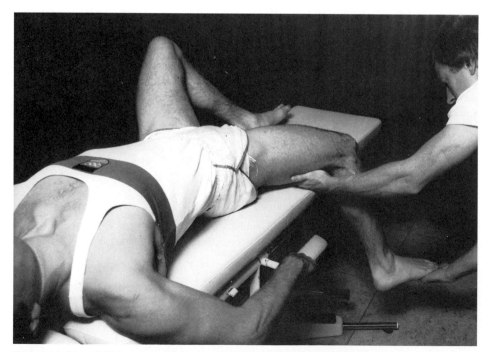

**Figure 14–38.** PNF training of leg muscles with slight bend in knees.

elevated. Further dynamic movements of both feet follow, then dynamic exercises along the axis of the leg for all leg muscles. Overextension of the knee should be avoided.

Remedial walking in water is followed by stepclimbing and other forms of stress. Minus training to full stress is another means of increasing performance (see *Meniscus Injury; Ligament Injury to the Knee*). About 10 treatments are necessary.

## SPECIAL NOTES

Supportive bandages should be used upon resumption of training. The physiologic sequences of movements in the knee should be observed closely. Athletic disciplines that require outward rotation of the knee, such as hurdles and breaststroke in swimming, should be avoided.

## CHAPTER 15

# Spinal Column and Torso

## WERNER KUPRIAN, HELMUT ORK, AND LUTZ MEISSNER

## Scheuermann's Disease

Scheuermann's disease, also known as kyphosis of adolescence or osteochondrosis, is a developmental and structural disorder of the spinal column that affects adolescents, boys more frequently than girls. Irregular contours of the inferior and superior articular surfaces of individual vertebrae, particularly the middle and lower thoracic vertebrae and more rarely in the lumbar vertebrae, are noticeable and can be confirmed with x-rays. This can result in a punctured superior articular surface, the formation of cuneiform vertebrae, Schmorl's cartilaginous nodules, and permanent hunchback. Patients complain of fatigue, tension, and hardening of the back muscles.

Causes may be hereditary, constitutional, and endocrine as well as disproportions between the amount of stress received and capacity for stress in adolescents. Scheuermann's disease occurs in approximately 30 per cent of the adult population. According to research by Riehle and Groh and Groh 40 per cent of 21 trampolinists, 51 per cent of 59 rowers, and 37 per cent of 74 gymnasts displayed Scheuermann's disease. The percentage of the disorder is therefore considerably higher in these sports. In a group of 320 general athletes, the percentage was approximately the same as for the average population. A study of 30 weight-lifters revealed no pathologic damage to the spine, however.

After osteochondrosis, spondylosis, displaced vertebrae, and pinched intervertebral disks, a high percentage of young competitive athletes complain of pain in the spine. Scheuermann's disease is the primary cause. It is, however, not rare for the disease to occur completely without pain. It is unclear as to whether the disease would have occurred without the stress of athletics, and whether the repeated traumatic stress on the spine during training and in competition for particular sports is a decisive factor in its occurrence.

In any case, the growing tissues of adolescents are particularly sensitive to mechanical stress, such as those that occur in gymnastics, trampoline, high diving, and wrestling. The fact that Scheuermann's disease is worsened through extreme athletic stress and from the trauma of an athletic injury can be considered indisputable.

## GOALS OF TREATMENT

Goals of treatment include loosening and relaxation of the usually tense shoulder, neck, and back muscles; strengthening of the stomach and back extensor muscles, and the muscular support around the spinal column; and correction of any increase in thoracic kyphosis and other spinal deformities.

## START OF TREATMENT

Begin treatment immediately after the diagnosis has been made.

## PASSIVE TREATMENTS

*Heat.*   Incandescent light, hot towels, and fango poultices for the back are good preparation for massage.

*Massage.*   Massage the shoulders, neck, and back muscles; underwater massage can also be used as preparation for remedial exercise.

*Hydrotherapy.*   Sauna and relaxing baths are helpful measures.

## ACTIVE TREATMENTS

*Physical Therapy and Remedial Exercise.*   Intensive remedial exercises should be done for the mobilization of the entire spinal column and strengthening of the muscles that support the spine. Other exercises to perform are stretching and loosening exercises for the spine, strengthening exercises for the stomach muscles, rectus abdominis, obliquus abdominis externus et internus, and transversus abdominis, as well as for the back muscles, erector spinal and the rhomboideus.

Remedial exercises begin in a position that relieves stress on the spine, with the athlete either prone or supine or kneeling on hands and knees. Mobilization of spine should be done using sling support.

Klapp's crawling exercises and stomach muscle exercises, performed while hanging from wall bars, are also recommended. Also begin breathing exercises, with emphasis on diaphragm breathing, and remedial exercise in an exercises bath. Corrective exercises performed in front of a mirror while standing and sitting should improve posture. Types of games that encourage stretching and backstroke supplement physical therapy. Therapy on horseback is also a good supplementary exercise for completely healed Scheuermann's disease.

The physical therapy treatment must be conducted over a period of several years, 2 to 3 times per week during adolescence. Periods of rest are necessary. The patient should have a daily exercise routine that can be performed at

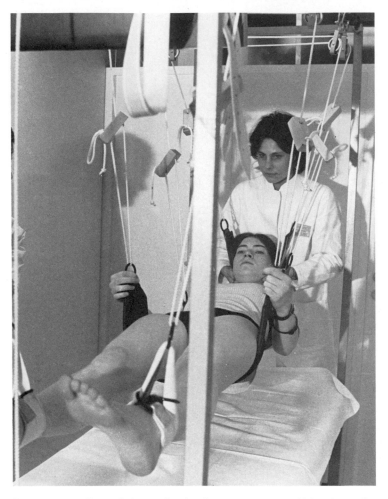

**Figure 15–1.**   Remedial exercise in sling support to mobilize the entire vertebral column with complete relief of body weight.

home. These programs of home exercise must be checked and corrected if necessary, so that no faulty movements develop.

## SPECIAL NOTES

All exercises that cause compression of the spine must be absolutely avoided. Unphysiologic motions, such as stress in a bent position of the spine, hard training for strenuous athletics, and extreme strength development, particularly before the age of 20 years, are also damaging. On the other hand, moderate strength work is permitted while lying down, such as with bench presses. It is important that the lumbar vertebrae be stabilized and that lordosis is not increased. Strength exercises and lifting work should be done primarily with the upper thighs and with the use of a ventral press. Warm

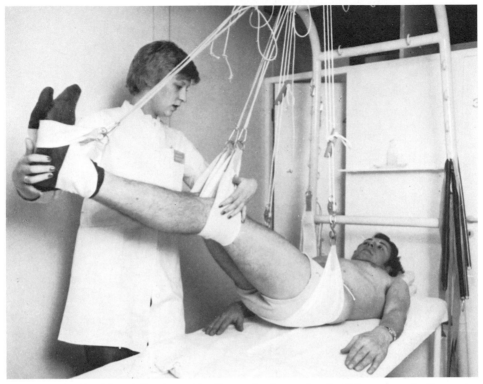

**Figure 15–2.**   Partial mobilization of the thoracolumbar region for Scheuermann's disease in a table-tennis player.

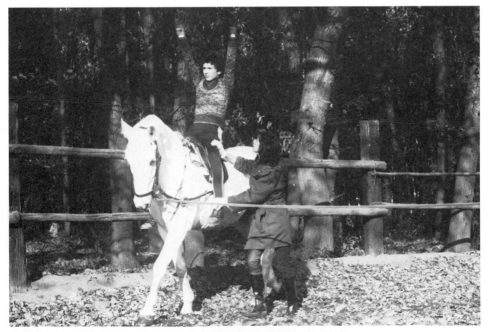

**Figure 15–3.**   Therapy on horseback for healed Scheuermann's disease.

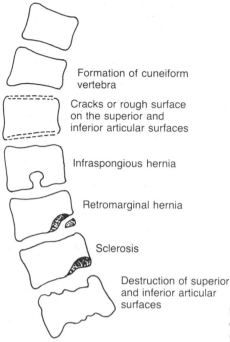

Formation of cuneiform vertebra

Cracks or rough surface on the superior and inferior articular surfaces

Infraspongious hernia

Retromarginal hernia

Sclerosis

Destruction of superior and inferior articular surfaces

**Figure 15–4.** Diagram of radiologic changes in osteochondritis deformans juvenilis dorsalis (Scheuermann's disease).

clothing, careful warm-ups, and local stretching and loosening exercises before training and competition are very important. Varied exercises and avoidance of all one-sided exercise and excessive long-term stress are important. Sports that encourage balanced muscular development are recommended. Regular x-ray checks and permanent observation and advice during training are necessary.

# Lordosis

Lordosis of the lumbar vertebrae is a widespread abnormal curvature of the spine that can become a permanent deformity. It involves an abnormally large arch in the ventral direction of the five lumbar vertebrae and the sacrum together with a forward tilt of the pelvis.

Although the basic posture of a person is inherited, external influences, such as age, disposition, sports, nourishment, illness, and working and living conditions have a considerable effect on posture and thus on spinal statics.

Faulty posture generally develops first in the growing years between ages 6 and 12. These posture defects are aggravated during high school years as the student is required to sit for many hours, thus being forced to remain immobile for long periods. Rapid growth can also have an adverse effect on posture; the development of the postural muscles does not keep pace with the rapid growth in height.

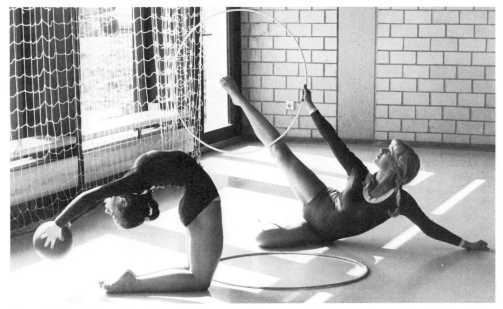

**Figure 15–5.**  Extreme back-bending movements in competitive gymnasts contribute to lordosis in the lumbar vertebrae.

Aside from the visible deformity, pain and tiring of the muscles of the lumbar vertebrae and often of the entire back are typical symptoms of lordosis. The back extensors and the insertions of the gluteus maximus on the edge of the pelvis, as well as the quadratus lumborum, are palpably tense and hardened.

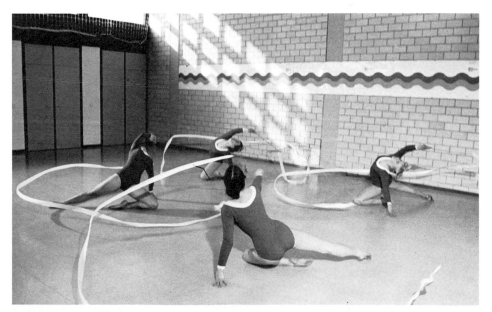

**Figure 15–6.**  Portions of a gymnastic exercise which develop lordosis (hollow back pattern).

The causes of lordosis can be varied: congenital deformities of the spine, postural weakness of the connective tissue and muscles, poor posture, paralysis and poor condition of the stomach muscles from sedentary life style in the office and at home. Lordosis is common in women. which may be due to overstretching of the stomach muscles during pregnancy.

Lordosis and its consequences are encountered in competitive athletics, particularly in those sports with movements and exercises that tend to involve an arched back position. This occurs primarily in gymnastics, as in performing handsprings, back somersaults, back handsprings, and swinging below the uneven parallel bars, in spiral movements for figure skaters, in javelin throwing, and in the butterfly stroke in swimming. In this case lordosis develops as a result of thousands of repetitions of the movement in training and competition.

Even if these sports and exercises are not necessarily the primary cause of formation of lordosis, they nevertheless increase the predisposition and aggravate the existing disorder. By placing improper stress on the articular surfaces and the intervertebral disks, lordosis generally leads to premature signs of aging and degenerative changes in the spine. Additional traumatization of the lumbar vertebrae, which do occur in competitive sports, could also contribute to premature attrition. Further deformities in the thoracic and cervical vertebrae can develop as a result of the lordosis.

Common in all cases of lordosis is weakness of the stomach muscles. Both the rectus abdominis and the diagonal stomach muscles are weakened and unable to perform the function of supporting the pelvis. On the other hand the extensors of the lumbar vertebrae are shortened. Patients with lordosis also generally lack good diaphragmic breathing. These factors govern the task of the physical therapist.

## GOALS OF TREATMENT

Treatment goals include strengthening of stomach muscles, correction of lumbar vertebrae, loosening and stretching of the lumbar extensor muscles, practice in proper pelvic and spinal posture, learning of diaphragmatic breathing, and creation of muscular balance between stomach and back muscles.

## START OF TREATMENT

Begin treatment immediately after diagnosis.

## PASSIVE TREATMENTS

*Positioning.*  A pillow must be placed under the stomach while the athlete is in the prone position. The size of the pillow depends on the extent of the lordosis, which must be corrected or overcorrected. The legs are bent in the supine position. Adjustable bands, "Trapex-positioning," and "Perlmann's apparatus" are particularly good at relieving stress for painful conditions.

**Heat.** Incandescent light, hot towels, and fango poultices on the lower back muscles are a good preparation for massage and remedial exercise.

**Electrotherapy.** Diadynamic currents are useful in the acute stages; also valuable are interference currents.

## ACTIVE TREATMENTS

*Physical Therapy and Remedial Exercise.* Therapy should include intensive exercise for strengthening of all the stomach muscles (the rectus abdominis, and the obliquus abdominis externus et internus) while stress on the back is relieved. The best position at the start of the treatment is the supine position. Afterward passive and active corrective or overcorrective exercises for the lumbar vertebrae follow. Kyphosing exercises on all fours, such as

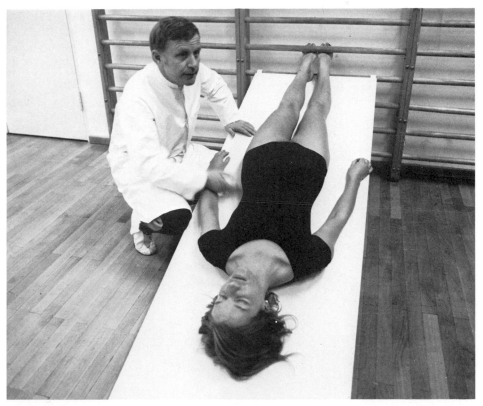

**Figure 15–7.** Physical therapy of lordosis on a slanted surface.

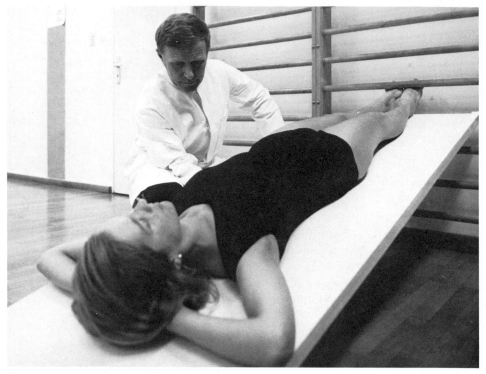

**Figure 15–8.** Lumbar vertebrae pressed down against therapist's hand.

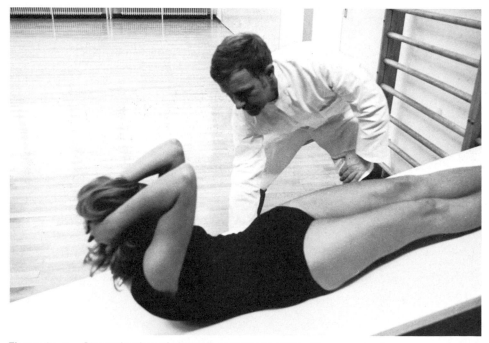

**Figure 15–9.** Strengthening of stomach muscles by lifting the upper body.

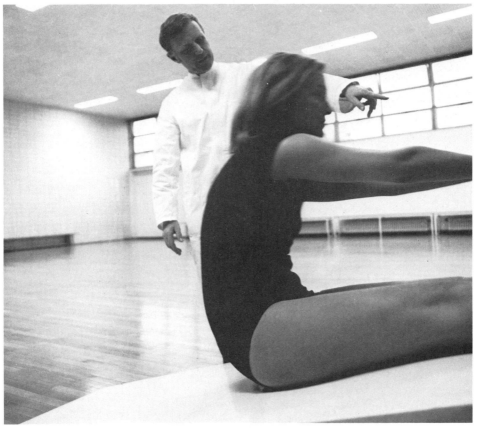

**Figure 15–10.** Overcorrection of lordosis by bending far forward.

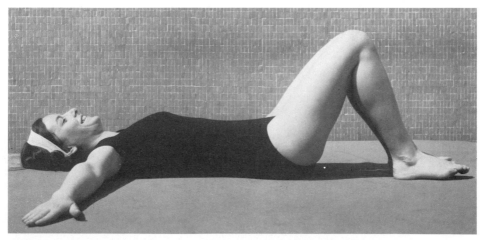

**Figure 15–11.** Lordosis exercises: supine position, both legs bent.

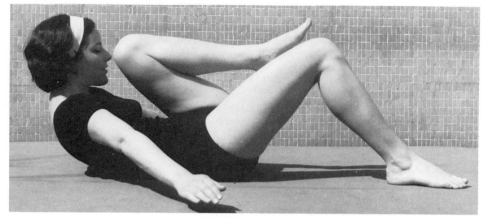

**Figure 15–12.**   Alternately bring knees up, lift head, and bring nose to knee.

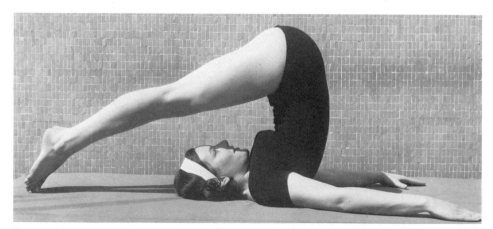

**Figure 15–13.**   Raise both legs together and place nose between legs.

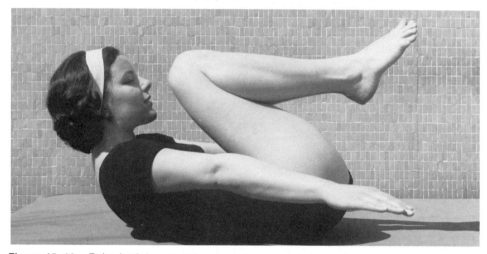

**Figure 15–14.**   Bend legs, then stretch them upwards and slowly extend toes, touching floor behind head.

bringing the knees up to the nose and arching the back like a cat, are recommended, together with stomach muscle exercises using wall bars, such as lifting the knees to the stomach, first individually and then together. Practicing diaphragmatic and sacral breathing is very important. Passive and active stretching of the shortened leg muscles, the hamstrings, is part of the standard treatment of lordosis. Hanging and swinging in a stretching position from the Perlmann apparatus serve to stretch and loosen the lumbar vertebrae. Further recommendations: Klapp's crawling exercises, correction of lordosis in front of a mirror, lordotic exercises in an exercise bath. After the treatment of the lumbar vertebrae in a position without stress, the corrected positioning is extended to a vertical position, in which there is stress on the spine. Exercises on a stool and with the patient standing and walking are helpful. The athlete should be taught self-checks. For example, he or she stands against a wall and checks to see if the spine touches the wall in all places from the lumbar and thoracic vertebrae to the cervical vertebrae. If the lumbar vertebrae do not touch the wall, they should be pressed against it by tensing the stomach and buttock muscles, without moving another part of the spine. This should feel as if the pelvis were being drawn underneath. Frequent checks and correction by walking in front of a mirror are necessary.

Therapy using the three-dimensional swinging rhythm of the horse for loosening and active correction of the lumbar vertebrae is a good means of treating lordosis.

The treatment of lordosis must take place 2 to 3 times weekly and can extend over several years, particularly for growing adolescents. Daily individual exercise of the patient is indispensable.

### SPECIAL NOTES

To be avoided or at least limited are all motions and exercises that lead to lordosis. Extreme weight-lifting and strength training in a standing position should also be avoided. On the other hand, varied movements and localized balancing exercises while stress on the spine is being relieved, particularly after training, should be recommended. Backstroke in swimming is a good equalizing exercise. High-heeled shoes should be avoided, as they contribute to a tilted pelvis. Permanent loosening and stretching of the tense and shortened lower back muscles, with heat, massage, and exercises are necessary. The trainer's supervision and advice are also required.

# Scoliosis

The bending of the spine to one side is called scoliosis. Lateral curvature is usually accompanied by a torsion of the vertebrae and permanent rotation.

The many causes, its progressive nature, and the resistance to therapy, which can lead to a complete deformation of the torso and corresponding effects

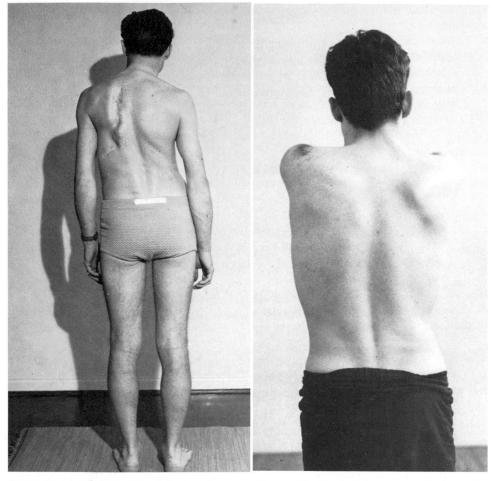

**Figure 15–15.**   Severe scar scoliosis; left convex scoliosis of thoracic vertebrae after automobile accident.

**Figure 15–16.**   Left convex scoliosis at the transition between lumbar and thoracic vertebrae.

on the heart and lungs have made scoliosis a classic orthopedic ailment. Most cases of scoliosis — at least in the early stages —are painless.

Both a postural scoliosis and a structural scoliosis can be distinguished. The postural scolioses are reversible, and active straightening is possible. Structural scoliosis, on the other hand, is permanent and cannot be completely corrected with active exercises.

Cobb and Scheier divide the causes into myopathic (muscular dystrophy), neuropathic (paralytic scoliosis), osteopathic (formation of cuneiform vertebrae), static (shortened leg), fibropathic (scar, skin), and idiopathic scolioses. Idiopathic scoliosis, which is by far the most common, is divided by Ponseti into infantile, juvenile, and adolescent scoliosis.

A clinical classification according to the degree of severity has been undertaken by Lindemann. Scoliosis of the first degree is a slight bending of

the vertebral column with slight but noticeable torsion, which can be corrected.

Scoliosis of the second degree is characterized by a noticeable bending of
the spine into an S or C shape, with beginning rib deformities and bulging
lumbar area. This type is no longer correctable. Scoliosis of the third degree
entails a severe deformation of the spine with pronounced deformity of the
thorax and lumbar region, as well as an overhang of the thorax on the convex
side of the primary bend.

Division according to the deviation from the axis of the primary bend
(Lipp, Cobb) is also common today.

Jenschura recorded the average frequency of scoliosis as 2 per cent. Krahl
and Steinbrück found 33.5 per cent slight and 1.6 per cent severe scolioses in

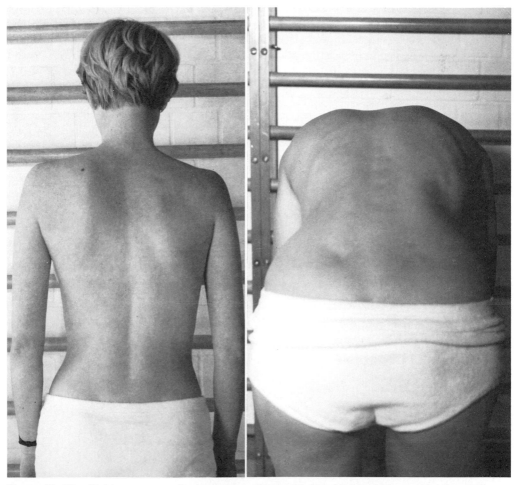

**Figure 15–17.** Right convex scoliosis at the transition between lumbar and thoracic verte-brae due to tilted pelvis in gymnast.

**Figure 15–18.** Humped rib-cage to the right of thoracic vertebrae while bending forwards.

the examination of 571 top athletes in the years 1974–1977. There was a noticeable concentration in athletes participating in sports that develop extreme torque in repetitive serving, throwing, and volleying motions, such as archers, javelin throwers, pole-vaulters, and table tennis players. These generally cause only slight damages when angles of less than 20 degrees are involved (Cobb). Certainly it is impossible to speak of scoliosis caused by athletics. Its frequency among athletes, particularly in times of accelerated growth, requires particular attention, as far as regular checkups, prevention, and early treatment are concerned.

Therapy for scoliosis consists of active remedial exercises, various braces and corsets, and, in serious cases, surgery (Harrington).

## GOALS OF TREATMENT

Treatment goals are strengthening of the postural muscles, primarily of the back and stomach, strengthening of respiration and enlargement of the vital capacity; correction and straightening of the nonfixed curvature; prevention of progression of scoliosis and muscular atrophy; relief of pain; and loosening of the generally tense muscles along the spine.

## START OF TREATMENT

Begin treatment immediately after diagnosis — for children, the sooner the better.

## PASSIVE TREATMENTS

*Positioning.*   In bed, the patient should lie flat on a hard surface, in prone position for several hours a day; then in a side position, allowing the concave side to sag; stretching; positioning on a slanted surface; extension in supporting slings, harness, or a running harness.

*Heat.*   Incandescent light, hot towels, fango poultices, and mud-paraffin poultices for the back are useful as a preparation for massage. Heat can also be applied while the patient is immobilized.

*Massage.*   Intensive massage of all the erector muscles of the torso, including back, shoulders, neck, pelvis, and stomach, as preparation for remedial exercise, should be done. Underwater massage and massage of scar tissue for scar scoliosis can be used as well.

*Electrotherapy.*   Use of electrogymnastic equipment, threshold current for paralysis scoliosis, and faradization is also of value.

## ACTIVE TREATMENT

*Physical Therapy and Remedial Exercise.*   Scoliosis has always been an area in which active physical therapy has been applied. Remedial exercises are the most important treatment for all forms of scoliosis and in all stages of the disorder, both while the patient is in a cast and brace and pre- and post-operatively. Passive treatments alone are of no success in treatment.

The primary exercises include isometric exercises for the torso and Niederhofer's exercise program, and strengthening of the stomach muscles from a supine position and back muscles from a prone position (known as arching exercises). Exercises in all positions that place stress on the spine, such as on hands and knees and Klapp's crawling, are recommended. Exercises performed using the wall bars are also recommended, particularly for scoliosis characterized by a large curvature. Symmetric strengthening of the back muscles is also suggested for mild scoliosis. Asymmetric exercises are added in severe cases. In particular, the muscles on the convex side are exercised. Besides strengthening exercises, mobilization and loosening are important. Manual therapy, particularly traction, should be employed for scoliosis. Patients with rigid scoliosis should not do mobilization exercises, however.

Breathing exercises are particularly important for scoliosis. Various exercise "systems" have been devised and propagated for scoliosis. Objective analysis, however, reveals that they usually cannot live up to their promises. Nevertheless, scoliosis is always accompanied by a more or less serious deformation of the thorax. Properly directed breathing exercises can be of considerable help as part of the remedial program. The primary goal is to bring air into side affected by the scoliosis. This should be stretched and enlarged. In general, the aims are to increase the vital capacity of the lungs and to develop the thorax. The strong breathing is a type of "inner antagonism" for the skeletal muscles. Breathing exercises should be conducted with the patient lying on the back or in a lateral or prone position at first, because it is easier to relax in these positions. At a later point in the treatment, the exercises can also be performed while sitting, standing, and walking.

An improvement of the respiratory function is also very important because of the damage to the respiratory and circulatory organs that results from the thorax deformity. As athletes are usually affected with only a slight scoliosis, running and other types of endurance sports are important for the balancing and improvement of breathing function.

The physical therapy takes place two to three times per week over an extended period of time, with interruptions for recuperation.

## SPECIAL NOTES

All exercises and movements that compress the spine should be avoided, as should exercises that require frequent repetition of torsion and sideward motion.

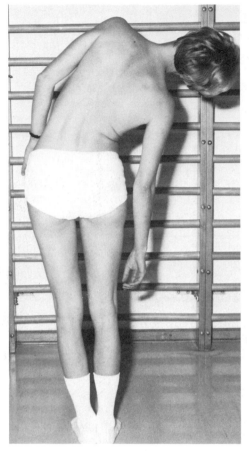 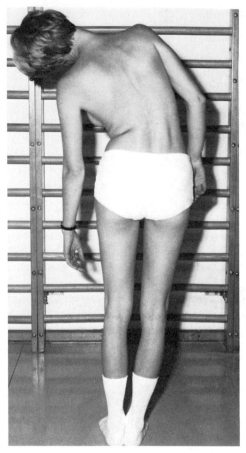

**Figure 15–19.** Flexion of vertebral column to the right is limited.

**Figure 15–20.** Flexion of vertebral column to the left is possible.

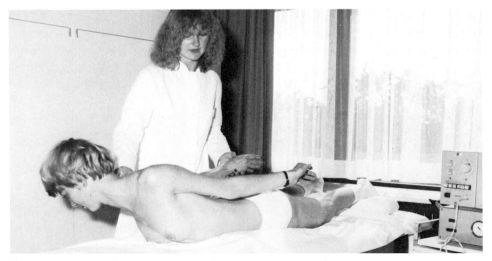

**Figure 15–21.** Arching exercises with sideward twist of vertebral column to the right in prone position which relieves stress on vertebral column.

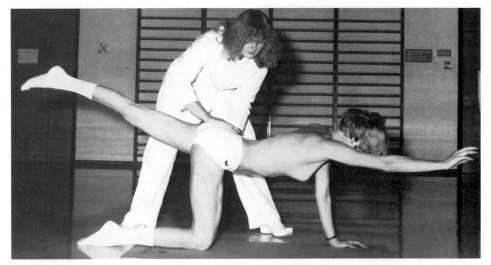

**Figure 15–22.**   Correction of scoliosis and strengthening of back extensors.

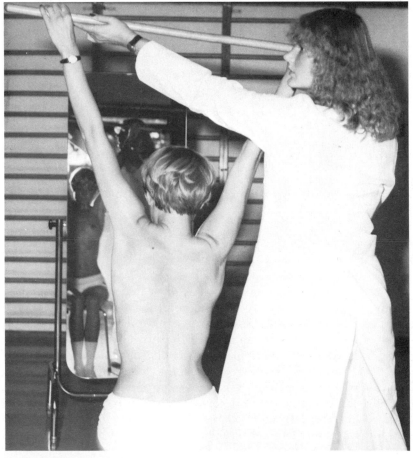

**Figure 15–23.**   Scoliosis correction in front of mirror with use of a staff.

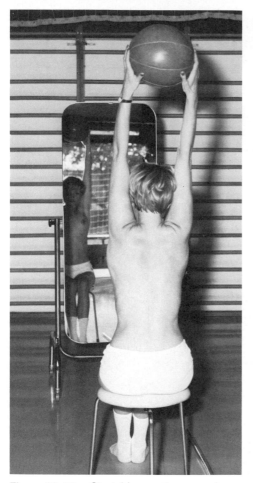

**Figure 15–24.** Stretching posture exercises for the entire torso with a medicine ball in front of a mirror.

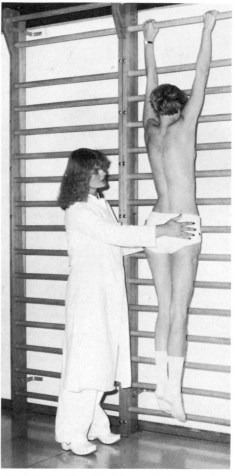

**Figure 15–25.** Stretching of the vertebral column with hanging exercises on the wall bars.

A corrective shoe should be considered for static scoliosis, which results in a shortening of a leg and thus postural deformity. Heel or sole inserts should be worn at all times during the physical therapy to equalize the difference in length. Swimming is strongly recommended as a sport that balances the body; the backstroke is particularly effective because it relieves the stress on the spine and respiratory organs. Additional therapy on horseback is recommended for mild cases of scoliosis. The horse used in therapy should permit a very gentle, swinging ride and the therapist must have special knowledge and experience with this method. Use of athletic shoes with soft soles and the avoidance of hard surfaces in training are also important.

Competition in particular sports may certainly be limited by even a slight case of scoliosis, if its progression is to be checked. This includes javelin-throwing, shot-putting, tennis, and other sports. A complete ban on all sports is not necessary, however. A school or hobby sport that uses varied movements

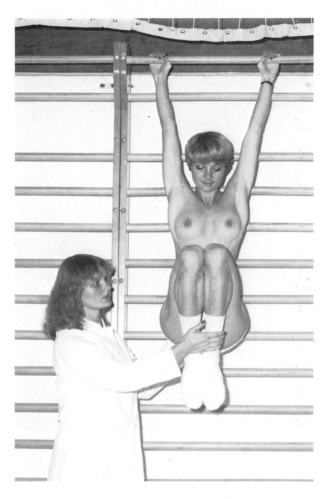

**Figure 15–26.** Stretching of the vertebral column while strengthening the stomach muscles on the wall bars.

is not contraindicated when scoliosis is present; indeed, it actually contributes to the strengthening and flexibility of the back and thus prevents worsening of the scoliotic curvature. Each case must be dealt with individually, according to its severity and the particular sport and its demands. Constant observation in training and regular medical checkups are absolutely essential.

# Spondylolysis and Spondylolisthesis

Spondylolysis involves the development of a crack in the articulation of the vertebral column. If spondylolysis is suspected, which can manifest itself as pain in the sacrum during motion and as tense muscles as well as a fixed lordosis, posteroanterior and lateral x-rays are taken as well as oblique views at an angle of 45 degrees to the axis of the body. The crack-like break is particularly visible from this angle.

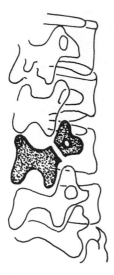

**Figure 15–27.** Diagnonal of lumbar vertebrae (schematic) showing "Scotty dog" described by Lachapèle.

Lachapèle noted that the diagonal x-rays of the spondylolitic crack had the appearance of a Scotty dog. The transverse process corresponds to the mouth of the dog, the superior process to the ears, and the inferior articular process to the feet. The neck is the intervertebral joint (lamina), and the body is the spinous process.

A shift in the vertebrae, so that one vertebra slides over another ventrally, is called spondylolisthesis. This slippage occurs most frequently between the fifth lumbar vertebra and the sacrum. The spondylolisthesis is clinically palpable as a gap in the row of spinal processes. The back extensor muscles are hypertensed, a reaction to guard against pain and further slippage.

Causes of spondylolysis and spondylolisthesis include both constitutional fatigue fractures and aseptic necrosis resulting from a disordered blood supply. The following percentages for various sports are listed by the authors named:

Javelin throwers: 40 per cent (Rompe)
High divers: 29 per cent (Groher)
Gymnasts: 26 per cent (Schwertner)
Trampolinists: 25 per cent (Riehle)

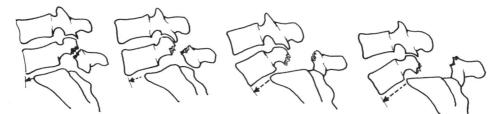

**Figure 15–28.** Degrees of spondylolisthesis from beginning to complete slippage (after Meyerding).

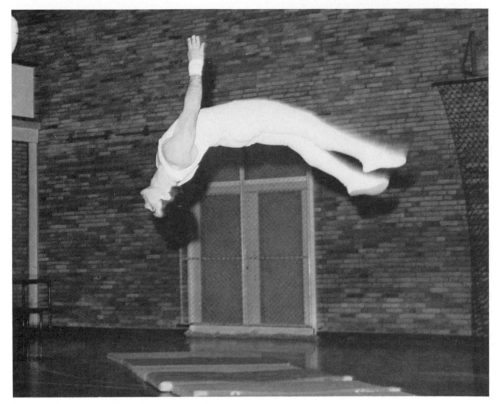

**Figure 15–29.**  Arching of the back with torsion.

As these percentages indicate, danger exists primarily in those sports which include a backwards curvature of the spine with simultaneous rotation in their motion as in javelin throwing and pole vaulting.

Spondylolysis or spondylolisthesis is likely to occur in 30 to 50 per cent of athletes involved in the increasingly complex patterns of movements and exercises in gymnastics, high diving, and trampoline.

## GOALS OF TREATMENT

Goals of treatment include loosening and relaxation of the usually tense back muscles, strengthening of the stomach and back muscles, and development of muscular support around the spine.

## START OF TREATMENT

Begin treatment immediately after diagnosis.

## PASSIVE TREATMENTS

*Heat.*   Fango poultices, incandescent light, and hot towels are used as preparation for massage.

*Massage.*   Massage the entire shoulder, neck, and back muscles; underwater massage is also helpful.

*Electrotherapy.*   Diadynamic currents, interference currents, and ultrasound are valuable treatment measures.

## ACTIVE TREATMENTS

*Physical Therapy and Remedial Exercise.*   The muscles responsible for the positioning of the spine must be strengthened with an intensive program of remedial exercise. Strengthening exercises for the stomach muscles (rectus abdominis, obliquus abdominis externus et internus, and transversus abdominis), as well as the erector spinal and all back muscles, should be prescribed. Remedial exercises in the exercise bath are also helpful.

At the start of the treatment, strengthening exercises should be performed while the spine is relieved of stress. Positions for major exercises include all fours, prone or supine position, along wall bars, or on a bench. Physical therapy using sling supports and weight-lifting following Brunkow's program help in stabilization. Corrective exercises done while sitting and standing improve posture.

A physical therapy treatment must be scheduled at least three times weekly to assure efficiency.

The previously described exercises should be given as homework assignments for the days without formal treatment. The treatment must extend over several years with pauses to aid recuperation.

## SPECIAL NOTES

Careful warm-up is absolutely necessary for training and competition. An increased lordosis should be avoided in this process, without neglecting stabilizing measures.

Equalizing exercises, such as backstroke, are good for the avoidance of extended stress. Sports and exercises that demand maximal backward curvature of the spine with a simultaneous rotation should be avoided, particularly by young athletes. X-rays and observation and advice in training are important.

# Groin Pain

Pain in the groin can be caused by strong tension. Other causes include tendopathy, known as gracilis syndrome. These pains can also be caused by the rectus abdominis impinging on the tuberculum pubicum, the adductor longus on the pectincus and the flexor groups on the tuber ischii. Pain, which often extends into the upper thigh and the abdominal wall, is caused by twisting motions, such as those that occur in gymnastics, soccer, and the throwing events in field athletics. Long jumpers and sprinters, particularly hurdlers and steeplechasers, are also affected. An additional cause is overstress together with frequently repeated minitraumas, particularly of the transverse stomach muscles and the adductor muscles, such as take place in continued painful play in soccer, with repeated forced straddle positions. Inguinal hernias and radiating irritations of the lumbar vertebrae should also be considered. Weakness in the group of stomach muscles with their diagonal connection to the muscles on the upper leg can also lead to groin pain.

## GOALS OF TREATMENT

Relief of pain by removing stress from the affected region and restoration and retraining to full athletic ability are the goals of treatment.

## START OF TREATMENT

Begin treatment immediately after the pain arises.

## PASSIVE TREATMENTS

*Positioning, Immobilization, and Bandages.*   A bandage immobilizes and relieves stress on the entire pelvic region, including the affected upper thigh. If pain is caused during outward rotation and abduction of the leg, the bandages are fixed for inward rotation on the adducted leg. Tape is also used for additional strengthening in the direction of adduction and inward rotation.

*Massage.*   Drainage massage in the acute stages, with later transition to friction on the muscle insertions, is valuable. The leg is bent and adducted somewhat over the center. In this way the affected muscle insertions are most relaxed.

*Cold.*   Apply ice in the acute phase around the groin and surrounding areas, also as preparation for remedial exercise.

*Heat.*   Fango poultices and hot towels are applied; these can be used as well in the area of pain for chronic conditions.

*Electrotherapy.*   Diadynamic currents, ultrasound, and other microwave and shortwave treatments are helpful.

## ACTIVE TREATMENTS

*Physical Therapy and Remedial Exercise.*    Remedial exercises focus on the affected muscle groups, in this case particularly the transverse stomach muscles and adductors, but in addition all other painful muscles.

Begin with isometric exercises and tensing large areas of muscle on the torso and upper leg. Make a gradual transition to dynamic exercises, at first without stress, with the athlete in the lateral position, later with resistance. Active exercises in the supine position follow, increasing in complexity to three-dimensional movements. Remedial exercises with complex motions constitute the final phase of treatment, in which the muscles of the torso are exercised with movements originating in the extremities. Later exercises with both extremities on one side of the body — that is, with the right arm and right leg or with the left arm and left leg — are performed. A further gain is possible by performing these exercises in a supine position but using opposite extremities. By bringing the right arm and left leg together or the left arm and right leg, the diagonal muscle groups in particular are strengthened. Additional diagonal movements, sideward movements made by crossing the legs forward and backward, running in place with an emphasis on high knee motion with the knee pointed toward or away from the midline or with both knees pointed toward either the right shoulder or the left shoulder. Ten to 12 treatments are necessary in the acute phase. A lengthy treatment is recommended for prevention and for instituting special strengthening exercises.

## SPECIAL NOTES

Preventive bandages should be used upon resumption of training. Active stretching should follow a thorough warm-up, together with strengthening exercises for the rectilinear and diagonal muscle groups.

*First Aid at Competition Site.*    Relieve pain with cold applications and thus prevent hematoma formation. Immobilizing bandages that bring muscle insertions and origins together are also recommended.

CHAPTER **16**

# Shoulder and Arm

*DORIS EITNER, HELMUT ORK,*
*AND LUTZ MEISSNER*

## Dislocated Shoulders

A dislocated shoulder occurs when the ball of the joint is violently wrenched out of the socket. This dislocation is usually a result of levering action in which the ends of the joint are extended beyond the natural limits.

Dislocated shoulders are characterized by a change in the size of the joint, a change in axis of the dislocated arm, and the unnatural position. Motion of the joint is limited or entirely restricted. The ball of the joint is jammed and held in place under pressure. Upon trying to correct this elastic forced position by bringing the arm toward the torso, the arm springs back into the unnatural position; this is known as an elastic fixation.

Dislocated shoulders are often accompanied by additional injuries, which occasionally are quite extensive. For example, tears and bruises of the plexus brachialis or paralysis of the axillary or musculocutaneus nerves can occur. The most frequent, however, is the combination of dislocation with chipping of the greater tuberosity.

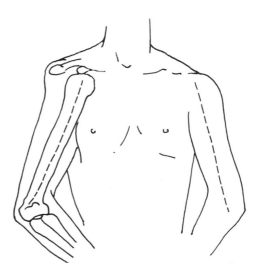

**Figure 16–1.** Dislocated shoulder.

A traumatically dislocated shoulder must be repositioned early and gently, within an hour of the accident, if possible. However, the repositioning should never be undertaken without having obtained x-rays. After the repositioning, immobilization in a sling is necessary. The immobilization can last up to 4 weeks, depending on the severity of the injury. Only in this manner is complete healing of the injury to the capsule-ligament apparatus and the torn muscles possible. It is extremely important that immobilization of a first traumatic shoulder dislocation be of the proper duration in order to prevent later chronic dislocations. Shoulders are frequently dislocated in sports by falling onto the joint, as in falling off a horse. Dislocation can also result from falling onto an outstretched arm, from throwing a ball, in gymnastics, from a powerful volley of the ball in handball when the arm is rotated far to the outside, and following overextension on the horizontal bar and in wrestling. In the 1972 Olympics a canoeist dislocated a shoulder when the canoe capsized.

## GOALS OF TREATMENT

Goals of treatment include relief of hematoma, strengthening of the muscle-ligament apparatus to prevent further dislocations, mobilization of the shoulder joint to prevent contractures, and attainment of normal function for all movements required in everyday life and in sports.

## START OF TREATMENT

Carefully controlled isometric exercises with cold treatments can begin with the joint in the abduction splint or in the "Desault bandage" even during the period of immobilization. The active program of exercises begins immediately after the immobilization is over.

## PASSIVE TREATMENTS

*Positioning.*   According to the type of dislocation, immobilize the shoulder in a Desault bandage or an abduction splint.

*Massage.*   Careful massage around shoulders and neck muscles, with exception of injured shoulder, can be carried out. Premature massage can very quickly make the situation worse. Adhesions are relieved in the later phases with deep friction and connective tissue massage.

*Cold.*   Apply cold, in form of ice packs, ice bandages, and ice massages after and during the immobilization.

*Electrotherapy.*   Use of diadynamic currents and electrogymnastic equipment for nerve damage, such as plexus paralysis or axillary nerve paresis, is helpful.

## ACTIVE TREATMENTS

*Physical Therapy and Remedial Exercise.*    After the period of immobilization ends, the emphasis is on active remedial exercise.

*Dislocated Shoulders or Bone Injury.*    Treatment begins during the immobilization period, with careful isometric exercises stressing the deltoids, biceps, and triceps. Active exercises of the hands and lower arm muscles should also begin during this period. Active dynamic exercises for abduction, anteversion, and flexion follow. Rotation, particularly in the outward direction, is contraindicated. Rotation is exercised carefully only in the late stages of the treatment. Be particularly careful during outward rotation because of the danger of a renewed dislocation.

*Shoulder Dislocation with Fracture of the Greater Tuberosity.*    Therapy begins after immobilization, also with isometric exercises. Abduction, anteversion, and flexion exercises without stress follow in a few days. The first exercises should begin with the patient in a supine position, which helps maintain the stability of the joint. It is imperative that the zero-rotation position be maintained. As an adductor-extensor contracture usually develops after immobilization, the mobilization of the shoulder with manual therapy

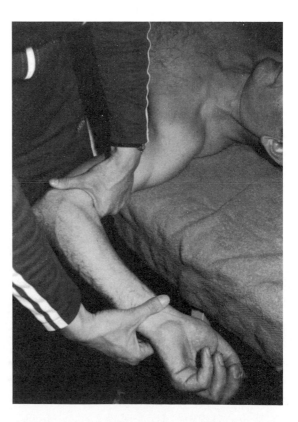

**Figure 16–2.** Stabilization of the shoulder in position of outward rotation. Treatment in late stages.

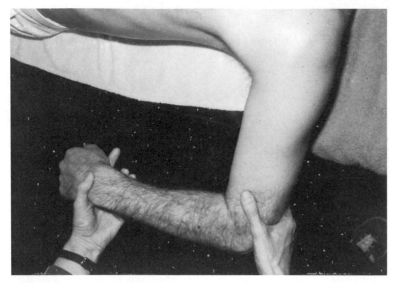

**Figure 16–3.** Stabilization of the shoulder in position of inward rotation. Treatment in late stages.

usually follows the healing of the capsules. Active exercises should be done in sitting, standing, or supine position. These movements are aided with devices such as sticks, ropes, Indian clubs, sling balls, wall bars (but not hanging exercises), or light dumbbells.

Active movement is improved with physical therapy in an exercise bath. Only light exercises are performed at first. If these exercises are satisfactory, complex motions in a diagonal direction are possible. At this point, the active stretching can be slightly forced. Swinging and pendulum motions follow, with or without helping devices. At the close of the physical therapy treatment exercises using practical and athletic movements are begun. Once these are under control, practice using the specific movement required by the athlete's sport can begin.

## SPECIAL NOTES

Massage and use of heat around the joint are forbidden because they may precipitate myositis ossificans. Early swinging exercises and outward rotation of the shoulders should be avoided because of the danger of a renewed dislocation. Passive motions, and pulling and lifting exercises, and hanging from wall bars should also be omitted.

Sports like handball, volleyball, basketball, or water polo should be avoided for a time; they should be resumed only after the muscles of the shoulder are completely restrengthened. As long as there are weaknesses in the muscles and overextended capsules in the shoulder, a renewed dislocation is possible. For this reason extreme stress, particularly in competitive sports, should be avoided.

*First Aid at Competition Site.*    The dislocated shoulder should be well padded, placed in a position without stress, and immobilized. Cold should be applied as an analgesic and to combat hematoma formation.

# Traumatic Humeroscapular Periarthritis

The strength and performance of the shoulder girdle is of great importance in many sports. Direct trauma to the shoulders and surrounding areas, such as a fall from an apparatus or a horse, or a judo throw, wrestling, boxing, a fall in handball, or through throwing motions of the type demanded by the throwing events of track and field, can lead to the development of traumatic humeroscapular periarthritis. It is characterized by a painful restriction of motion, particularly in abduction and inward and outward rotation. Pressure also causes pain in the shoulder joint and the surrounding tissues. The guarding position assumed against the pain leads to a contracture of the shoulder. Athletic stress on the shoulder therefore is not possible for a time. The traumatic humeroscapular periarthritis can also result from degenerative damage to the neck vertebrae, throwing damage to the neck vertebrae, and calcium deposits, particularly on the supraspinatus and long biceps tendon. The latter can be confirmed radiologically.

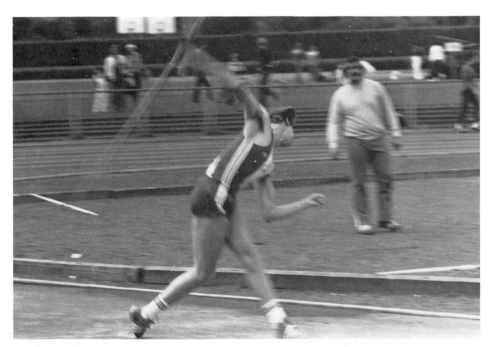

**Figure 16–4.**  Throwing motion of javelin thrower at point of release.

## GOALS OF TREATMENT

Treatment goals include relief of pain, prevention of muscular atrophy, restoration and preservation of the mobility of the joint, and attainment of full strength.

## START OF TREATMENT

In the acute stage, begin treatment immediately after the trauma occurs.

## PASSIVE TREATMENTS

*Position, Immobilization, and Bandages.* The arm should be placed on sandbags or in an abduction splint with flexion of the elbow to prevent contracture. For smaller traumas with less pain, use an immobilizing shoulder bandage with padding for the abduction.

*Massage.* Massage the cervical shoulder and neck region, with the exception of the painful area of the joint; also massage the arm muscles.

*Cold.* Cold treatments with cold towels and ice packs will relieve pain; later they are used as a preparation for active remedial exercise, particularly for treatment of contractures.

*Heat.* Apply heat, such as fango poultices, hot towels, and incandescent light, to the area above the segment and to the affected shoulder area in the chronic stages.

*Electrotherapy.* Diadynamic currents, ultrasound, and shortwaves are helpful treatments.

## ACTIVE TREATMENTS

*Physical Therapy and Remedial Exercise.* Loosening exercises for the entire shoulder girdle are introductory measures. Remedial exercises follow for the strengthening of the shoulder and arm muscles, particularly the deltoids, the biceps, and the triceps, and for strengthening the outer and inner rotation of the shoulder joint. Manual therapy for the improvement of the limited joint play along with active and passive stretching, particularly of the shrunken joint capsule, is also recommended. The newly developed range of motion must be reinforced with active exercises, also performed in the exercise

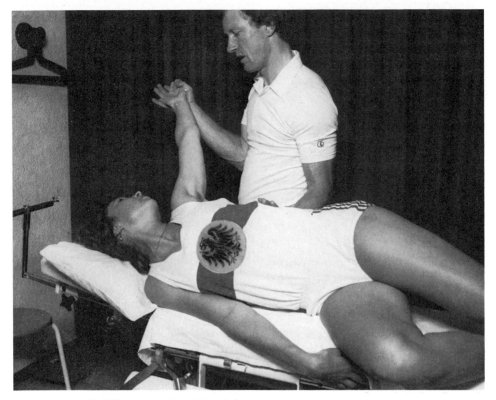

**Figure 16–5.** Stabilization of shoulder girdle.

bath. The use of dumbbells, the "Bali-device," chest expanders, and medicine balls is recommended in the final stages of the treatment. Hanging on wall bars for the stretching of the capsules and arm exercises on a Universal Gym are preparations for special exercises for the athlete's particular sport. The treatment takes a long time and requires at least 20 sessions, three times per week.

## SPECIAL NOTES

Heating modalities, such as hot air, incandescent light, or fango, should be avoided for the shoulder area during the acute stages. These treatments are recommended for chronic illnesses, however, for the support of joint mobilization and to improve blood supply. The humeroscapular periarthritis tends to relapse; all violent movements and leverage motions must be avoided. Be careful to avoid irritation during the physical therapy.

*First Aid at the Competition Site.*    Ice treatment and immobilization with shoulder bandage are helpful.

# Tennis Arm and Thrower's Elbow

Injuries and soreness in the area of the elbow and the lower arm occur frequently to tennis players and throwers as a result of a disproportion between the stress endured and the stress tolerance of the affected muscles, tendons, and ligaments. The cause lies in the excessive tension on the extensor muscles, the tendon insertions, the joint capsules, and the ligaments. If the process is chronic, clinically and radiologically verifiable microtraumas can be caused by the excessive stress. Two forms can be distinguished — the considerably more frequent radiohumeral epicondylitis or tennis elbow, and medial epicondylitis or thrower's elbow, such as occurs in javelin throwing and other throwing disciplines, and also in cross-country skiing, from the stress of thrusting with the ski poles. Blockage syndromes around the cervical vertebrae in these tendopathies are also frequent, because of the slipping of the seventh cervical vertebra to the side, particularly when serving in tennis, owing to the twisting motion of the spine and head. The sixth and seventh cervical and the first thoracic vertebrae are usually affected. Pain radiating to the entire arm can result. Ensuing problems are limitations in the motion of the elbow, in which full extension is often no longer possible; of the wrist, with limitation of both extension and flexion movements; and an additional disability in the shoulder. The last-mentioned can result in the so-called capsulary symptoms, in which abduction and outward and inward rotation of the shoulder are limited. Additional adhesions around the shoulderblades and the back can occur. Conservative treatment is preferred; operation should be necessary only in severe cases.

## GOALS OF TREATMENT

Treatment goals are reduction of painful condition to complete freedom from pain and restoration of normal movements up to complete ability to perform sports.

## START OF TREATMENT

Begin treatment immediately after the disorder arises.

## PASSIVE TREATMENTS

*Positioning, Immobilization, and Bandages.*    The arm is placed in a comfortable position, with a slight bend in the elbow and the lower arm muscles completely relaxed by immobilizing the hand and finger joints. Bandages are used to immobilize and relieve stress on the painful muscles of the lower arm.

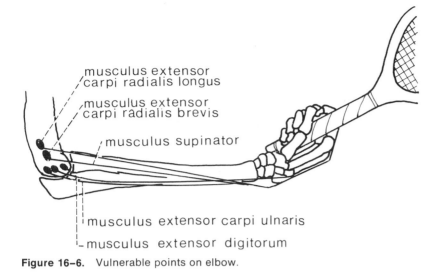

**Figure 16-6.**  Vulnerable points on elbow.

***Massage.***    Perform segmental massage during the acute stages; particular attention should be paid to the shoulder girdle and the neck. The painful elbow region should not be massaged. Later massage can be performed on the lower arm also, to break down possible deposits in the lower arm muscles. At first use light friction, then deeper friction, using a stylus, if necessary. The muscle insertions on the epicondyle are treated with diagonal friction. Soft

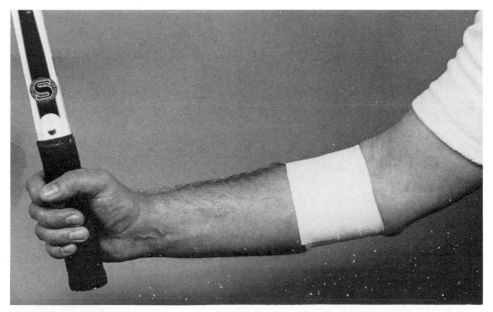

**Figure 16-7.**   Tape bandage to relieve stress on epicondyles for tennis elbow.

tissue techniques for the stretching of muscles and connective tissue can also be used.

*Cold.* Apply cold, such as ice packs, cold towels, and ice massage, in the acute stages; later, cold can be applied in the entire region of the elbow and lower arm as a preparation for remedial exercises.

*Heat.* Fango poultices and hot towels can be applied in different sectors of the arm and also around the elbow for chronic conditions.

*Electrotherapy.* Ultrasound, diadynamic currents, and microwaves have proved helpful.

## ACTIVE TREATMENTS

*Physical Therapy and Remedial Exercise.* Manual therapy for the cervical vertebrae and upper thoracic vetebrae is valuable for relieving segmental radiation of pain. Manual therapy is also used to treat restricted motion in shoulders, elbows, and wrists. Active physical therapy begins with isometric exercises for the affected muscles. Do not go beyond the pain threshold. In order to protect the strained extensor and flexor muscles, all active exercises for movement of the elbow are conducted without hand motion at first. Exercises for the wrist follow for flexion and extension, also for supination and pronation in one-, two-, and three-dimensional form. Later, active exercises of the entire arm and shoulders are performed. The primary exercises in this case are stretching the elbow by flexing or extending the wrist. Complex motions with increasing resistance and range of motion bring the athlete to readiness for regular athletic stress. The various tennis strokes are practiced (without hitting balls). If no new complaints arise, training for the sport can resume. Twelve treatments, with two to three sessions per week, are sufficient.

## SPECIAL NOTES

There are recognized preventive methods for the avoidance of elbow disorders. The arm and shoulder area can be massaged to avoid deposits. Correct stroke technique, use of proper rackets (including a larger racket if necessary), and a light rather than too tight grip all relieve stress on the elbow. Prolonged tension of the lower arm muscles from gripping the racket has an adverse effect on the flexibility and elasticity of the muscles. The flexion and extension of these muscles can be improved by frequently relaxing the muscles, that is, by relaxing the grip or opening the fist after every stroke, if possible. Relaxation of the lower arm muscles by flexing the fingers and shaking the entire area during pauses between play is also a good method of avoiding tension. Massage the elbow with an ice cube before the game and use general loosening exercises and massage; also stretch the muscles of the lower arm by extending the elbow, with maximal extension or flexion of the wrist as well. This should be done for 2 to 3 minutes. Additional bandages can also be used to lessen the stress on the muscle insertions on the epicondyles.

*First Aid at Competition Site.*    Stop the game immediately, apply cold for acute pain, and surround the elbow with a bandage and immobilize it.

# Sprained Wrist and Fingers

Sprained wrists are caused by falling on the hand. Handball and volley-ball players, wrestlers, and goalies in soccer are particularly at risk. Fingers are often dislocated in volleyball, handball, and downhill skiing. In addition to exceeding of the physiologic range of motion of the joint, small tears of the capsule also frequently occur. The affected area swells painfully.

## GOALS OF TREATMENT

Restoration of normal function and prevention of contractures around the joint are the goals of treatment.

## START OF TREATMENT

Treatment begins immediately after the sprain occurs. After swelling has been relieved with ice, a period of immobilization for 10 to 14 days can shorten the irritation, which otherwise can be of long duration.

## PASSIVE TREATMENTS

*Positioning, Immobilization, and Bandages.*    The hand or finger is relieved of stress. Compression bandages are suited for immobilizing affected joints if there is swelling; later, immobilizing bandages can be used after the swelling has died down.

*Cold.*    Apply cold, together with compression bandages; use measures to enhance rapid reabsorption of effusions; and relieve pain.

*Electrotherapy.*    Ultrasound, diadynamic currents, and microwaves are helpful.

## ACTIVE TREATMENTS

*Physical Therapy and Remedial Exercises.*    Perform manual therapy for the affected joints. At first, only traction is used, then gliding in the joint.

Active remedial exercises reinforce the range of motion developed and restore normal function. At first, only isometric exercises are performed if motion causes pain; pure axial motions follow, advancing to complex motions. A cushion or beanbag is good for these treatments; the hand is placed so it can hang over the bag or cushion. Grasping and supporting exercises with and without apparatus help in achieving normal function. Twelve to 20 treatments two to three times per week are necessary.

## SPECIAL NOTES

Preventive measures include applying a supportive bandage, use of wrist-support, and taping of the fingers. Training in proper falling techniques and exercise with small dumbbells are recognized methods of avoiding sprains.

***First Aid at Competition Site.***    Apply cold with compression bandages and immobilize the hand or wrist (or both).

# PART IV Treatment for Training and Competition

Treatments to supplement training and competition are those that improve the general health and fitness of the athlete, prevent athletic injury and damage, and "warm-down" and restore the athlete after great physical and psychic stress. The task of supporting the actual training, which will prepare the athlete optimally for competition and permit him to increase his athletic performance by safe means, is important. These supplementary measures for training and competition are not therapy. They are an important part of a regular training program and make use of physical therapeutic methods and treatments. Athletic massage, for example, is not for the purpose of healing an injury or improving a pathologic condition; rather, its goal is clearly increased performance (see Chapter 1, *Athletic Massage*). Other supplementary measures for training and competition have the same goal. Besides athletic massage, these measures include warm-ups, stretching, special exercises, warm-downs, relaxing baths, self-massage, sauna baths, balancing sports and exercises, and forms of rehabilitative training. Functional bandages and first aid treatments are also included. These will be described in the following chapters.

There are additional measures that supplement training and competition, which are capable of increasing athletic performance. Examples include a balanced diet, mineral supplements, proper hygiene and skin care, use of functional clothing and shoes, and the proper, well-adjusted athletic apparatus. Finally, mention should be made of the extremely important psychologic care of athletes and teams in this connection. This involves either individual or group meetings between the trainer and the athlete(s) for the purpose of regulating the athlete's state of mind, to improve motivation, or give emotional support to the athlete in various stressful situations. Group dynamics and autogenic and mental training can support and improve psychologic care. Cooperation among trainer, athletic psychologist, physician, and therapist is of increasing importance in this area.

The latter measures are only mentioned in passing here. They have been discussed in many publications in the literature. Experienced trainers and attendants know how to use them correctly; it is not the purpose of this book to examine them individually.

All measures that supplement training and competition help protect the health of the athlete and improve his athletic performance, provided that they are coordinated properly and applied at the right time, with sound professional knowledge.

Doping, shots, and pharmacologic manipulation of all types, including stimulants to improve performance, are to be condemned in all cases. They are capable of temporarily improving performance, to be sure, but they repress the natural protection against excessive stress and exhaustion and can thus cause severe damage to the athlete. The use of anabolic steroids can lead to disproportion between muscular strength and tendinous strength, to impotence, and to other harmful effects. A disruption of the hormone balance in female athletes can bring about a change in secondary sexual characteristics and also a change in personality. "Muscle pills" can create "muscle monsters," which have nothing to do with health and esthetics in sports. Many skills that can be achieved through training, such as motor skills, technique, tactics, and so forth cannot be achieved through drugs anyway. Furthermore, the temporary improvement in condition and endurance can result in a more rapid decline and collapse.

Treatments to supplement training and competition that are professionally applied and therapeutically sound work organically with the actual training. They are safe and capable of improving performance.

CHAPTER **17**

# Preparation for Competition

*LUTZ MEISSNER*

## Warm-up

In most sports, athletes prepare for training and competition by warming up. For example, general warming up for distance runners and many other sports begins with jogging; swimmers swim warm-up laps; riders break in their horses. Extent and intensity are gradually increased, and circulation and metabolism are thus stimulated. Warm-ups last about 20 to 30 per cent of the entire training time. In preparation for competition, the warm-up takes substantially longer. For sprinters and dressage riders, the warm-ups take considerably more time than the competition itself.

The goal of warm-ups is to achieve optimal conditioning before training or competition. The danger of injury is decreased as a result of the increase in muscle temperature and the effect on the nervous system. Muscles contract more quickly, blood supply to the muscles is improved, muscles become more elastic and flexible, and nerve reflexes are more rapid. In addition to the preventive effects of warm-ups, they can also increase performance.

The general warm-up is supplemented by stretching or loosening exercises. Specific warm-ups follow the general warm-up. The goal is to remove any difficulty in the transition from warm-up to regular training or competition by increasing the extent and the intensity of the warm-ups with further exercises and coordination exercises. The exercises are performed intensively and are targeted for the particular demands of each sport. The warm-up time is proportionally longer for sports that are of short duration. Unfortunately, these preparations for training and competition are still often neglected.

Alongside the physiologic effects of the warm-up and preparation for competition, a simultaneous psychic preparation is also important. The athlete should be inwardly calm and relaxed. His expectation and readiness for competition should reach the point where he says: "It is time to begin. I am completely ready." This condition is reached through the coordination of physical and psychic factors. Mental simulation of the upcoming event can work together with the physical preparation to achieve optimal readiness. The warm-up is important not only for competitive athletes; weekend athletes, particularly older ones, are also in need of sufficient preparation for their sports. Warm clothing protects the muscles from injury. This should be worn in all cases to prevent loss of warmth and too rapid cooling. Clothing that is too warm, however, particularly when it is worn on the upper body, can lead to a buildup of heat and have a negative influence on the performance. Clothing damp with sweat should be exchanged for dry clothing before competition. When weather conditions are poor during a game, it should also be possible to change clothing during halftime.

In sports that require repeated interruptions and resumptions of activity, it is necessary to warm-up each time before beginning play. Exercises for the particular discipline supplement the general warm-up. The warm-up program should be based on general principles, but it should also take into account the demands of particular disciplines.

Light trotting is not a sufficient warm-up for soccer. The warm-up must be supplemented by stretching exercises, short sprints in different directions, and running in circles, in serpentine lines, forward and backward. In the final phase of the warm-up, include sprints and stops, further coordination exercises, and practice with the ball.

Warm-up time varies for different sports. Sprinters prepare for up to an hour, middle distance runners up to 45 minutes, and soccer players up to 30 minutes before the start of the game.

Passive warm-ups by means of applying heat or massage or use of electrogymnastic equipment can only be considered supplements to active warm-ups. Be cautious of hyperemic muscle salves, as these usually warm only the skin and not the deep-lying muscles. Proper warm-ups guard against injury and prepare the body for optimal performance in training or in competition.

# Stretching

The stretching of the muscle-ligament apparatus is an important supplement to the general warm-up in preparing for training and competition. Muscles and soft tissues undergo primarily active stretching. Stretching makes the distance between the muscle origins and insertions greater, up to the point of maximal extension. A thorough program of stretching minimizes the danger of injury under maximal stress. Various positions affect the muscle-tendon transitions and improve the stretching. Overly tense muscles are particularly prone to injury. Active stretching has proved to be effective in these cases. No stretching exercises should ever extend beyond the limits of movement for either the joint or the muscles. Passive stretching should only follow sufficient active warm-ups and stretching, if at all.

Exercises with a partner must never be jerky or cause injury to the muscles. General stretching supplements other preparations for training and competition. The particular stretching motions are geared to the demands of the particular sports. Thus, sprinters should stretch the upper leg muscles and keep them supple; soccer players stretch the adductors and quadriceps muscles; weight-lifters the back muscles; and wrestlers and judo participants the stomach muscles.

## Special Exercises

Calisthenics are usually geared toward a specific purpose, and are known as functional exercises or as training or conditioning exercises. Specific calisthenics follow the warm-up period and stretch the muscles in preparation for training or competition. The exercises are primarily specific but can also include balancing and rhythmic exercises. Specific movements required by the various sports are prepared for in this way. Thus, the exercises vary for skiers and swimmers, hurdlers and riders. Each particular sport is prepared for by imitating the movements required by the sport itself. General fitness and special conditioning are thereby improved. General conditioning, such as in mobility, agility, and strength, is also trained in this process.

Exercises for the entire body today are more and more frequently replacing the traditional form of the warm-up. Experience and observation has shown that a special program of exercise has many advantages. Time is saved, and the athlete is prepared properly for training and competition.

Work by Klümper and Keydel in the area of track and field athletics questions the value of traditional warm-ups with running, calisthenics, and games on the basis of their frequently superficial nature. Both authors propose ways and means of warming up with specific exercises for the entire body. As the cardiovascular stimulation through calisthenics is only slight, however, general running exercises should not be omitted.

The warm-up concludes with the use of the individual apparatus for the particular sport. Ball players warm-up with the ball, gymnasts on the apparatus, and throwers with the javelin, discus, or shot. In this way the athlete is optimally prepared for training and competition.

CHAPTER **18**

# Relaxing Warm-Down

*WERNER KUPRIAN*

## Warming Down

Active warming down has been proved to be an effective means of decreasing the effects on the musculoskeletal system of the stimuli of training and competition in many sports. These effects are reduced by, for example, slow jogging on soft surfaces, such as on grass or in woods. Active loosening and shaking of the extremities and torso are also included as warming-down modalities. Light jumping, hopping, and knee lifts improve the active warm-down, such as for track and field athletes. A warm-down period of 10 to 20 minutes should follow every workout or competition. When the warm-down can be made more interesting, as in tossing a ball, psychic relaxation can take place with the physical relaxation. Properly relaxed muscles demonstrate at most only a slight reaction to the stress of training or competition in the form of sore muscles and similar effects.

The development of reactions to competition or training is also decreased in other sports by performing light activity, such as slow swimming or skiing after the event. The primary goal here is also the loosening and relaxing of muscle by means of active warm-down. Ball games and other types of sports can form the mainstay of active warm-downs. Proper warm-down can also be a preparation for the next training session or the next competition.

## Relaxing Bath

A relaxing bath is used like a sauna bath, after hard training or competition involving great muscular, circulatory, or psychic stress, for relaxation, loosening, and the removal of metabolic wastes.

This includes loosening exercises in water and also exercises that relieve the stress on the spine and other joints; the athlete can perform these exercises alone, with a partner, or in small groups. Games should also be included. Athletes can also take a relaxing bath in a large tub. A pool that can hold an entire team is more effective for the group dynamic aspects.

The buoyancy and resistance of the water are exploited in these exercises. Apparatus such as waterballs, buoyant devices, rings, and so forth, can be used. The water should be between 28° and 30°C; water colder than this is not suitable. The relaxing bath should not last longer than 15 to 30 minutes. It should be conducted in a way that also encourages psychic relaxation after the stress of competition. Its aims are fun, pleasure, and relaxation following the pressure of competition.

Cold showers and an extended period of relaxation, or sleep, if possible, should follow.

# Self-Massage

Self-massage, that is, the athlete's massaging of parts of his own body, can also be used for relaxation purposes. It is particularly suited for combination with a relaxing bath or a sauna bath. A short self-massage can also be used in connection with warm-ups as a preparation for competition. Heat, such as a hot shower or a hot sitdown bath, helps prepare for the self-massage. The body should not cool down during the self-massage.

Of course, there are great limitations to self-massage in comparison with the massage by a therapist. The athlete must do the work himself, in particular using the muscles in his arms and shoulders, which does not relax these parts of the body.

The self-massage is primarily suited for the large muscle groups of the upper leg — that is the extensor muscles on the front, the flexors on the back, and the internal adductor groups. Calf muscles can also be relaxed with self-massage. The best position for this is sitting on a bench or on the ground.

The lower and upper arms and the hand muscles are also accessible for a self-massage; the back and shoulders are difficult to reach. As these are always partial massages, 5 to 10 minutes is sufficient.

Suitable techniques include stroking the extremities from the periphery toward the center of the body, gentle kneading, rubbing, and loosening massage. A good skin oil should be used, but sparingly. Brushes, loofa sponges, or other aids can enhance skin and muscle circulation. These objects can also be used through training clothing. A therapist should demonstrate the basics of self-massage for the athlete.

Self-massage must not be considered a means of healing or as a remedial tool, but solely as a loosening massage for athletics. Remedial massage should be left to an experienced therapist, because of the danger of causing injury. Self-massage is strongly advised against when an athlete has been injured. As a means of preparing for competition or of relaxing following performance, however, it is one of the most effective treatments, which the athlete can be encouraged to perform, and which he is able to carry out himself if there is no therapist at hand.

# Sauna Bath

The sauna bath can no longer be ignored as an adjunctive measure in training and competition. It is primarily a means of relaxing after the stress of

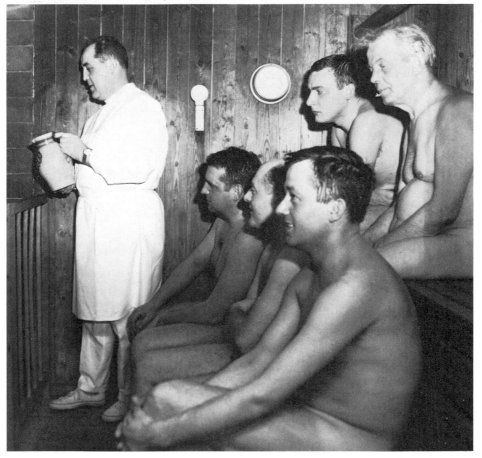

**Figure 18–1.**    In the sauna; water is poured onto hot stones of the sauna oven.

training and competition, aiding in the removal of metabolic wastes, relaxing the body, and assisting in regeneration.

This ancient Scandinavian bath, which originated in Finland, has been used in athletics since as early as the 1936 Olympics in Berlin. In 1972, during the Olympic Games in Munich, several sauna baths were available to the athletes. Many thousands of sauna baths were taken there by the athletes of many nations.

The physiologic effects of the sauna bath include an increase in body temperature ("healing fever"), an intensive stimulus to metabolism and the circulation, and considerable perspiration, thus aiding in the removal of metabolic wastes. The psychic components of the sauna bath include relaxation, regeneration, and a feeling of general well-being. This modality is popular among many athletes. The sauna bath not only relieves muscular stress, but in addition its meditative nature relaxes the entire person and helps him completely forget the stress of competition. It is a nonspecific means of maintaining health and well-being and of encouraging regeneration, and thus it improves performance. It enhances the body's defenses against colds and helps prevent infections of the upper bronchial tubes as well as other illnesses.

The contractile elements of the muscles are also positively influenced in athletes who take regular sauna baths along with their usual programs for increasing muscular strength. The bone-ligament system, which has poor circulation, is also improved. The reduction of muscle tension, improved reabsorption of waste materials in the relaxing phase, and the replacement of glycogen in the muscles are among the useful effects the athlete can derive from the sauna bath. The idea that the sauna bath could replace active training is erroneous, however; the sauna can only aid general fitness and increase athletic performance in connection with other active training.

In contradistinction to the steam bath, a sauna is a dry hot air bath, in which the air temperatures are between 60° and 90°C. The relative humidity of the air should be between 5 and 10 per cent. This is maintained by short bursts of steam from pouring water with fir or pine extracts on the hot stones of the sauna oven. The essential oils and the burst of steam serve to deepen the breathing.

The sweat-bath portion is conducted in a room paneled with ash, fir, or hemlock. The wood paneling of the room rapidly absorbs the humidity from the air and restores dryness to the sauna room.

Sauna rooms used to be heated by wood ovens. Today industrially manufactured saunas are in use, which use heated sauna stones or heating slabs. Good air circulation should be ensured in all saunas. A thermometer to gauge room temperature and a hygrometer to measure humidity are also necessary.

Showers, changing rooms, and relaxation area, as well as an open-air room with a cold water pool and hose, are necessary.

A thorough cleansing of the body with warm water is necessary before the sauna to open the pores. Two or three alternations between sweating and cooling phases are usually recommended.

The phase in the sauna bath itself last 10 to 20 minutes, depending on the individual. Begin by sitting on the lower benches and only gradually move up to the higher ones. There should be a strong outbreak of perspiration over the entire body. Between 400 and 1000 grams of water are usually lost in the course of a sauna bath. This loss of weight is quickly regained by a corresponding intake of fluids. The idea that one can lose weight in a sauna is still a widely held misunderstanding. The use of sauna by boxers, wrestlers, and jockeys to control weight is a very questionable practice; it generally causes more harm than good. The athlete should control his weight by other means.

The sweating phase is followed by a cooling phase, which is an important part of the sauna. Begin with cool air, then take a cold shower, and finally take a short plunge into a cold pool of water. This is best done in an open-air room. The goal of cooling is to close the pores and the vessels of the skin, so that the heat accumulated within the body remains, although the perspiration has stopped. Cooling should begin on the legs and move toward the head. To avoid headaches owing to heat buildup in the neck, always include the head in the

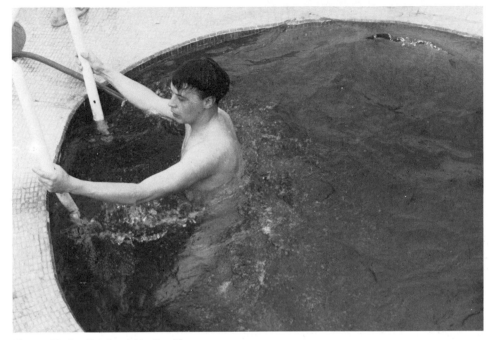

**Figure 18-2.** Brief cold bath after sauna.

cooling process. Cooling should not last too long. The length of the cooling period depends on the time of year and the outside temperature when conducted outdoors. In winter, brief rubdowns with snow are a refreshing means of cooling. Dry toweling follows immediately.

Excessive cooling must be avoided. If shivering develops or the feet become cold, warm footbaths are necessary between the periods in the sauna, which last about 10 minutes. Strenuous exercises are not recommended in the intervals because of the strain on the cardiovascular system. However, loosening and relaxing exercises are possible. Lying in a relaxed position with the legs elevated is best.

The sauna room is reentered after a pause of 10 to 15 minutes. After two or three periods in the sauna, a rest period of at least 30 minutes is absolutely necessary for the physiologic effects to wear off. Thirst can now be quenched also, with mineral water, herb tea, or fruit juice. Alcoholic beverages are absolutely forbidden. A full stomach before a sauna and a heavy meal afterward are likewise advised against. Light foods, such as fruit, salad, yoghurt, and so forth, are best. The sauna is a good way to relax immediately after strenuous training or competition. Because of the stress on the circulatory system, a sauna should not be taken within 3 days preceding competition.

CHAPTER **19**

# Balanced Exercises

## *LUTZ MEISSNER*

The purpose of the balanced exercises is to counteract one-sided stress, such as occurs in many sports. In addition, weakness of the muscles and poor posture can be corrected or improved. In competitive sports, the repeated patterns of certain movements increase with the stress of training and competition. One-sided exercises strengthen particular muscle groups but often lead to a muscular imbalance. Balanced exercises are necessary to limit or equalize this imbalance. All parts of the body are exercised, and thus the one-sided stress on the body is counteracted. Such exercises also contribute to the lessening of motor dysfunction and help prevent injuries, as well as normalize motions.

All these exercises begin with the athlete in a supine position. A blanket constitutes sufficient padding, but grass or a mat is also a good base for the exercises. The movements are carried out slowly and evenly. They begin with the head and the neck vertebrae and progress to include the entire body. Up to 10 repetitions of the individual exercises are possible. Each series of exercises is followed by an equally long pause, so that tension and relaxation last for the same amount of time. Afternoon and evening hours are good times for these to

*Text continued on page 316*

STARTING POSITION FOR ALL EXERCISES
IS SUPINE POSITION

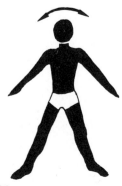

**Figure 19–1.** Position for all exercises: incline head alternately to right and left shoulders.

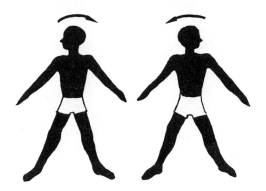

**Figure 19–2.** Twist head alternately to the left and right shoulders.

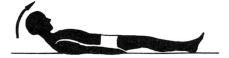

**Figure 19–3.** Alternately lift head (chin to chest) and relax (extend chin).

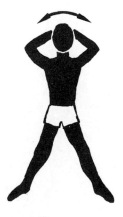

**Figure 19–4.** Fold hands behind head, incline shoulders and head alternately to right and left.

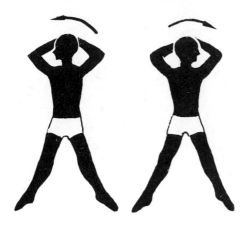

**Figure 19–5.** Fold hands behind head, twist shoulders and head alternately to right and left.

**Figure 19–6.** Fold hands behind head, alternately lift head and shoulders (chin to chest) and relax (extend chin).

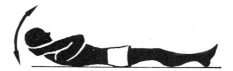

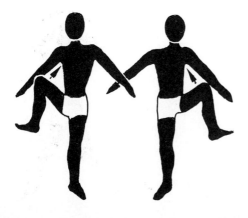

**Figure 19–7.** Alternately lift right and left knees diagonally toward the opposite shoulder and return.

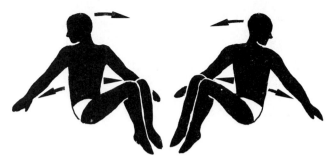

**Figure 19–8.** With legs bent, twist to either side; head twists in opposite direction.

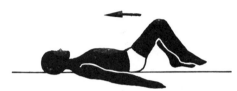

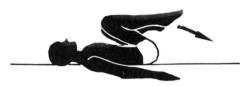

**Figure 19–9.** With legs bent, lift both towards left or right shoulder and return them while still bent.

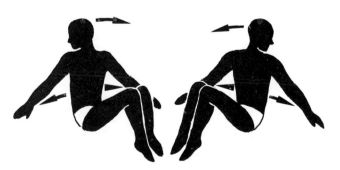

**Figure 19–10.** With legs bent, twist both legs to either side, twisting the head in the opposite direction.

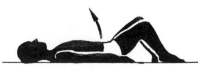

**Figure 19–11.** With legs bent, bring hips to full extension and relax.

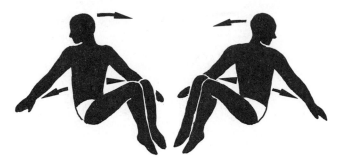

**Figure 19–12.** With legs bent, twist to either side; head twists in the opposite direction.

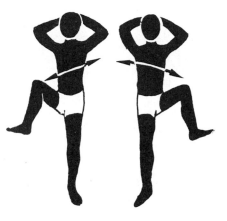

**Figure 19–13.** Fold hands behind head, bring left elbow and right knee together; then do the same with right elbow and left knee.

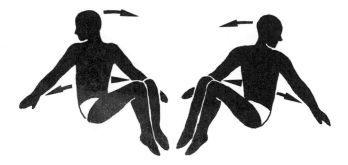

**Figure 19–14.** With legs bent, twist to either side; head twists in the opposite direction.

**Figure 19–15.** Fold hands behind head, bend legs, bring knees and elbows together and relax.

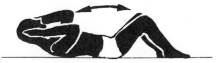

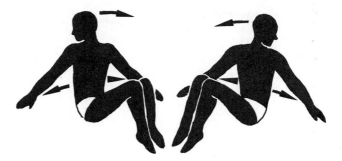

**Figure 19–16.** With legs bent, twist to either side; head twists in the opposite direction.

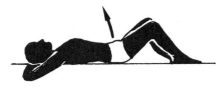

**Figure 19–17.** Fold hands behind head, lift and extend hips, relax.

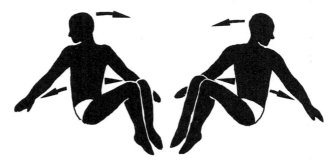

**Figure 19–18.** With legs bent, twist to either side; head twists in opposite direction.

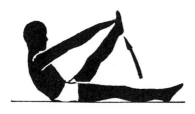

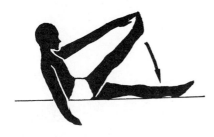

**Figure 19–19.** Bring extended left arm and extended right leg together, lifting head, then do the same with the opposite limbs.

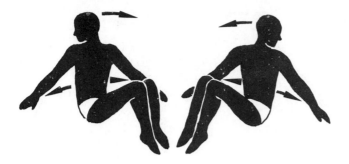

**Figure 19–20.** With legs bent, twist to either side; head twists in opposite direction.

**Figure 19–21.** Bend knees, bring extended arms and legs together in air, return legs to the bent position.

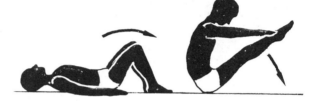

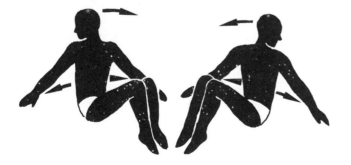

**Figure 19–22.** With legs bent, twist to either side; head twists in the opposite direction.

**Figure 19–23.** Fold hands behind head, left leg bent, right leg extended; lift hips to extension and relax; then do the same with other legs.

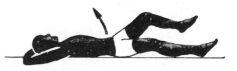

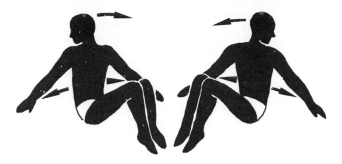

**Figure 19–24.** With legs bent, twist to either side; head twists in the opposite direction.

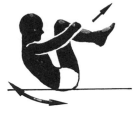

**Figure 19–25.** With both hands grasping the knees, roll body back and forth, until nape of neck and feet alternately touch ground.

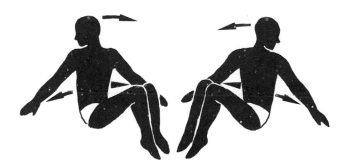

**Figure 19–26.** With legs bent, twist to either side; head twists in the opposite direction.

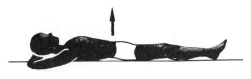

**Figure 19–27.** Fold hands behind head; with both legs extended, lift hips slightly and relax.

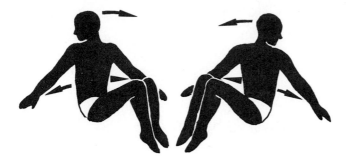

**Figure 19–28.** With legs bent, twist to either side; head twists in the opposite direction.

be done. Sidewards inclination, rotation, flexion, and extension motions follow one another, producing spiral- and diagonal-shaped patterns as the exercises progress. Alternate with opposing exercises; this results in the favorable contraction and extension of the entire musculature.

The initial position taken for the balanced exercises depends on the type of stress encountered in the individual's sport. For athletic disciplines that increase lordosis, such as javelin throwing and butterfly stroke in swimming, the legs are bent to correct the curvature of the lumbar vertebrae. The balanced exercises are carried out in the form of holding work for stabilization in those sports that tend to produce excessive mobility of the spine, such as gymnastics and synchronized calisthenics. For these sports, the final position of the exercises is held for up to 7 seconds. Athletes who perform sports with little motion, such as weight-lifters, are helped to increase their range of motions with balanced exercises, in this way relieving stress. The increase in the range of motion also aids in general mobility.

CHAPTER **20**

# Balanced Sports

*LUTZ MEISSNER*

Balanced sports represent a way for the athlete to keep fit without the stress of training and competition in his particular specialty. Balanced sports maintain function while the athlete is not actively competing, as in the off-season. For those athletic disciplines that place a high degree of stress on the musculoskeletal system, such as combative sports, ball games, and gymnastics, balanced sports such as swimming, particularly using the backstroke, bicycling, and cross-country skiing are recommended. The joints, the vertebral column, and the muscles are not as severely taxed and receive balanced, usually symmetric, stress. Injuries from excessive stress are rare in sports that place relatively low demands on the musculoskeletal system, such as swimming and cross-country skiing. When they do occur, ball games, such as indoor soccer, basketball, or volleyball, are recommended. The intensity of the games should be kept low because of the danger of injury.

Participating in balanced sports is also psychologically relaxing for the athlete, representing a break from the rigors of training for competition. Thus, soccer players like Sepp Maier and Gerd Müller play tennis for relaxation. The sprinter Jutta Heine rode horses in the off-season.

Physicians and therapists have long recognized that sports and exercise can bring balance to working environments as well. Thus, managers and factory workers, for example, in industrialized nations are encouraged to participate in athletic activities. Exercise should maintain or improve general physical conditioning. Running is a good exercise for people in sedentary professions.

It seems justified to suggest a parallel between stresses in the work environment and the stress encountered by the top competitive or professional athlete. He too can be helped by relief from the stress of his normal work — namely, competitive sport — in the form of other exercises for the relaxation of mind and body.

## CHAPTER 21

# Rehabilitation Training

### *LUTZ MEISSNER*

Rehabilitation training after injuries should return the athlete to his normal performance level. It must be geared to the process of healing. The primary consideration is freedom from pain; the pain threshold must not be exceeded. The various possible physical therapy treatments and remedial exercises for specific injuries were discussed earlier (Part III). The athlete can make use of the possibilities listed in this chapter along with the treatments described earlier during his rehabilitation training to systematically accelerate his recuperation. They can also be built into the exercise program upon resumption of normal training.

## Minus Training

Minus training involves the complete or partial relief of body weight. This can be accomplished with a running harness, sling supports, a strength machine, an exercise bath, or an exercise bicycle.

When movements are permitted again after an injury, an athlete usually returns to his or her normal exercise regimen. The training program for the particular sport is resumed gradually, but it is not specially prepared for the convalescing athlete. This can lead to a relapse and permanent damage, which can put an end to the athlete's career. However, such an unfortunate occurrence can be avoided with the gradual increase in stress permitted by minus training.

*Example:* An athlete was given first aid and physical therapy for a sprained ankle. Remedial exercise permitted the restoration of normal function. The joint was painless while at rest, but as soon as the athlete even began to walk, pain set in.

The following schedule sketches a program of gradually increasing stress. It can also be used as a guideline for treating other athletic injuries.

*Day 1:* Walking in water up to the neck.
*Day 2:* Walking in water up to the shoulders.
*Day 3:* Walking in water up to the chest.
*Day 4:* Walking in water up to the abdomen.
*Day 5:* Walking in water up to the hips.

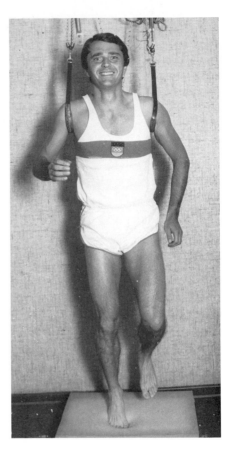

**Figure 21–1.**  Minus training in harness on soft mats.

*After day 5:* Walking in supportive harness with relief of one third of body weight alternating with exercise bicycle.

*After day 9:* Running in supportive harness with relief of one third of body weight alternating with exercise bicycle.

*After day 13:* Running on 6 to 8 soft mats alternating with exercise bicycle; remove one mat daily.

*After day 20:* Normal stress and running.

Stress of the muscles is increased by 1 minute daily; begin with 2 minutes.

# Complex Training

Complex training is a special form of training. It is used in both the rehabilitative and the preventative phases of training. The basic concept is derived from the book by Knott and Voss, *Complex Motions — Motion Facilitation After Dr. Kabat* (see Chapter 7).

Three-dimensional patterns of motion are trained particularly by exploit-

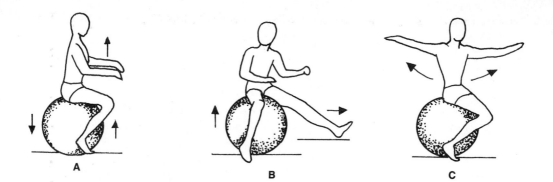

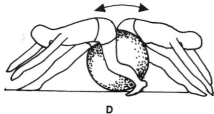

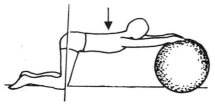

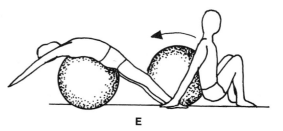

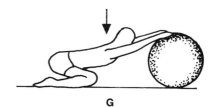

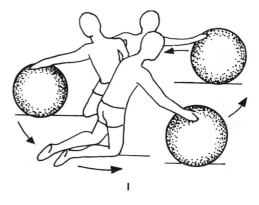

**Figure 21–2.** Complex training with Pezzi ball.

*Illustration continued on opposite page*

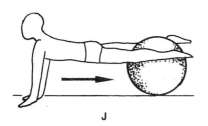

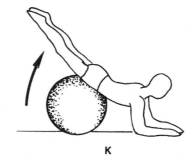

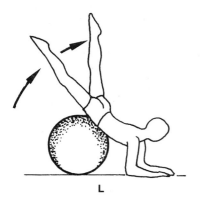

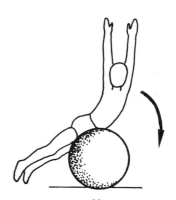

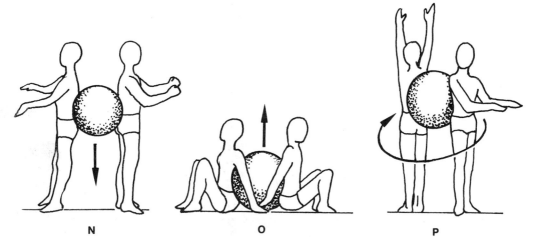

**Figure 21–2.** *Continued.*

ing various surface conditions and running techniques with the help of various additional devices, such as balls, mats, trampoline, and others.

The exercises are intended to simulate the stress of training and competition and of extreme situations, and to prepare the body specially for them. Examples:

*Running patterns:* Running in serpentine lines, circles, figure-eights, and sideward, backward, and forward is possible. This is the simplest form of complex training.

*Running barefoot:* Running on a thick mat, bouncing on a trampoline, running movements while balancing on a medicine ball.

*Running on various surfaces:* Running on the beach, on hard and soft sand, into and out of knee-deep water. Running along the bed of a stream or jumping over rocks.

*Running on slopes:* Running back and forth, up and down an incline, in serpentine lines, in circles, in figure-eights, and forward, backward, and sideward.

*Exercises with partner:* Partners jostle one another while standing, kneeling, sitting, or lying, and try to knock each other out of the initial position. This is good for improvement of coordination and balance.

*Pezzi ball exercises:* These improve stabilization, coordination, and equilibrium and can be performed alone or with a partner.

CHAPTER **22**

# Functional Bandages

*LUTZ MEISSNER*

## History

Bandages for injuries and for the support and relief of stress on parts of the body are as old as medicine itself. The application of bandages in athletics is known to have taken place in ancient Greece. Many of the techniques for compensation, stabilization, and immobilization remain unchanged in principle today. Bandaging techniques such as the spica (literally, ear of grain) and testudo (tortoise shell) remain in use today and testify to their effectiveness. Since antiquity, bandages have been held on to the skin with natural materials, such as pitch and honey. Ancient bandaging systems reveal that what are sometimes regarded as modern techniques were already being taught in classic medical schools.

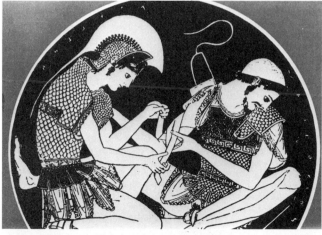

**Figure 22–1.** Achilles binds Patrocles, 500 B.C.

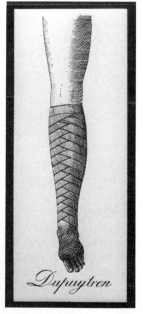

**Figure 22–2.** Classic lower-leg bandage—spica ascendens.

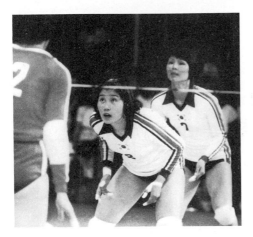

**Figure 22–3.** Tape bandages for volleyball players.

# Use of Functional Bandages

Further developments in functional bandages for athletic injuries have been made in recent years with the availability of better bandaging materials and evolution of more refined techniques. Experience has shown that compression, immobilizing, and stabilizing bandages, together with additional physical therapy treatments, are capable of accelerating the healing process and preventing traumas or relapses. Bandages supplement training and competition by immobilizing, supporting, and guiding the movements of joints and muscles. The following classifications are made on the basis of the time of application, the type of bandage, bandaging techniques, and bandaging materials.

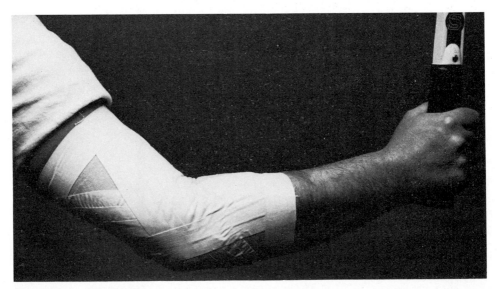

**Figure 22–4.** Elbow bandage with strips of adhesive tape.

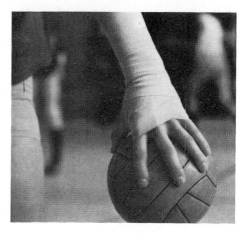

**Figure 22–5.** Wrist bandage for German handball.

# Classification According to Time of Application

1. *First bandage.* First aid bandage for open wound (see Chapter 23). Use a compression bandage for the initial treatment of a hematoma.

2. *Second bandage.* After the wound has closed or the hematoma is reabsorbed, a second bandage is applied to aid in the healing process.

3. *Later bandage.* This bandage is for support and the relief of stress.

4. *Prophylactic bandage.* Traumas, relapses, and athletic damages are avoided or minimized with this bandage.

# Classification According to Type of Bandage

1. *Open wound.* Cuts are treated with first aid measures (see Chapter 23).

2. *Compression bandage.* Strong compression prevents or minimizes swelling or hematoma. Cold, foam rubber, and materials that encourage reabsorption improve the effect. Large areas of swelling, such as in the lower leg, are completely contained with a circular bandage around the leg. So-called "varicose bandages" are suited for this purpose. Compression bandages tightened with string are good for fingers and toes and also for the backs of the hands and feet. String that has been dipped in cold water can be fitted more closely and also provides cooling.

3. *Immobilizing bandage.* The immobilization of joints or muscles after injury permits a quicker and better healing. The possibility of static stress is maintained.

4. *Supportive bandage.* The range of motion is restricted for muscles and joints by a supportive bandage. Extreme movements are avoided and relapses are prevented.

# Classification According to Bandaging Techniques

1. *Circular bandage (dolabra ascendens or descendens)*. This circular bandage can spiral either upward or downward and is used for the neck, torso, thigh, calf, upper arm, or lower arm.

2. *Testudo reversa or inversa*. This bandage, which begins on either the inside or the outside of the knee or elbow, is wrapped in figure-eights around the joint.

3. *Spica ascendens or descendens*. The bandage can be wrapped in either an ascending or a descending direction and is used for immobilizing large areas, such as the shoulder, hip, or ankle.

4. *Head bandage (mitra reversa or inversa)*. This bandage is wrapped around the head like a cap.

# Classification According to Bandaging Material

1. *Elastic bandage*. Use elastic materials of differing compressions and elasticity (50 to 200 per cent). The less elastic the material is, the greater pressure that can be exerted.

Slight elasticity: strong compression.

Moderate elasticity: normal compression.

Great elasticity: gentle compression.

2. *Adhesive bandage*. Use adhesive bandages that stretch lengthwise (60 per cent) and crosswise (30 per cent). Apply these primarily for support, relief of stress, and guiding movements.

3. *Cloth tape*. Inelastic, strong, tearable tape with or without adhesive tape.

4. *Self-sticking bandage (adhesive bandage, Band-Aid)*. Use this adhesive bandage for small wounds. The bandage also sticks to perspiring skin. Primary uses are for slight injuries; as a protective covering; and as dressing beneath adhesive bandages.

The various materials permit combinations that are more effective than use of a single type alone. Thus, strips of adhesive tape increase the pressure of an elastic bandage. An elastic adhesive bandage, when reinforced with nonelastic adhesive tape, is similarly improved in its effectiveness.

# Indications

Functional bandages are applied as first aid, as after-treatment, and in remedial care.

The following athletic injuries or damages can be treated with functional bandages:

Contusions                    Injured ligaments
Sprains                       Injured joints
Injured muscles               Deformities
Injured tendons               Luxations (dislocations)
Injured capsules              Fractures

# Contraindications

Contraindications to use of bandages include the following:

Recent, complete fractures
Completely ruptured tendons
Completely ruptured ligaments
Large open wounds

# Basic Principles in the Application
# of Functional Bandages

*Care of wounds.* Give first aid treatment to open wounds; only then is a bandage applied.

*Padding.* Cover condyles, tendons, and nerves, or other pressure points, with padded bandages.

*Bandages with holes.* Surround kneecaps, ankles, and other protruding parts of the body with foam rubber cut to form to protect them.

*Skin protection.* Protect the skin with a light adhesive bandage. This also serves to stabilize additional padding or bandaging that may be necessary and facilitates their application.

*Positioning.* Joints are relieved of pain and stress before proper bandage is applied. Muscles are positioned so that the origins and insertions are brought together. In this way pain from traction and stretching will diminish as the scar decreases in size. Preventive bandages are applied to the legs while the patient is standing and to the arms while he or she is sitting.

*Improvement of effectiveness.* The compression by a bandage is increased with underlying wadding, gauze, or foam rubber. Additional strips of adhesive tape improve the stability of the bandage.

*Length of application.* Nonelastic adhesive bandages for prevention are applied only for training and competition and removed afterward. Bandages for rehabilitative purposes are constantly checked and frequently changed to avoid further damage. If swelling develops distal to the bandage or if the blood supply is restricted, the bandage is loosened or, if necessary, cut up the side, or it is removed and renewed. The entire period of application depends on the extent of the injury and the rate of healing.

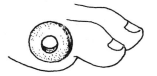

**Figure 22–6.** Bandage with hole for little toe.

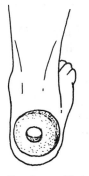

**Figure 22–7.** Bandage with hole for heel.

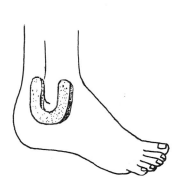

**Figure 22–8.** Bandage with cut out area for ankle.

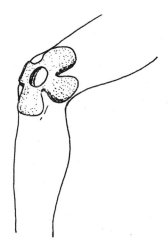

**Figure 22–9.** Bandage with hole for knee.

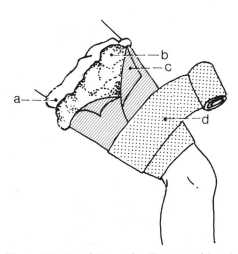

**Figure 22–10.** Schematic diagram of bandage. *a,* Layer next to wound; *b,* padding; *c,* fixation bandage; *d,* elastic bandage.

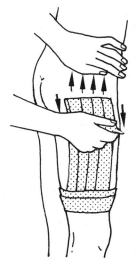

**Figure 22–11.** Removal of tape with traction and pressure.

*Removal of bandage.* The application of a light bandage underneath the main bandage simplifies the removal. Adhesive bandages come off better in a shower or bath. Pressing against the skin eases the removal or change of a bandage.

# Materials

*Bandaging materials.* Plaster and bandages for wounds are the most common materials used.

*Padding.* Wadding, fleece, foam rubber, and varicose bandages may be used for padding.

*Underlying bandages.* These may be made of mull, gauze, clinging material, "Snöggbind" bandage, "Sporty-Quick" bandage, or "Underwrap" bandages.

*Fixation bandages.* These are made of mull, netting, tube bandage, gauze, or clinging material.

*Elastic bandages.* Elastic bandages can have slight, moderate, or great elasticity.

*Adhesive bandages.* These can be elastic, with 60 per cent elasticity lengthwise and 30 per cent sideways, or inelastic tape, which is strong and can be torn lengthwise and laterally.

*Adhesive bandages (Band-Aid type).* These are made of clinging material, "Snöggbind" bandage, or "Sporty-Quick" bandage.

*Additional materials* include scissors, spray adhesive, and cords of various thicknesses.

# Application

Functional bandages are most effective when they achieve proper care of the wound, compression, supportive and holding functions, relief of stress, guidance of motion, and freedom from pain. If a part of a movement is painful, the functional bandage must support the joint or muscle in such a way that all of the above factors are considered. Supportive strips are usually applied to a tape bandage to improve the adhesion of the subsequent lengthwise or diagonal strips of tape.

*Examples:* If flexion of the hip causes pain, the affected area is immobilized with a bandage that limits movement so that it does not go beyond the point of pain.

If abduction and outward rotation of the leg causes pain, the affected area is immobilized with a bandage for adduction and inward rotation, so that abduction and outward rotation of the leg do not go beyond the point of pain.

*Text continued on page 348*

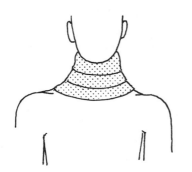

**Figure 22–12.** Supporting and extending bandage for cervical vertebrae after whiplash injury and compression fracture of the cervical vertebrae.

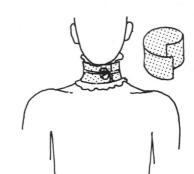

**Figure 22–13.** Schanz's wadding bandage, neck cravat.

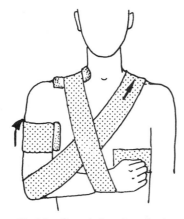

**Figure 22–14.** Sayre's bandage for immobilization of shoulder girdle after broken collarbone or dislocated shoulder.

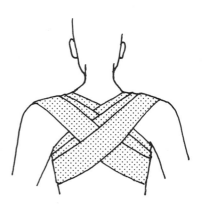

**Figure 22–15.** Spica dorsi bandage for immobilization after broken collarbone.

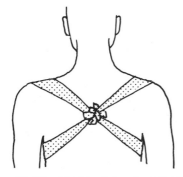

**Figure 22–16.** Rucksack bandage for immobilization after broken collarbone.

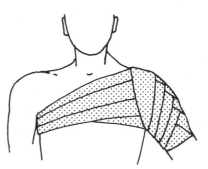

**Figure 22–17.** Spica descendens bandage for the immobilization of the shoulder.

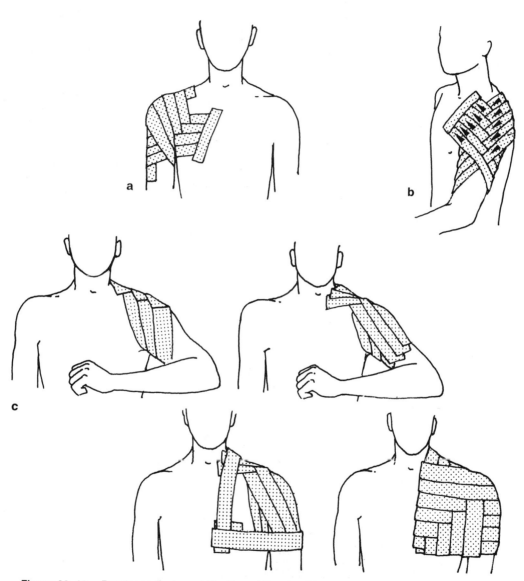

**Figure 22–18.**   Bandages for immobilization of the shoulder.

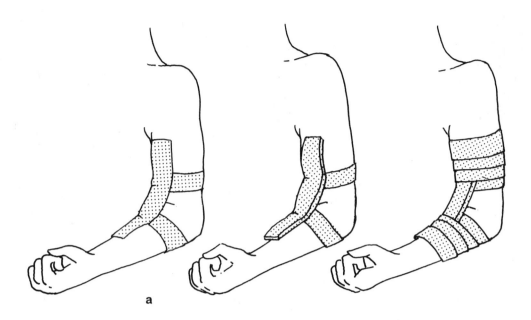

a

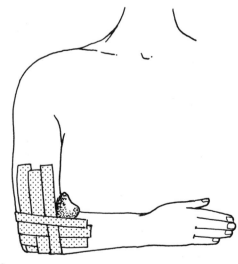

b

**Figure 22–19.**  Bandages for immobilization of the elbow.

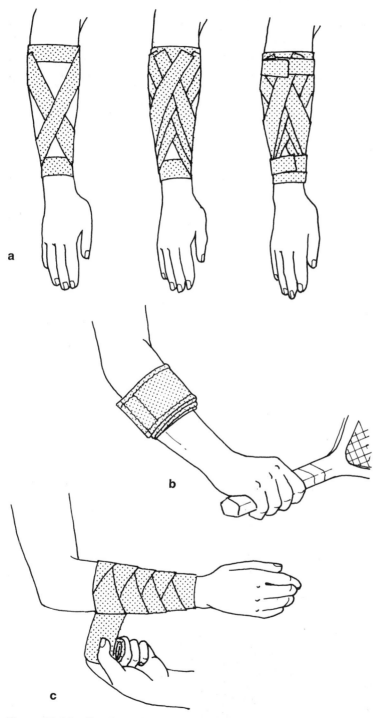

a

b

c

**Figure 22–20.** Bandages for immobilization of the lower arm.

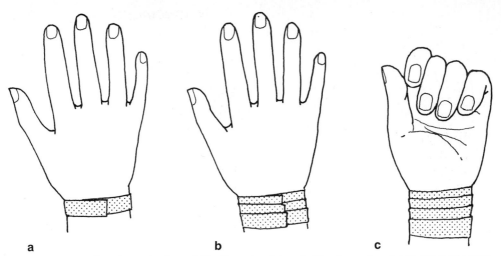

**Figure 22–21.** Bandages for immobilization of wrist. *a*, *b*, Bandages for stabilization of wrist; *c*, strengthening wrist band.

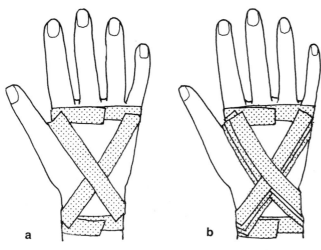

**Figure 22–22.** Bandages for immobilization of the hand.

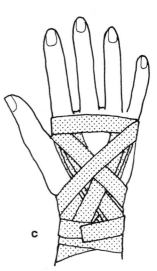

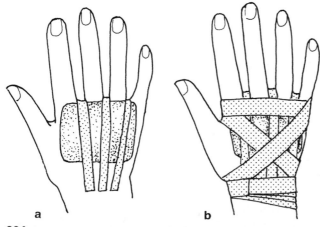

**Figure 22–23.** Compression bandages for hand.

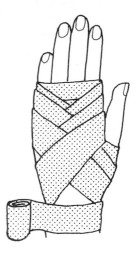

**Figure 22–24.**  Bandages for immobilization of the wrist and hand.

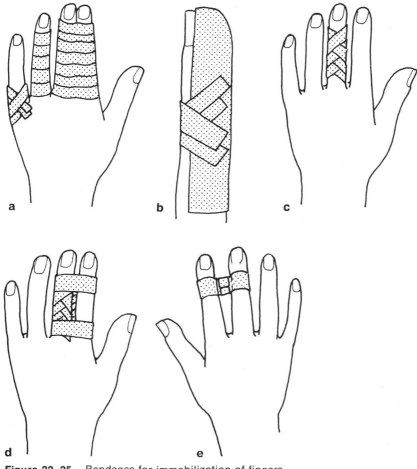

**Figure 22–25.**  Bandages for immobilization of fingers.

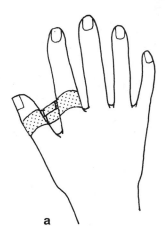

a

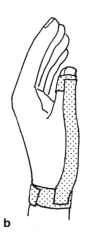

b

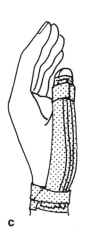

c

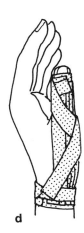

d

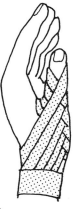

e

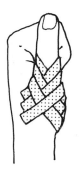

f

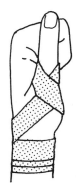

g

**Figure 22–26.**   Bandages for immobilization of the thumb.

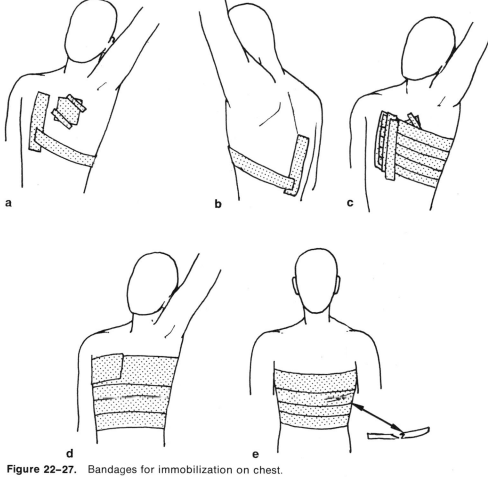

**Figure 22–27.** Bandages for immobilization on chest.

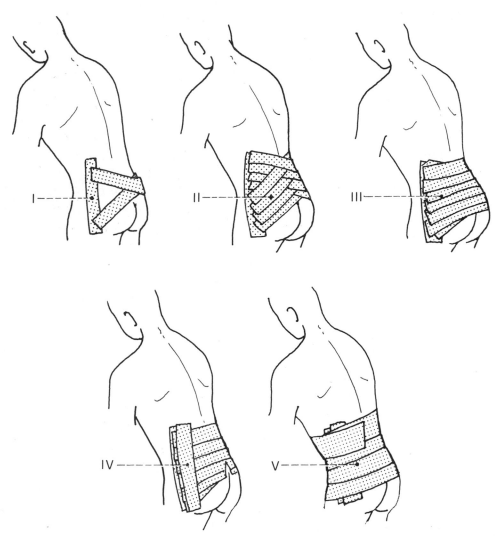

**Figure 22–28.** Bandages for immobilization of the lumbar vertebrae. *I,* Holding strips; *II,* diagonal strips; *III,* cross strips; *IV,* reinforcing strips; *V,* circular wrappings.

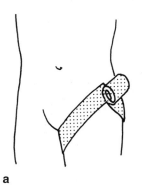

**a**

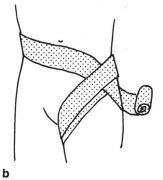

**b**

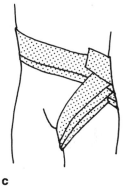

**c**

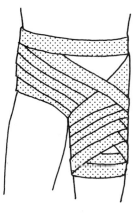

**d**

**Figure 22–29.** Bandage for immobilization around hip.

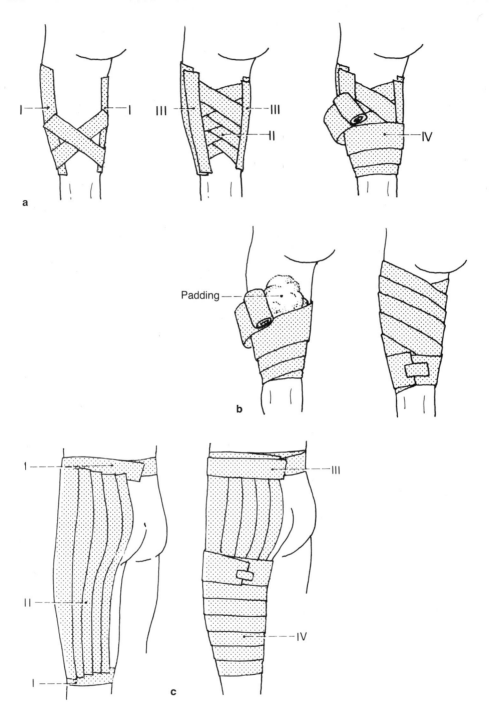

**Figure 22–30.** Bandages for immobilization of thigh (dorsal side). *a, I,* Holding strips; *II,* diagonal strips; *III,* reinforcing strips; *IV,* circular wrappings. *b,* Padding. *c, I,* Holding strips; *II,* long strips; *III,* reinforcing strips; *IV,* circular wrappings.

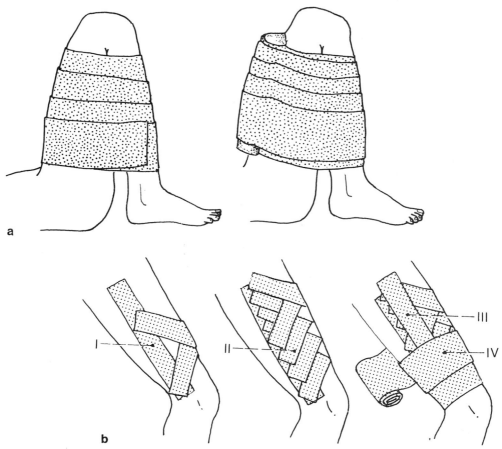

**b**

**Figure 22–31.** Bandages for immobilization of the thigh (lateral and ventral). *a*, Compression bandage with and without Cool Pac. Efficiency is improved by extending muscle and bending knee. *b*, Quadriceps bandage. *I*, Holding strips; *II*, diagonal strips; *III*, reinforcing strips; *IV*, circular wrappings.

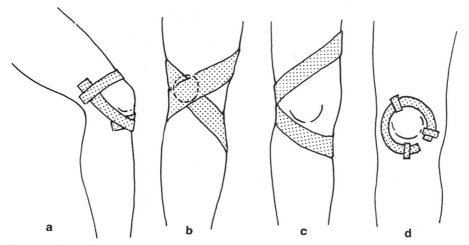

**Figure 22–32.** Bandages for immobilization of knee. *a–d*, Fixation of the patella.

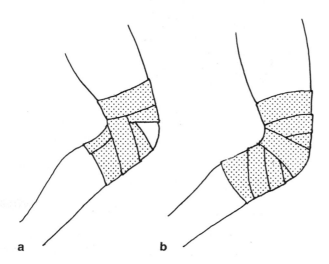

**Figure 22–33.** Testudo bandage on knee. *a,* Reversa; *b,* inversa.

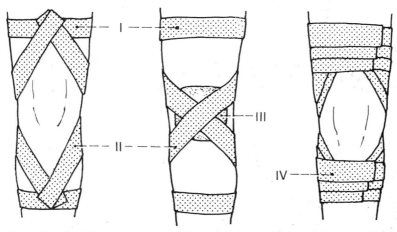

**Figure 22–34.** Bandage for immobilization of knee (dorsal side). *I,* Holding strips; *II,* diagonal strips; *III,* padding; *IV,* reinforcing strips.

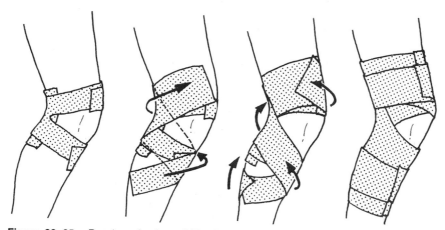

**Figure 22–35.** Bandage for immobilization of knee after rotation injury. Traction is from outside to inside for injuries to the inner ligaments, from inside to outside for injuries to outer ligaments.

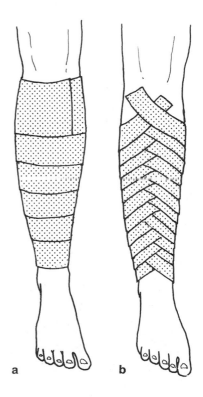

**Figure 22–36.** Bandages for immobilization of lower leg. *a*, Circular wrapping; *b*, spica.

a        b

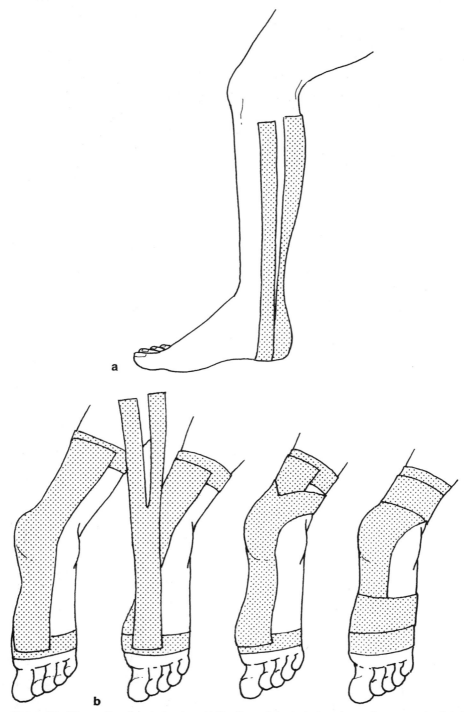

**Figure 22–37.** *a,* Bandages for immobilization of foot; *b,* bandages for support of Achilles tendon.

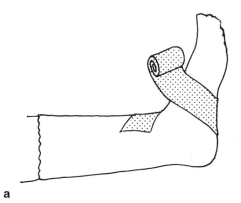

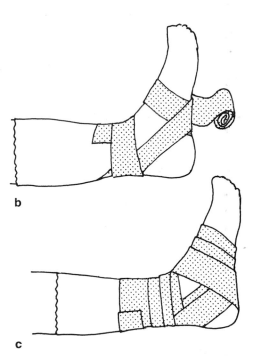

**Figure 22–38.** Ankle bandage limits supination and increases pronation.

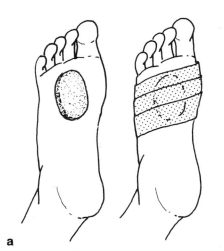

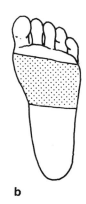

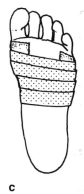

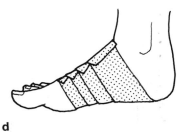

**Figure 22–39.** Bandages for the correction of foot deformities (splayfoot, fallen arches, flatfoot).

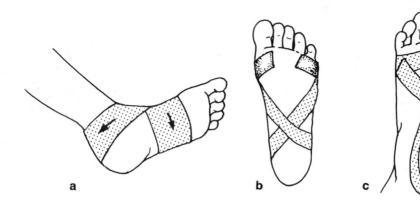

**Figure 22–40.** Heel bandages for support of heel.

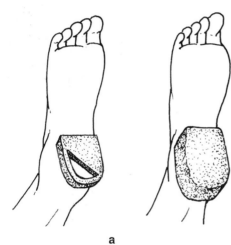

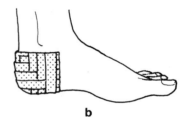

**Figure 22–41.** Bandage for bruised heel.

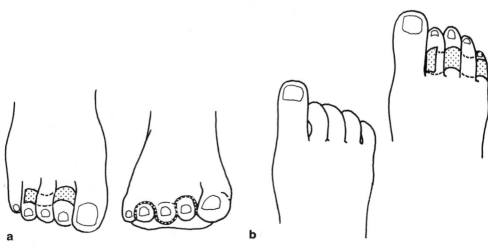

**Figure 22–42.** Bandage for correction of toe deformities (hammer toes).

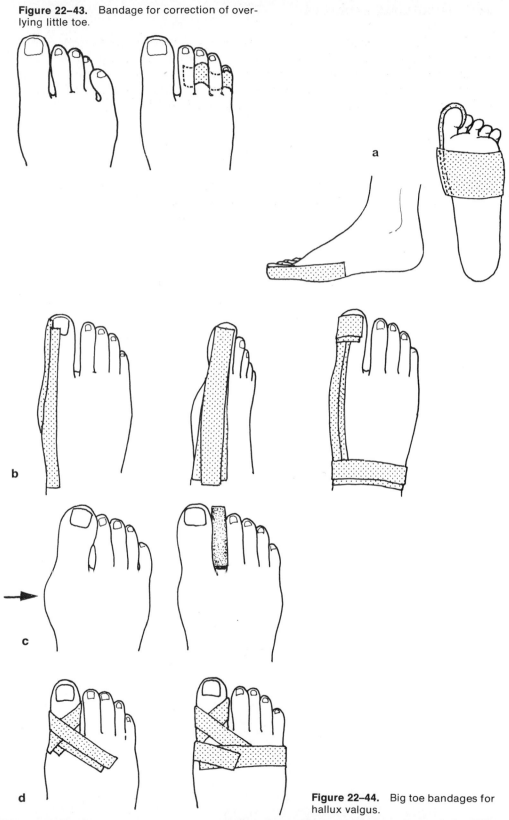

**Figure 22–43.** Bandage for correction of overlying little toe.

**Figure 22–44.** Big toe bandages for hallux valgus.

Following a sprained ankle there is frequent pain in supinating movements of the foot. The foot is immobilized in a medial position with a bandage so that flexion and extension are permitted, but supination is possible only to the point where pain occurs. The bandage is applied from the inside of the foot to the outside, thus placing the foot in a pronated position.

# Summary

The proper use of functional bandages in athletics depends not only on knowledge of athletic injuries and damages, but also on the nature, function, and manner of working of the various bandaging materials.

CHAPTER **23**

# First Aid

*LUTZ MEISSNER*

## History

In prehistoric times natural products, such as plants, leaves, bark, roots, wood fibers, earth, resin, and similar materials, were used in the treatment of wounds. A pot from the Bronze Age was found that suggests that wounds were covered with leaves and shredded linen.

The earliest known documents from Egypt relating to the treatment of wounds provide information about their methods of treatment, which even today retain their validity: "Immobilize the wound and bandage it." In this time the earliest known physician, who was also a priest, architect, writer, and astronomer, Im-hotep (ca. 2600 B.C.) particularly distinguished himself.

The techniques of spinning and weaving permitted the early development of bandages for wounds. Linen bandages of the type found on mummies lead us to suspect that similar bandages were also used to treat injuries. Hippocrates (460–377 B.C.) provides a detailed description of treatments for injured people in his writings. His basic criteria for bandaging materials are still valid today: "The material of the bandage should be clean, light, soft, and thin, and correspond in both length and width to the size of the wound."

The famous doctors of Imperial Rome, such as Galen (A.D. 129–199) and Celsus learned about the care of wounds from the Greeks, and wrote down their directions for treating wounds on the basis of their work.

In the Middle Ages barber-surgeons treated wounds with tinctures; magic and sorcery were also used. Not until Paracelsus (1493–1541) were there significant new developments in medicine. Paracelsus first recognized the infectious nature of disease.

Felix Würtz (1518–1575) and Ambroise Paré (1510–1592) made new methods known in the 16th century. They were successful for the first time in treating wounds with certain aseptic substances.

Heister, Bass, Bernstein, Moore, Hunter, and Cooper are known for their work in modern bandaging techniques. Professor Victor von Bruns (1812–1883) from Heidelberg and the surgeon Joseph Lister (1827–1912) from Glasgow introduced a new development into modern bandaging techniques.

With Lister's work, and after Louis Pasteur (1822–1895) had formulated the principles of asepsis, antisepsis began to be generally accepted. Ernst von Bergmann (1836–1907), a German-Baltic physician, continued Lister's work. Gradually a new antiseptic method, as it is still practiced today, developed.

# Need for First Aid

The danger of accidents, particularly in sports, make it necessary for first aid to be available. This means being able to give the injured person the proper care. Life-saving techniques, such as are required after traffic accidents or accidents at work, are rarely required in sports. In sports, the goal is to treat wounds and injuries in the best way possible. This entails relieving or limiting pain after a serious injury by proper positioning, treatment, and other means, such as applying cold. Training or competition must be interrupted if additional injury is possible and there is still risk to the athlete. Complete treatment must follow within approximately 6 hours. As a preventive measure, every athlete should be inoculated against tetanus.

# First Aid for Wounds

Wounds are caused by external factors. Cover the wound with a sterile bandage to prevent infection. Do not touch the wound, wash it out, or treat it with salve, powder, or disinfecting materials; do not remove foreign bodies. Light bleeding can be disregarded, but heavy bleeding involves danger to life and limb. Sufficiently strong manual pressure will stop this bleeding.

### SPRAY PLASTER

Spray plaster is good for the quick and uncomplicated care of small wounds. It guards against infection and creates a highly elastic, air-permeable protective film. It is watertight and falls off of its own accord after a few days. Spray plaster is used where other adhesives will not stick, such as during heavy perspiration, on the elbow, between the fingers, and on the knee.

### ADHESIVE BANDAGE

Cover small wounds with sterile bandage. Injuries to the fingertips and nails, such as occur in handball and basketball, are treated with finger-tip bandages. If these are not available, two wedges may be cut from a rectangular bandage and the injured finger placed on the lower part of the bandage; the two upper corners are then folded over the finger and taped into place.

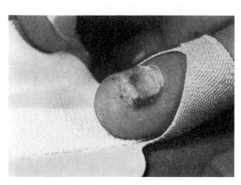

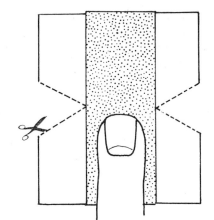

**Figure 23–1.**  Fingertip bandage.

**Figure  23–2.**  Homemade  fingertip bandage.

## BANDAGE FOR WOUNDS

A bandage for a wound consists of a sterile pad, such as gauze, and padding material, such as wadding or cotton. This serves for larger wounds. Strips of adhesive tape, netting, or cloth hold the padding in place. A first aid kit contains all the necessary materials. In the first aid of athletic injuries, netting bandages and tubing are a good means of holding the padding in place, particularly for the head, arms, and legs. Such bandages remain in place even under stress. For a jaw bandage, place the entire webbing over the head to the neck, and then cut out the area around the face. A netting bandage or a tubing bandage permits easy changing of the bandage. A bandanna can be used to hold the bandage in place if necessary.

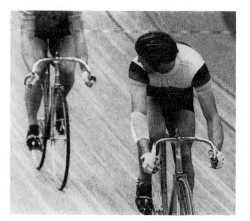

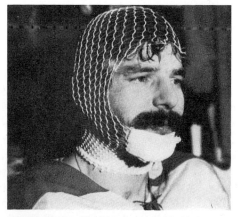

**Figure 23–3.**  Net bandage on arm.

**Figure 23–4.**  Net bandage on head.

## ARTERIAL BLEEDING

Severe arterial bleeding from an open wound is extremely serious. The loss of 1 liter of blood creates the risk of bleeding to death. Shock can set in. The blood vessel leading to the wound must be compressed with strong manual pressure. If an extremity is affected, the arm or leg is elevated and a compression bandage is applied. Most arterial bleeding can be stopped in this manner. Only if bleeding continues through the compression bandage should a tourniquet be applied, using a scarf or a tie. Rope or wire should never be used. The tourniquet must be released from time to time to prevent stoppage of the circulation. Details of the time of injury and personal data must be supplied to the physician.

## NOSEBLEED

For slight nosebleed, the person affected should sit with his head tilted back, while his neck is cooled with cold towels or ice. Serious nosebleeds require the patient to lean forward with his forehead in his hands to prevent suffocation.

# Treatment of Skin Damage

## EXCORIATION OF THE SKIN

The skin is sometimes irritated by the rubbing of clothing against body parts. Irritated skin is covered with oil, cream, talcum, or salve, which can also be used as preventive measures. Clothing made of artificial fabrics has a greater tendency to cause irritation. Women should wear a well-fitting bras-sière.

## BLISTERS

Mechanical pressure or friction on the foot or hand can cause blisters. Closed blisters are covered with adhesive for protection. Open blisters are cleaned and treated like a wound. Surround open or closed blisters with a felt ring to relieve pressure. The felt ring must be held in place with adhesive tape or other adhesive material. Small, unopened blisters dry up on their own.

Continuation of training or competition is possible after this care. Prevention includes good foot and nail care, better shoes, well-fitted wool socks, application of talcum powder of the feet before training or competition when there is a tendency to heavy perspiration, and rubbing the areas of the shoes that cause blisters with softening ointments. For blisters on the heel, foam rubber or celluloid inserts are placed in the shoe. Long distance runners can make do with leaves, grass, moss, or paper until the end of training. Blisters between the toes can be treated or avoided by wrapping the toes in adhesive material. Adhesive tape is also wrapped around the fingers to prevent blisters, but it should not be wrapped too tightly. The bandages are applied while the fist is tightened to prevent later constriction.

## SKIN BURNS

Falls in the gymnasium, on the track, or on hard surfaces can cause skin burns. These are treated like a wound.

## SUNBURN

Intense irradiation from the sun may cause sunburn. In this condition, the skin reddens deeply. Affected areas are covered with soothing creams. Sunburn can be prevented by using sunscreens, wearing protective clothing and a hat, and remaining in the shade.

# Other First Aid Treatments

## SUNSTROKE

Sunstroke results from excessive exposure of the uncovered head to direct sunlight. The head becomes hot and extremely red. Headaches, nausea, vomiting, and dizziness frequently result. Unconsciousness can develop. The affected person is brought to a cool, shady area and positioned with the head slightly elevated. Clothing is loosened and the neck and chest are rubbed with ice or cold water.

## HEAT STROKE

Breakdown of the sweating mechanism results in a buildup of heat, termed heat stroke. Circulation is disturbed. The head becomes extremely red and there is high temperature and dizziness. Unconsciousness can develop, and the condition can be fatal. A physician should be called immediately. The affected person must be taken to a cool, shady area and positioned in a stable side position if he is unconscious. While waiting for emergency treatment, the clothing should be loosened and cool towels should be laid on the person; the victim should also be fanned.

## HYPOTHERMIA

Physical overexertion while wearing clothing dampened by perspiration or rain can cause hypothermia after long exposure to cold temperatures. This can be accelerated with improper clothing and shoes. The victim should be brought into an area at room temperature, rubbed with dry towels, supplied with dry clothing, and kept warm. He or she should drink something warm, such as tea, but alcohol is forbidden.

## EXHAUSTION

Exhaustion can develop in athletic competition. Buildup of heat and the surpassing of one's physical limits are the causes. For recovery, support the exhausted athlete with the help of another person and walk up and down in a shaded area. Rub the neck and chest, and also the legs, with cold water, and encourage the athlete to breathe deeply. For heat exhaustion resulting from extensive water and salt losses, supply mineral water without carbonation with 1 teaspoon of salt dissolved in one liter. Poor circulation is aided with oxygen. Unconsciousness and stopped breathing require other treatments.

## UNCONSCIOUSNESS

Unconsciousness can result from a blow to the head, from overheating, or from overexertion. It can be fatal. The victim is moved out of danger and placed in a stable side position. In this way the head is the lowest part of the body, permitting the drainage of fluids. In the case of stopped breathing, artificial respiration must begin immediately. Mouth-to-mouth or mouth-to-nose respiration is used to make the patient start breathing again. The patient is placed in a supine position with the chin extended. The attendant kneels beside the victim, placing one hand on the forehead, the other under the chin. Depending on the method of artificial respiration conducted, either the mouth

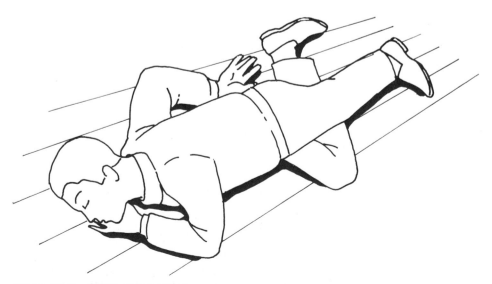

**Figure 23–5.**  Stable side position.

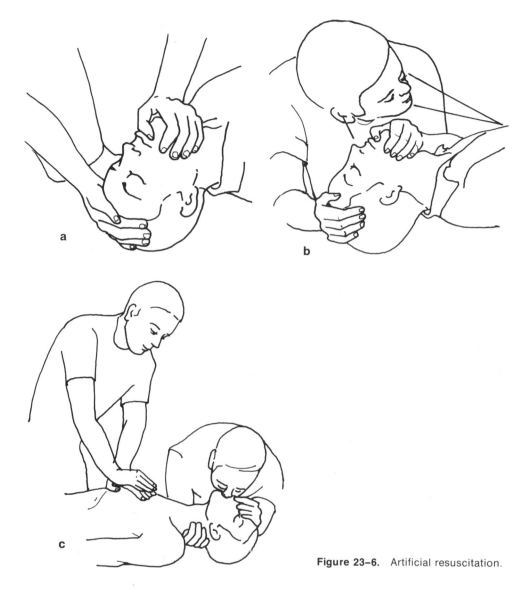

**Figure 23–6.** Artificial resuscitation.

or the nose of the patient is closed. Keep the patient breathing in a natural rhythm until he or she regains consciousness.

## SHOCK

Shock frequently accompanies severe injuries and extensive loss of blood. It can be fatal. The greater the loss of blood, the less the available blood in circulation and the deeper the shock. The pulse becomes weaker and faster. The victim is placed supine while the legs are elevated slightly, called shock positioning. Pulse and respirations are watched closely. Should breathing stop,

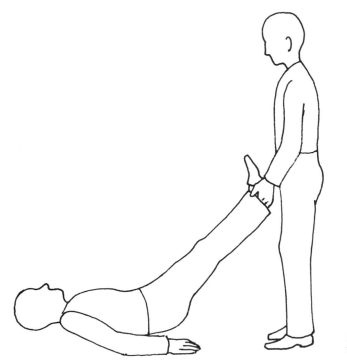

**Figure 23–7.** Shock position.

artificial respiration is necessary (see *Unconsciousness*). Loss of warmth is limited with blankets and towels covering and underneath the victim.

## STITCH IN THE SIDE

A stabbing, cramp-like pain can develop in the area of the lower ribs. Frequent causes include cramping of the abdominal muscles or the diaphragm, or cramps in the area of the spleen or liver. Training too hard or running too fast can be the cause; also, improper breathing can contribute. Insufficient preparation for competition or exercising directly after eating can likewise play a role. The running pace or the stress of training must be reduced, and often a pause is necessary. Deep breathing, in which the body is erect when inhaling and bent forward while exhaling, is often effective in relaxing the affected area. Severe cramping requires that the victim lie on his back or side, in which position easier breathing and massage may relieve the pain.

## SERIOUS INJURIES

Injured athletes with fractures or damaged organs are removed from danger, positioned correctly, and have the injury splinted or treated with other necessary first aid measures; they are then taken to a hospital or physician's office as soon as possible.

Every athlete, trainer, and attendant should be capable of giving first aid, and at least the following materials should be at hand in a separate kit for this purpose:

Band-Aids
Adhesive tape
Gauze
Assorted gauze bandages
Disposable cleaning towels

Scissors
Safety pins
Elastic cloth bandages
Rubbing alcohol, surgical spirits

# First Aid Kit

The therapist who attends athletes and teams needs a well-stocked and well-organized first aid kit with the following contents:

## BANDAGING MATERIALS

Band-Aids
Larger adhesive bandages
Spray plaster
Fingertip bandages
Adhesive tape
Cloth tape
Mull
Compresses
Wadding

Disposable towels
Cellulose
All-purpose bandage
Foam rubber (covered)
Netting
Bandanna
Splints (also inflatable)
Self-adhesive foam rubber,
    which can be cut to form

## BANDAGES

Elastic bandages ("Ideal bandages")
Mull bandages
Padded, cotton, fleece, and foam rubber
    bandages
Gauze bandages
Light adhesive bandages
Varicose bandages

Underwrapbind
Adhesive bandages
Netting bandages
Tubing bandages
Compression bandages
Snöggbind Bandage
Sporty-Quick Bandage

## MEDICATIONS

Massaging oil
Massaging balsam
Rubbing alcohol
Ice packs
Cool Pac
Freezing spray
Chlorethyl

Powder
Petroleum jelly
Disinfecting spray
Hydrogen peroxide
Spray adhesive
Salve to encourage reabsorption
    (also liquid)

## ADDITIONAL MATERIALS

Scissors (cloth and bandaging)
Safety pins
Nail clipper
Tweezers
Tongue depressors
Massage stylus
Joint supports

Universal support
Small bucket
Sponge
Soap
Hand towel
Bottle opener
Cords (various lengths and thicknesses)

Keep a list of contents with the first aid kit to make checking the materials easier.

# Concluding Remarks

*WERNER KUPRIAN*

The German Association for Physical Therapy–Central Association of Remedial Therapists is an association of physical therapists who concern themselves with the problems of athletic medicine. In clinics, private practice, and sporting associations they gain experience in the treatment of athletic injuries and damages. This work on the problems of physical therapy for sports goes back to 1969. In this year, a committee was formed by the Central Association of Remedial Therapists, which worked with the organizational committee of the XXth Olympic Games to organize the group of physical therapists at the games. In 1972, an organized group of physical therapists was present for the first time as a unit at the Olympic Games. During the games, 23 physical therapists treated over 7000 sports injuries to athletes of all nations.

Between 1970 and 1980, the Association for Medicine in Sports sponsored 30 continuing education courses. These courses focused on prevention, rehabilitation, and therapy for injuries and damages in various athletic disciplines as well as discussed means of improving athletic performance. In addition to the programs for track and field, games, gymnastics, trampoline, and swimming, which were held at various local athletic centers and professional clinics, there were also week-long programs for skiing and winter sports on the Winklmoosalm and in Klosters, Switzerland.

New methods of treatment as well as current theory and practice in the individual athletic disciplines were taught and discussed at these meetings. The members of the Association for Medicine in Sports have a wide range of personal experience in competitive sports, and were also granted an instructor's license of the German Athletic Association.

Respected German sports physicians and instructors and trainers took part in these courses as advisors and lecturers. The authors of this book are closely connected with the work of the Association for Medicine in Sports and in the Central Association of Remedial Therapists. They thank all lecturers, advisors, and the athletes who took part in these courses in the methods of physical therapy for athletics. Special thanks to Dr. D. Böhmer, the director of the Association of German Physicians for Sports in Hessen, Dr. W. Heipertz, the director of the Orthopedic University Clinic, "Friedricksheim," Frankfurt am Main, Dr. W. Pfeifer, the Director of the Association of German Physicians for Sports, Rheimland-Pfalz, Dr. H. Schoberth, the Director of the Damp Ostsee Clinic, and Dr. H. Stoboy of the Orthopedic Clinic of the free university "Oskar Helene Heim," Berlin, for their interest and support. And finally the authors thank the instructional centers for remedial therapy and massage at the Orthopedic University Clinic, "Friedricksheim," Frankfurt am Main, at the University Clinic of Cologne, and at Berlin-Charlottenburg for the opportunity to learn the basics of physical therapy and remedial exercise.

# The Authors

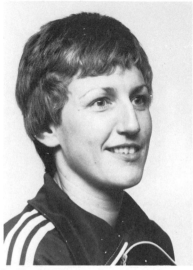

## Doris Eitner

Born 1949, education and degree at the Institution for Physiotherapy of the Orthopedic University Clinic in Cologne, active at the center for operative medicine at the city hospital in Leverkusen and in private practice. Physiotherapist at the Olympic Games in Munich, 1972, member of the Association for Medicine in Sports within the German Association for Physiotherapy—Central Association of Remedial Therapists. Physical therapist to the German national women's basketball team since 1973 as well as to the "A-team" of the German track and field association. Active pentathlete, basketball player, and trainer for track and field. Several times national champion in javelin throw, second place in junior national championship.

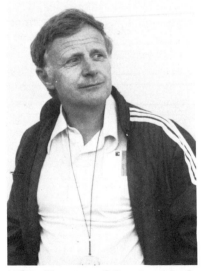

## Werner Kuprian

Born 1929, education and degree for instruction in athletics and gymnastics in Frankfurt/Main; education and degree in physiotherapy at the center for physiotherapy at the Orthopedic University Clinic in Frankfurt/Main. Licensed to instruct riding at the Westphalian Riding and Driving School in Münster. Distinguished with silver medal in riding. Active for many years as instructor for gymnastics and riding, as a trainer and physiotherapist. After clinical experience and private practice director of the department of health at Braun AG. The leader of the group of physiotherapists employed at the Olympic Games in Munich, 1972; director of the Association for Medicine in Sports; member of the board of directors of the German Association for Physiotherapy–Central Association of Remedial Therapists; member of the executive committee on the governing body for therapeutic riding; awarded medal of honor by the president of Germany in 1978; instructor and writer in the fields of physiotherapy sport, riding, and Hippo-therapy.

## Lutz Meissner

Born 1948, education and degree as physiotherapist at the Institution for Physiotherapy and Massage in Berlin-Charlottenburg. Active as physiotherapist at the Rheuma-clinic, Leukerbad, Switzerland; at the Kabat Kaiser Institute, Vallejo, California; in Bergen, Norway; and in private practice. Physiotherapist at the Olympic Games in Munich, 1972. Member of the German Association for Physiotherapy–Central Association of Remedial Therapists; licensed athletic instructor; active as trainer for middle distance running and in both alpine and nordic skiing; attendant for many years for the regional handball team of

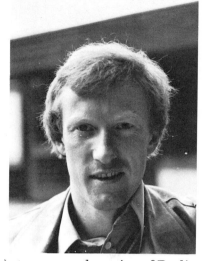

Borussia Fulda. Active in track and field and skiing, twice champion of Berlin in middle- and long-distance running, second place in Hessian 800 m run, and second place in Hessian slalom.

## Helmut Ork

Born 1947; education and degree at the Institution for Physiotherapy of the Orthopedic University Clinic in Cologne, active at the center for operative medicine at the city hospital in Leverkusen and in private practice. Physiotherapist at the Olympic Games in Munich, 1972, member of the Association for Medicine in Sports within the German Association for Physiotherapy–Central Association of Remedial Therapists. Attendant of track and field athletes and handball players at the Bayer sport club 04 in Leverkusen; functionary in the league of handicapped athletes in Nordrhein-Westphalia; active track and field athlete.

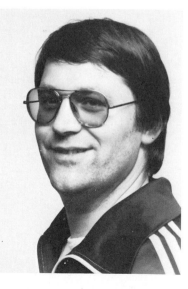

# References

*References*

# Part I

## Passive Treatments

Bear, K.H.: Beobachtungen in Mexiko, Ausblick auf die Olympischen Spiele 1972, München. Der deutsche Badebetrieb, Otto Haase Verlag, Lübeck

Brauchle, A.: Naturheilkunde. Bertelsmann Verlag 1965

Bruhin, A.: Elektrotherapie. ORTHOPÄDIE 7/78. Springer Verlag

Callies, R.: Differenzierte Ultraschalltherapie und ihr Einsatz in der Sportmedizin

Deuser, E.: Schnell wieder fit. Verlag Bintz/Dohany, Offenbach 1973

Deuser, E.: Das japanische Massagestäbchen. Verlag: Fitneß Vertrieb Olpe 1971

Deuser, E.: Die Gesundheit des Sportlers. Econ Verlag, Düsseldorf–Wien 1977

Diem, C.: Weltgeschichte des Sports und der Leibeserziehung. Cotta-Verlag, Stuttgart 1960

Eitner, D.: Sportverletzungen. Sonderdruck zur KRANKENGYMNASTIK. 29. Jg/77. Richard Pflaum Verlag, München

Gadomski, M.: Elektrotherapie bei Sportverletzungen. KRANKENGYMNASTIK 73/8. Richard Pflaum Verlag, München

Gierlich, K.: Elektrotherapie im Sport. ELEKTROMEDICA 3/72

Gierlich, K., A. Jung: Die kombinierte Anwendung von Ultraschall und Reizströmen Sonderdruck Physikalische Medizin und Rehabilitation 9/68. Medizinisch-Literarische Verlagsgesellschaft, Uelzen

Gillert, O.: Niederfrequente Reizströme. Aus Theorie und Praxis der Krankengymnastik 1974. Richard Pflaum Verlag, München

Gillert, O.: Hydrotherapie und Balneotherapie aus Theorie und Praxis der Krankengymnastik. 5. Aufl. 1973. Richard Pflaum Verlag, München.

Groh, H., P. Groh: Sportverletzungen und Sportschäden. Luitpold-Werk München 1975

Hamann, A.: Massage in Bild und Wort. Gustav Fischer Verlag. Stuttgart–New York 1976

Heipertz, W.: Sportmedizin. Georg Thieme Verlag, Stuttgart 1976

Hoffa, A., H. Gocht, U. Storck, H.S. Lüdke: Technik der Massage. Ferdinand Enke Verlag. Stuttgart 1978

Hüter, A.: Deutscher Verband für Physiotherapie – Zentralverband der Krankengymnasten ZVK e.V. KRANKENGYMNASTIK 5/1979. Richard Pflaum Verlag, München

Kirchberg, F.: Sportmassage. Weidemann Verlag, Berlin

Koppelmann, J · Die Eisbehandlung orthopädischer Erkrankungen. KRANKENGYMNASTIK 3/1972. Richard Pflaum Verlag, München

Koppelmann, J.: Eisanwendung als Ergänzung zur krankengymnastischen Behandlung. Zentralverband Krankengymnastik e.V., München, Juli 1974

Kraus, H.: Periostbehandlung. V.P. Vogler, Leipzig 1953

Krummrei, J.: Kälteanwendungen bei Sportverletzungen. Vortrag beim Deutschen Sportärztebund – Landesverband Rheinland-Pfalz

Kuprian, W.: Krankengymnasten im Einsatz bei den XX. Olympischen Spielen in München. KRANKENGYMNASTIK 11/1972. Richard Pflaum Verlag, München

Kuprian, W.: Sportmassage. KRANKENGYMNASTIK 7/1972. Richard Pflaum Verlag, München

Kuprian, W., Gräfin L., Hendrikoff: Gruppendynamik, Skilauf und Sportmedizin. KRANKENGYMNASTIK 1977 S. 483–490. Richard Pflaum Verlag, München

Kuprian, W., G. Süßmeyer: Wintersportlehrgang des Deutschen Sportärztebundes In Klosters 1979. KRANKENGYMNASTIK 6/1979. Richard Pflaum Verlag, München

Kuprian, W.: Fortbildung auf sportmedizinischem Gebiet. KRANKENGYMNASTIK 5/1971. Richard Pflaum Verlag, München

Lampert, H.: Physikalische Therapie. Verlag Theodor Steinkopff. Dresden-Leipzig 1954

Lange, H.: Eis zur Unterstützung krankengymnastische Behandlung. KRANKENGYMNASTIK 4/69. Richard Pflaum Verlag, München

List, M.: Eisbehandlung in der Krankengymnastik. Zentralverband Krankengymnastik e. V., München–April 1978

List, M.: Krankengymnastische Behandlungen in der Traumatologie. Springer Verlag, Berlin–Heidelberg–New York 1978

Lindemann, K., H. Teirich-Leube, W. Heipertz: Lehrbuch der Krankengutgymnastik Band I, II, III und IV 1959–1965. Georg Thieme Verlag, Stuttgart

Mülmann, A. v.: Krankengymnastik bei Verletzungsfolgen am Bewegungsapparat. Richard Pflaum Verlag, München 1970

Pulc, W.: Die Kryotherapie. KRANKENGYMNASTIK 11/1975. Richard Pflaum Verlag, München

Sperling, O. K.: Indikationen zur medizinischen Massage und deren Wirkung. Der Kassenarzt 18/78

Steinbach, M.: Medizinisch-psychologische Probleme der Wettkampfvorbereitung. Verlag Bartels & Wernitz KG. Berlin 1971

Storch, U.: Technik der Massage. Ferdinand Enke Verlag, Stuttgart 1978

Strohal, R.: Grundbegriffe der Massage. U + S Fachbuch. München–Berlin–Wien 1975

Teirich-Leube, H.: Grundriß der Bindegewebsmassage. Gustav Fischer Verlag, Stuttgart 1968

Thomson, W.: Lehrbuch der Massage und manuellen Gymnastik. Georg Thieme Verlag, Stuttgart 19490

Tittel, K.: Beschreibende und funktionelle Anatomie des Menschen. Gustav Fischer Verlag, Stuttgart–New York 1976

Tranzky, G.: Kryotherapie. KRANKENGYMNASTIK 4/1978. Richard Pflaum Verlag, München

Treumann, F.: Die Behandlung der Peratenonitis Achillea. Orthopädische Praxis 10/1971

Vogler, P.: Physiotherapie. Georg Thieme Verlag, Stuttgart 1964

Schoberth H.: Sportmedizin. Fischer Taschenbuch-Verlag, Frankfurt am Main, 1977

Zielke, K.: Taschenbuch für krankengymnastische Verordnungen. Gustav Fischer Verlag, Stuttgart 1969

# Part II

## Active Treatments

Bartmess-Kohlhaußen, B.: Propriozeptive Neuromuskuläre Fazilitation – PNF – ein Grundelement der Krankengymnastik. KRANKENGYMNASTIK 10/1979. Richard Pflaum Verlag, München

Baumeister, H.: In der Badewanne fängt es an. Copress-Verlag, München 1972

Beineke, H.: Nutzen komplexer Bewegungsmuster zur gezielten krankengymnastischen Behandlung. KRANKENGYMNASTIK 1/1979. Richard Pflaum Verlag, München

Beitel, H.: Komplexe Bewegungsübungen bei Schmerzzuständen der Wirbelsäule. KRANKENGYMNASTIK 10/1977. Richard Pflaum Verlag, München

Berlin, I.: Die Behandlung nach Kabat-Praxis und Grundlagen. KRANKENGYMNASTIK 10/1975. Richard Pflaum Verlag, München

Bold, R. M., A. Grossmann: Stemmführung nach Brunkow. Enke Verlag Stuttgart 1978

Brenke, H., J. Weber, L. Dietrich: Rehabilitationstraining nach operativ behandelter Achillessehnenruptur bei Sportlern. Medizin und Sport 12/1974. VEB Verlag Volk und Gesundheit Berlin

Brokmeier, A. A.: Einführung in die Orthopädische-Manuelle Medizin. Brokmeier, KRANKENGYMNASTIK 4/1979. Richard Pflaum Verlag, München

Daniels, L., M. Williams, C. Worthingham: Muskelfunktionsprüfung. Gustav Fischer Verlag, Stuttgart

Derbolowsky, U.: Manuelle Medizin und Chirotherapie. Verlag für Medizin. Dr. Ewald Fischer, Heidelberg

Deutscher Sportbund – Bundesausschuß Leistungssport: Das sportmedizinische Untersuchungssystem. Limpert Verlag Frankfurt am Main. 4. Okt. 1975

Dumont, W.: Die Behandlung von Wirbelsäulenbeschwerden durch den Krankengymnasten. KRANKENGYMNASTIK 10/1977. Richard Pflaum Verlag, München

Dumont, W.: Die krankengymnastische Behandlung der Schulter. KRANKENGYMNASTIK 9/1977. Richard Pflaum Verlag, München

Eitner, D.: Sportverletzungen. KRANKENGYMNASTIK 6/1977. Richard Pflaum Verlag, München

Forstreuter, H.: Gymnastik. Limpert Verlag, Frankfurt am Main

Frisch, H.: 5 mal 5 – Untersuchungsschema nach H. Frisch

Frisch, H.: Manuelle Therapie in der Krankengymnastik. KRANKENGYMNASTIK 3/1976. Richard Pflaum Verlag, München

Gardiner, M. D.: Grundlagen der Übungstherapie. Georg Thieme Verlag, Stuttgart 1968

Gekeler, I.: Schwimm- und Wassertherapie. J. McMillan, Theorie und Praxis. KRANKENGYMNASTIK 11/1974. Richard Pflaum Verlag, München

Groh, H., P. Groh: Sportverletzungen und Sportschäden. Luitpold-Werk München 1975

Grosser, M.: Zweckgymnastik des Leichtathleten. Verlag Karl Hofmann, Schorndorf

Groves, R., D. N. Camaione: Bewegungslehre in Krankengymnastik und Sport. Gustav Fischer Verlag, Stuttgart

Heipertz, W.: Sportmedizin. Georg Thieme Verlag, Stuttgart 1976

Hettinger, Th., G. Kaminsky, H. Schmale: Ergonomie am Arbeitsplatz. Kiehl Verlag, Ludwigshafen 1976

Hettinger, Th.: Isometrisches Muskeltraining. Georg Thieme Verlag, Stuttgart 1972

Hettinger, Th.: fit sein – fit bleiben. Georg Thieme Verlag, Stuttgart 1965

Hirschfeld, P.: Die Sportverletzung und ihre Behandlung. I. Das Knie. Schwareck-Verlag München 1976

Hollmann, W.: Sportmedizin. Springer Verlag, Berlin–Heidelberg–New York 1977

Jonath, U.: Circuit-Training. Verlag Bartels & Wernitz KG, Berlin

Jonath, U.: Die biologischen Grundlagen des Trainings. RK Sportgeräte Vertriebs GmbH, Stadthagen

Kaltenborn, F. M.: Manuelle Therapie der Extremitätengelenke. Olaf Norlis Bokhandel Oslo 1979

Kemmer, V.: Sinn und Bedeutung der Manuellen Therapie – Ausführung und Anwendung zur Mobilisation von Gelenkkontrakturen. KRANKENGYMNASTIK 4/1979. Richard Pflaum Verlag, München

Kendall, H. O. und F. P., G. E. Wadsworth: Muscles Testing and Function. Williams and Wilkins Company, Baltimore 1971

Klein-Vogelbach, S.: Funktionelle Bewegungslehre. Springer Verlag 1966

Knott, M., D. E. Voss: Komplexbewegungen. Bewegungsbahnung nach Dr. Kabat. Fischer Verlag Stuttgart 1962

Krejci, V., P. Koch: Muskelverletzungen und Tendopathien der Sportler. Georg Thieme Verlag, Stuttgart 1976

Kuprian, W.: Muskelfunktionstest bei Lehrlingen. Die Leibeserziehung 2/1964. Verlag K. Hofmann, Schorndorf

Kuprian, W.: Krankengymnastik und XX. Olympische Spiele München 1972. KRANKENGYMNASTIK 7/1972. Richard Pflaum Verlag, München

Kuprian, W.: Postoperative krankengymnastische Behandlung der Achillessehnenruptur. KRANKENGYMNASTIK 10/1973. Richard Pflaum Verlag, München

Kuprian, W.: Fortbildung auf sportmedizinischem Gebiet. KRANKENGYMNASTIK 5/1971. Richard Pflaum Verlag, München

Kuprian, W., G. Süßmeyer: Wintersportlehrgang des Deutschen Sportärztebundes in Klosters 1979. KRANKENGYMNASTIK 6/1979. Richard Pflaum Verlag, München

Lehmann, G.: Praktische Arbeitsphysiologie. Georg Thieme Verlag, Stuttgart 1953

Lewit, K.: Manuelle Medizin im Rahmen der medizinischen Rehabilitation Urban & Schwarzenberg 1977. München–Wien–Baltimore

Lindemann, K., H. Teirich-Leube, W. Heipertz: Lehrbuch der Krankengymnastik, Band I. Georg Thieme Verlag Stuttgart

List, M.: Krankengymnastische Behandlungen in der Traumatologie. Springer Verlag Berlin–Heidelberg–New York 1978

McMillan, J.: Schwimmtherapie. Scriptum

Marées, H. de: Medizin von heute. Sportphysiologie. Troponwerke, Köln

Meissner, L.: Die krankengymnastische Betreuung im Hallenhandball. KRANKENGYMNASTIK 11/1975. Richard Pflaum Verlag, München

Meissner, L.: Gründung der krankengymnastischen Arbeitsgruppe für Manuelle Therapie (AGMT). KRANKENGYMNASTIK 2/1978. Richard Pflaum Verlag, München

Mülmann, A. v.: Krankengymnastik bei Verletzungsfolgen am Bewegungsapparat Richard Pflaum Verlag, München 1975

Neumann, G. D.: Scriptum zum Informationskurs der Deutschen Gesellschaft für Manuelle Medizin. 2. Aufl. 1978

Nöcker, J.: Physiologie der Leibesübungen. F. Enke Verlag, Stuttgart

Ozarcuk, L., C. Brod: Zum Tode von Margaret Knott. KRANKENGYMNASTIK 3/1979. Richard Pflaum Verlag, München

Papadopulos, J. S.: Holotopometer. Byk Gulden Pharmazeutika. Konstanz 1973

Politzer, A.: Verletzungsrückstände und ihre krankengymnastische Behandlung. KRANKENGYMNASTIK 7/1972. Richard Pflaum Verlag, München

Sachse, J.: Manuelle Untersuchung und Mobilisationsbehandlung der Extremitätengelenke. Verlag für Medizin Dr. Ewald Fischer

Schauer, U.: Manuelle Therapie an Extremitätengelenken im Rahmen der krankengymnastischen Behandlung. KRANKENGYMNASTIK 7/1975. Richard Pflaum Verlag, München

Schmid, H. J.: Seminar für Medizinische Trainigstherapie in Moss/Norwegen 8/1978. KRANKENGYMNASTIK 11/1978. Richard Pflaum Verlag, München

Schmidt, K.: Sonder- und Heilschwimmen. Verlag Theodor Steinkopff, Dresden 1975

Schmidt, H.: Orthopädie im Sport. Joh. Ambrosius Barth, Leipzig

Schüler, H.: Schwimm- und Wassertherapie bei mehrfach behinderten Kindern. KRANKENGYMNASTIK 11/1973. Richard Pflaum Verlag, München

Schoberth, H.: Sportmedizin. Fischer Handbücher 1977

Stoboy, H.: Neurophysiologische Grundlagen der Krankengymnastik. Der Kassenarzt 18/1978 Heft 35

tum Suden, A.: Unterwassergymnastik. KRANKENGYMNASTIK 8/1972. Richard Pflaum Verlag, München

Zielke, K.: Taschenbuch für krankengymnastische Verordnungen. Gustav Fischer Verlag, Stuttgart 1969

# Part III

## Possible Treatments with Physical Therapy and Remedial Exercise for Particular Athletic Injuries and Damage

### *General*

Apel, J., R. Metze: Ermüdungsfrakturen bei Gewichthebern. Medizin und Sport 10/1975. VEB Verlag Volk und Gesundheit, Berlin

Baetzner, W.: Sportunfall und Erste Hilfe. Ruhrländische Verlagsgesellschaft mbH, Essen, Band 5/1965

Becker, W., H. Krahl: Tendopathien. Georg Thieme Verlag, Stuttgart 1978

Brenke, H.: Rehabilitationstraining nach operativ behandelter Achiellessehnenruptur bei Sportlern. Medizin und Sport 12/1974. VEB Verlag Volk und Gesundheit, Berlin

Burri, C., A. Rüter: Verletzungen des oberen Sprunggelenkes. Springer Verlag 1978

Cotta, H.: Orthopädie. Georg Thieme Verlag, Stuttgart

Cotta, H., H. Krahl: Das verletzte Kniegelenk des Sportlers – moderne diagnostische und therapeutische Verfahren. Deutsches Ärzteblatt 15, April 1978

Einsingbach, T.: Trainingsanleitung nach Meniskusoperation bei Leistungssportlern. KRANKENGYMNASTIK 5/1979. Richard Pflaum Verlag, München

Exner, G.: Kleine Orthopädie. Georg Thieme Verlag, Stuttgart

Groh, H., P. Groh: Sportverletzungen und Sportschäden. Luitpold-Werk, München 1975

Franke, K.: Indikationen und Methoden der operativen Behandlung von Sportverletzungen und Sportschäden am Bewegungsapparat. Medizin und Sport 7/1974. VEB Verlag Volk und Gesundheit, Berlin

Franke, K.: Muskelverletzungen und Überlastungsfolgen am Oberschenkel. Medizin und Sport 6/1975. VEB Verlag Volk und Gesundheit, Berlin

Franke, K.: Traumatologie des Sports. VEB Verlag Volk und Gesundheit, Berlin 1977

Hackenbruch, W., P.M. Karpf: Kapselband-Verletzungen des Sprunggelenkes. Fortschritt der Medizin. 95. Jahrg. 6/1977

Heiss, F.: Unfallverhütung beim Sport. Karl Hofmann Verlag, Schorndorf Band 57

Hirschfeld, P.: Der Schulterschmerz und seine Behandlung. Schwarzeck-Verlag München

Hirschfeld, P.: Sportverletzungen und ihre Behandlung. Teil I: Das Knie. Schwarzeck-Verlag München

Hort, W.: Ursache, Klinik, Therapie und Prophylaxe der Schäden auf Leichtathletik-Kunststoffbahnen. Leistungssport 1/1976

Jonas, B.: Meniskus- und Kreuzbandverletzungen. Luitpold Information 29/1977

Kaltenborn, F.M.: Manuelle Therapie der Extremitätengelenke. 5. Aufl. Olaf Norlis Bokhandel, Oslo 1979

Krämer, J.: Bandscheibenbedingte Erkrankungen. Georg Thieme Verlag, Stuttgart 1978

Krejci, V., P. Koch: Muskelverletzungen und Tendopathien der Sportler. Georg Thieme Verlag, Stuttgart 1976

Krüger, A.: Kleiner Ratgeber für Leichtathletik-Verletzungen. Verlag Bartels und Wernitz KG, Berlin, 1. Aufl. 1975

Kuprian, W.: Postoperative krankengymnastische Behandlung der Achillessehnenruptur. KRANKENGYMNASTIK 10/1973. Richard Pflaum Verlag, München

Kuprian, W., Gräfin L. Hendrikoff: Gruppendynamik, Skilauf, Sportmedizin KRANKENGYMNASTIK S. 483–490 Richard Pflaum Verlag, München

Kuprian, W.: Das Hohlkreuz. KRANKENGYMNASTIK 9/1979. Richard Pflaum Verlag, München

Lewit, K.: Manuelle Medizin im Rahmen der medizinischen Rehabilitation. 2. Aufl. 1977. Urban & Schwarzenberg, München–Wien–Baltimore

Lindemann, K., H. Teirich-Leube, W. Heipertz: Lehrbuch für Krankengymnastik, Band III. Georg Thieme Verlag, Stuttgart

List, M.: Krankengymnastik in der Traumatologie. Springer Verlag Berlin

Mang, W., P. M. Karpf: Scheibenmeniskus. Fortschritte der Medizin. 96. Jahrg. 10/1978

Marées, H. de: Sportphysiologie. Medizin von heute. Troponwerk, Köln 1976

Mülmann, A. v.: Krankengymnastik bei Verletzungsfolgen am Bewegungsapparat. Richard Pflaum Verlag, München

Nirschl, R. P.: Diagnose und Behandlung des Tennisellenbogen. Zeitschrift TENNIS

Rolf, G., G. Kaeppel: Das Schlingengerät in der Praxis der Krankengymnastik. Verlag W. Kohlhammer, Stuttgart 1971

Schmidt, H.: Orthopädie im Sport. Joh. Ambrosius Barth, Leipzig 1972

Schönberger, M.: Diskussionsbemerkungen: Die «Epicondylitis humeri» und andere Insertions-Tendopathien von der Manuellen Medizin her gesehen. Manuelle Medizin 3/1977. Verlag für Medizin Dr. E. Fischer GmbH, Heidelberg

Schoberth, H.: Funktionelle Verbände

Schoberth, H.: Sportmedizin. Fischer Taschenbuch Verlag 1978

Schoberth, H.: Die kleine Sportverletzung und ihre Behandlung. KRANKENGYMNASTIK 7/1972. Richard Pflaum Verlag, München

Schoberth, H.: Die Leistungsprüfung der Bewegungsorgane. U + S 1972

Stein, W., H. Krahl: Die funktionelle Anatomie als Schlüssel zur Diagnostik und Therapie von Kapselbandverletzungen des Kniegelenkes. KRANKENGYMNASTIK 5/1979. Richard Pflaum Verlag, München

Steinbrück, K.: Der Tennisellenbogen. Physiotherapie. 67. Jahrg. 11/1976

Steinbrück, K., H. Krahl: Sportschäden und Sportverletzungen an der Wirbelsäule. Deutsches Ärzteblatt 19/1978

Steinbrück, K., G. Rompe: Sportschäden und Sportverletzungen. Deutsches Ärzteblatt. G 1043 CX – 17. 2. 1977

Steinbrück, K., G. Rompe: Sportschäden am Ellenbogen. Luitpold Informationen 29/1977

Stohr, A., W. Jelinek, D. Wilkens: Intraartikuläre Injektionsbehandlung bei Chondropathie des Kniegelenkes. Medizin und Sport 11/1979. VEB Verlag Volk und Gesundheit, Berlin

Thiel, A.: Achillessehnenschmerzen – Ein Vorschlag zur Prophylaxe und Therapie. Leichtathletik 38, 30. Jahrg. 9/1979

Treumann, F.: Die Behandlung der Paratenonitis Achillea. Orthopädische Praxis 10/1971

Werding, M.: Tennisarm. Physiotherapie. 70. Jahrg. Heft 10/1979

Wietoska, B.: Was ist eigentlich Muskelkater. Sportmedizin 12/1979. Deutscher Ärzte Verlag, Köln

Zielke, K.: Taschenbuch für krankengymnastische Verordnungen. Gustav Fischer Verlag, Stuttgart

# Part IV

## Treatment for Training and Competition

Baetzner, W.: Sportunfall und Erste Hilfe. Ruhrländische Verlagsgesellschaft mbH, Essen, 6. Aufl.

Baumann, S., K. Zieschang: Handbuch der Sportpraxis. BLV Verlagsgesellschaft, München–Bern–Wien

Beiersdorf AG: Elastofix Netzverbände. Verbandstechnik. Medical-Programm

Beiersdorf AG: Geschichte, Herstellung, Eigenschaften, Anwendungsgebiete, Ausgabe 1978. Medical-Programm

BG-Ausgabe: Anleitung zur Ersten Hilfe bei Unfällen. 10/1973

Bottke, M., W. Günthner: Atemgymnastische Übungen und abhärtende Maßnahmen zu Hause. Boehringer Mannheim

Brauchle, A.: Naturheilkunde. Bertelsmann Verlag, 1965

Deuser, E.: Schnell wieder fit. 6. Aufl. Bintz-Verlag GmbH, Offenbach/Main

Deutsches Rotes Kreuz: Erste Hilfe Fibel. Ausgabe 1973

Diem, C.: Wesen und Lehre des Sports. Weidmann'sche Verlagsbuchhandlung, Berlin 1960

Dumont, W.: Die Behandlung von Wirbelsäulenbeschwerden durch den Krankengymnasten. KRANKEN-GYMNASTIK 10/1977. Richard Pflaum Verlag, München

Fabian, D.: Bader. Verlag G. D. W. Callwey, München 1960

Fresenius, H.: Sauna. Rowohlt Sachbuch 1974

Hanebuth, O.: Grundschule zur sportlichen Leistung. Limpert-Verlag, Frankfurt am Main 1956

Hartmann, P. AG: Verbandstoffe und moderne Wundversorgung. Ausgabe Oktober 1977

Hartmann, P. AG: Verbandstoffe und moderne Wundversorgung. Schriftenreihe der Paul Hartmann AG, 1–5 Ausgabe 10/1977

Heipertz, W.: Sportmedizin. Georg Thieme Verlag, Stuttgart 1967

Jensen, H. P.: Bewegungsübungen für die Wirbelsäule. Friedrich & Kaufmann, Hannover

Johnson u. Johnson: 79 Athletic Products Information, Catalog – 501 George Street. New Brunswick – 08903 New Jersey

Kaganas, G.: Physiotherapie bei degenerativ-rheumatischen Erkrankungen der Wirbelsäule. DOCUMENTA Geigy – Acta Rheumatologica Nr. 23, Basel

Keydel, H.: Ganzkörpergymnastik als Aufwärmprogramm. Leichtathletik 1/2, 8. Jan. 1980/31. Jahrg., Verlag Bartels & Wernitz, Berlin

Klafs, C. E., D. D. Arnheim: Modern Priciples of Athletic. Training. Fourth Edition. The C. V. Mosby Company. Saint Louis 1977

Klaus, E. J., H. Noack: Frau und Sport. Georg Thieme Verlag, Stuttgart 1961

Klümper, A.: Wirbelsäulengymnastik. Briefreihe: Tip für den Athleten

Kötschau, K.: Leistung und Gesundheit. Verlag Wissenschaft, Wirtschaft, Technik, Bad Harzburg 1963

Krämer, J.: Bandscheibenschäden. Goldmann, Medizin-Band 9035

Kraus, H.: Rückenschmerzen. Goldmanns Gelbe Taschenbücher Band 1887

Krejci, V., P. Koch: Muskelverletzungen und Tendopathien der Sportler. Georg Thieme Verlag, Stuttgart 1976

Krüger, A., H. Oberdieck: Kleiner Ratgeber für Leichtathletikverletzungen. Verlag Bartels & Wernitz, Berlin–München–Frankfurt 1975

Kuprian, W.: Arbeitsbewegungsuntersuchungen in einem Betrieb der Elektroindustrie 1959/60. KRANKEN-GYMNASTIK 12/1961. Richard Pflaum Verlag, München

Kuprian, W.: Erfahrungen aus dem Saunabad eines Industriebetriebes. Der Deutsche Badebetrieb. 8/ 1965. Verlag O. Haase, Lübeck

Kuprian, W., G. Süßmeyer: Wintersportlehrgang des Deutschen Sportärztebundes in Klosters 1979. KRAN-KENGYMNASTIK 6/1979. Richard Pflaum Verlag, München

Laabs, W.: Selbstbehandlung bei Rückenschmerzen und Bandscheibenbeschwerden. Haug Verlag, Heidelberg

Lampert, H.: Physikalische Therapie. Verlag Theodor Steinkopff, Dresden–Leipzig 1954

Lang, E., V. Mair: Sport und Freizeit. SANDOZ

Lenk, H., S. Moser, E. Beyer: Philosophie des Sports. Verlag K. Hoffmann, Schorndorf 1973

Lindemann, K., H. Teirich-Leube, W. Heipertz: Lehrbuch der Krankengymnastik, Band I. Georg Thieme Verlag, Stuttgart

Lohmann, KG: Stütz- und Entlastungsverbände. 1968, 3. Aufl. Lohmann KG Fahr/Rhein

Mallow, J., H. Papst: Alles übers Laufen. Moderne Verlags GmbH, München 1979

Mengershausen, J. v.: Bewegungsübungen und Selbstmassage. Quellen der Gesundheit. Bircher-Benner-Verlag Bad Homburg

Nöcker, J.: Die biologischen Grundlagen der Leistungssteigerung durch Training. Verlag K. Hoffmann, Schorndorf 1960

Röder, H.: Salbenverbände bei Sportverletzungen sport + enelbin 7-Cassella-Riedel. Pharma GmbH, Frankfurt am Main 61

Rothig, P.: Sportwissenschaftliches Lexikon. Verlag K. Hoffmann, Schorndorf/Stuttgart

Ringopharm Sportverzorging: Tapen – Wolphaertsbocht 276 Postbus. 51100 Rotterdam

Scheid, K. P.: Sauna. Verlag G. D. W. Callwey, München 1962

Schilling/Bichlmeier: Gymnastische Bewegungsübungen für Ihre Rheumapatienten. Siegfried GmbH, Säckingen

Schlevogt, E.: Sauna. Hippokrates Verlag, Stuttgart 1966.

Schoberth, H.: Funktionelle Verbände, Indikationen, Anwendung, Verbandstechnik – 4. Aufl., Verlag Beiersdorf AG, Hamburg

Stolzenberg, G.: Gesund durch Sport und Lebensreform. H. G. Müller Verlag, Krailling/München

Vogler, P.: Physiotherapie. Georg Thieme Verlag, Stuttgart 1964

Wöllzenmüller, F., B. Grünewald: Die Gesundheitskarriere durch Ausgleichssport. Bertelsmann Ratgeber,
 München

# Index

Page numbers in *italic* type indicate illustrations; *t* indicates table.